HERBAL PRESCRIPTIONS FOR HEALTH AND HEALING

Your Everyday Guide to Using Herbs Safely and Effectively

DONALD J. BROWN, N.D.

PRIMA HEALTH
A Division of Prima Publishing
3000 Lava Ridge Court · Roseville, California 95661
(800) 632-8676 · www.primahealth.com

The PRIMA HEALTH logo is a registered trademark of Prima Communications Inc.
Prima Publishing and its colophon are trademarks of Prima Communications, Inc.

ILLUSTRATIONS BY HELENE D. STEVENS

Library of Congress Cataloging-in-Publication Data on File
ISBN 0-7615-2410-X

00 01 02 03 DD 9 8 7 6 5 4 3 2 1
Printed in the United States of America

HOW TO ORDER

Single copies may be ordered from Prima Publishing, 3000 Lava Ridge Court, Roseville, CA 95661; telephone (800) 632-8676 ext. 4444. Quantity discounts are also available. On your letterhead, include information concerning the intended use of the books and the number of books you wish to purchase.

Visit us online at www.primahealth.com

To
GABY, MILES, AND ARI
for their love,
encouragement,
and reminding me
where I left the ginkgo.

It was suggested that I used unconventional methods and there is nothing a professional group mistrusts so nervously as it does anything that appears unconventional, and that has not been thoroughly written up in journals. It may be quackery. Worse still, it may be effective. And if it is both quackery and effective it is utterly hateful.

—ROBERTSON DAVIES, *The Cunning Man*

Contents

Contents

PART 6

HERBAL PRESCRIPTIONS FOR
COMMON HEALTH CONDITIONS   241

Contents

ix

Contents

x

Contents

xi

Preface

MY HERBAL ODYSSEY

HERBS and I didn't get off to a good start during my early childhood. While playing outside our house in Buena Park, California, I managed to run a rather substantial sliver of wood under a thumbnail. My mother, after failing to get the intruder out with tweezers, called her mother, who was working as a nurse at the time. I was whisked to maternal grandmother's abode and promptly set up in the kitchen among some stainless steel utensils not commonly associated with eating and a ton of gauze.

Four hours later, after my screams had exhausted her, grandmother declared that amputation was the only rational option. Shielded by my equally hysterical mother, I was transported to my paternal grandmother, whose primary claim to fame was her pot roast. She calmly informed my mother that all my ill-fated thumbnail needed was a healthy application of herbal salve. The herbal salve, according to grandma, would draw the splinter out from under the nail. After telling me to shut up (which was anesthesia that could rival morphine), she proceeded to anoint my finger with salve and then wrap it with gauze. She then proclaimed that the pot roast was calling and that we should hit the road. Instructions were given for replacing the salve and wrap every day.

The salve didn't work and three days later my infected thumb felt as though a two-by-four was embedded under the nail. My mother sat me down on the couch with a root beer float and we shared a Kodak moment—watching *The Ozzie and Harriet Show*. Empowered by Ricky Nelson's song at the end of the show (which always had mom chirping like a bird), she grasped my thumb, subdued me with a forearm stranglehold, and removed the splinter.

It took a good ten years for me to develop a truce with herbs. My initial interest grew out of my study of American Indians and their healing systems. Two years later, I was given a copy of *Back to Eden* by Jethro Kloss. I began brewing exotic herbal teas and identifying local plants that had medicinal properties. An herbal student was born!

A number of divergent paths have contributed to my current interest in herbal medicine. Studies in Jungian psychology led to further exploration of the healing systems of different cultures. Work with emotionally disturbed children and adults led to critical thinking regarding drug therapy and the limitations of our health care system. My studies in naturopathic medicine took the tradition and mysticism of herbal medicine and paired it with modern scientific scrutiny. This was a wonderful discovery and helped decide the path I'm currently pursuing.

This book represents my development in herbal medicine to date. The primary focus is on safe and responsible use of herbal medicines. The secondary focus is on herbs that have a track record of modern clinical studies or a reliable history of clinical use to ensure their effectiveness in the treatment of human illness. Because I'm a naturopathic doctor by training and not an herbalist, my focus is one based on the impatience of what works and what doesn't. Last, but not least, I hope the book inspires you to become a more critical consumer and student of herbal medicine.

Thanks for reading. I'm off to perfect grandma's herbal salve!

Acknowledgments

Helene Stevens, for the wonderful illustrations and for fostering my interest in herbs; Nick Gallo, for working his magic with the text; Michael Danko, for reminding me when it was soda time; Freddie Yudin for his contributions to my non-herb library; Linda Moss, for trying out many of the herbs covered in the book; Kevin Kim for the Knicks tickets; Joe Pizzorno, N.D., and Steve Austin, N.D., for providing a model of natural health care education that has successfully merged science and tradition; David Springer for teaching me to be a better doctor; Skye Lininger, Loren Israelson, and Mark Blumenthal for their contributions to my professional growth; Steven Foster for all the free advice he's given me over the years; my students at Bastyr University for assisting my growth as a teacher and student of natural medicine; Natasha Kern, the best agent any wacky herbal guy could ask for.

Introduction

A QUICK GLIMPSE AT THE HISTORY OF HERBS IN MEDICINE

2000 B.C. *"Here, eat this root."*

1000 A.D. *"That root is heathen. Here, say this prayer."*

1850 A.D. *"That prayer is superstition. Here, drink this potion."*

1940 A.D. *"That potion is snake oil. Here, swallow this pill."*

1985 A.D. *"That pill was ineffective. Here, take this antibiotic."*

2000 A.D. *"That antibiotic doesn't work anymore. Here, eat this root."*

—Author unknown

The first edition of this book led off with a section entitled "Health Care Consumers Speak Out!" Now, five years later, I'm here to tell you that your voice was heard! Consumer demand for herbs has caused the herbal supplement industry in the United States to double in size since 1994.[1] Primarily because of consumer demand and supplement industry feedback, the Food and Drug Administration (FDA) has actually expanded the scope of claims that can be made on herbal supplement labels. The Office of Alternative Medicine at the National Institutes of Health (NIH) began in the early 1990s with a yearly budget of $2 million for research. Now known as the National Center for Complementary and Alternative Medicine, the yearly budget for research has ballooned to $68 million. Three of their studies are on herbal medicines. Finally, the face of medicine in the United States is changing because of you. Medical schools are incorporating classes on herbs and other "alternative" therapies,[2] and health care providers are increasingly including coverage of alternative medicine practitioners.[3]

Let's look at the wild and crazy world of herbs since last we met.

TRENDS IN THE USE OF HERBS

Back in 1993, Dr. David Eisenberg and his colleagues rocked the medical community when they reported that, according to a survey completed in 1990, an estimated one-third of the U.S. adult population was using some form of alternative (they called it "unorthodox") medicine.[4] Of the rather extensive list of therapies, herbs ranked somewhere in the middle of the pack.

Dr. Eisenberg and his colleagues decided to repeat their survey in 1997.[5] Compared to 1990, estimated expenditures for alternative medicine services increased by 45.2 percent in 1997 and were estimated at $21.2 billion (a number Dr. Evil could be proud of!). Of this rather large sum of money, over one-half was paid out of pocket! Compared with 1990, the largest increase in use for any therapy was herbal medicine, which now ranked second. Two other interesting findings in the survey deserve mention. First, persons using alternative therapies such as herbs were no more likely to discuss their choice with their doctor in 1997 than they were in 1990. Second, the survey suggests that an estimated fifteen million adults in the United States are using herbal or nutritional supplements together with prescription medications.

HERBS GO TABLOID

Coverage of herbal medicine in the mainstream press has exploded since 1995. Herbal experts who had been living in peaceful obscurity suddenly found themselves thrust in front of television cameras or being interviewed for *Time* or *U.S.A. Today*. While issues about quality control and safety were mentioned, the media were largely focused on the exploding herbal supplement market and profiling the herbal supplement user. Unprecedented coverage of herbs such as St. John's wort, ginkgo, and saw palmetto cast a largely favorable view on herbal medicine.

Things took a rather abrupt about-face toward the end of 1998. The media suddenly shifted to reporting on what was wrong with herbal supplements. While some stories responsibly covered problems with quality control and consistency in some herbal products, many ended up sounding as if they were straight out of tabloids such as the *National Enquirer.* Reporting on a Loma Linda University test tube study looking at how St. John's wort, ginkgo, saw palmetto, and echinacea affect the ability of human sperm to fertilize a hamster oocyte, Jane Brody released a story in the *New York Times* entitled "Herbal Remedies Tied to Pregnancy Risks."[6] The study found that human sperm was less likely to fertilize the hamster oocyte if St. John's wort, ginkgo, or echinacea were directly added to the test tube.[7] While the ability of these herbs to block the unsightly child that might result from this union should be celebrated, the coverage by Ms. Brody made it sound as if men might become infertile if they took the herbs! Fortunately in this case, the scientific community roundly criticized the study and its conclusions about these herbs potentially causing infertility.[8]

While media reporting isn't always this silly, remember that your self-education and working with a health care professional who is experienced in herbal medicine will allow you to cut through some of the confusion created by news stories on herbs.

REGULATION OF HERBS

Another event contributing to the growth of the herbal supplement market was the passage of the Dietary Supplement and Health Education Act (DSHEA) at the end of 1994. DSHEA marked a profound change in government policy toward the regulation of herbal and nutritional supplements, which had previously been regulated as mere foods. DSHEA actually created a new category for these products known as *dietary supplements.*

DSHEA was a real boon for both the supplement industry and consumers. Suddenly, labels were able to make claims that told you what an herb actually does in the body. Known as *structure and function claims,* they describe the way an herb or herbal constituent influences or supports a bodily structure or function. Suddenly consumers were seeing ginkgo labels that claimed improved mental sharpness and memory, saw palmetto labels claiming support for normal urinary flow, and valerian products promising a restful night's sleep. DSHEA is adamant that herb companies must not promise treatment or prevention of disease and that structure-function claims are based on sound scientific evidence and not someone's impression of the ancient Greek application of a particular herb.

Life under DSHEA has been a mixed bag. Although a boon to herb companies and consumer education, it has led to a lot of products on the shelf making similar claims. Company A can actually give you the world's best-researched ginkgo extract that has been used in over 90 percent of the completed research but find that its extract is on a shelf next to Company B's generic ginkgo product that makes the same claims. Worse yet, Company B's generic ginkgo product uses the data from Company A's ginkgo research to support its claims. We'll look more closely at this issue in Part 1.

DSHEA continues to evolve. In a rather startling about-face, an FDA ruling on February 7, 2000, actually expands the scope of structure-function claims that can be made for herbal and nutritional supplements. The ruling allows structure-function claims to encompass common conditions associated with normal passages of life. Examples include acne in adolescence, premenstrual syndrome, hot flashes associated with menopause, and age-related memory loss.

Stay tuned: I'm sure more changes are coming. As health care professionals learn more about the medicinal application of herbs such as St. Johns' wort, ginkgo, kava, saw palmetto, and horse chestnut, it is going to be difficult to rationalize the constraints of DSHEA on these products.

THR EXPANDING ROLE OF HEALTH CARE PROFESSIONALS

Herbal medicine seems to have fallen into a new category these days, namely, *complementary and alternative medicine* (CAM). While access to information on herbs and CAM therapies has exploded in the past decade, a similar trend has been noted in publications for health care professionals. About 1,500 articles are being published yearly on CAM in mainstream medical journals.[9] Over two-thirds of all U.S. medical schools have courses on CAM aimed at helping doctors answer patient questions.[10] Pharmacy schools and continuing education programs for practicing pharmacists are following suit.

While naysayers claim that CAM and herbal medicine have no place in mainstream medical practice,[11] increasingly larger numbers of medical doctors, osteopaths, chiropractors, physician assistants, nurses, and pharmacists are becoming more qualified and willing to discuss use of herbal medicines with their patients. In fact, polls suggest that many doctors and pharmacists feel that herbal medicine will be an integral part of their practice in the next five years.[12]

As mainstream medicine becomes more interested in herbal medicine, one of the payoffs will be increased opportunities for clinical studies. As mentioned earlier, the National Center for Alternative and Complementary Medicine at NIH has already started the ball rolling. A study looking at the use of St. John's wort to treat depression began in 1999 at Duke University, and studies looking at the use of ginkgo for preventing Alzheimer's disease and echinacea for treating the common cold are set to begin in 2000. Studies such as these will give health care professionals greater insight into the role that herbs may play in their clinical practice.

Last but not least, don't forget those health care professionals who are trained and actually licensed in some states to practice herbal medicine. Naturopathic physicians are trained in four-year, postgraduate institutions that combine orthodox medical science (pathology, microbiology, and physical diagnosis) with clinical training in nutrition, herbal medicine, homeopathy, and hydrotherapy. In the "Herbal Medicine Resources" section at the back of the book, I've given you the number of the American Association of Naturopathic Physicians (AANP) as well as the accredited postgraduate schools that train naturopathic physicians. While naturopaths are licensed in only some states currently (Alaska, Arizona, Connecticut, Florida, Hawaii, Maine, Montana, New Hampshire, Oregon, Utah, Vermont, Washington), the AANP can direct you to a qualified naturopathic physician in your area who can help guide your use of herbal medicines in your health care and wellness programs.

Navigating the Future of Herbal Medicine

As we begin a new millennium, it's ironic that one of our most ancient healing systems is poised to jump back into the mainstream with both feet. The next decade is a crucial one for the growth of herbal medicine in the United States. It's in its adolescence, and all the factors are in place to continue the maturation process and reach adulthood. Many of the trends mentioned earlier are critical to this process—particularly integration into medical practice and increased clinical research.

The onus, however, is not just on health care practitioners. Companies making and selling herbal supplements must reach for new standards of excellence in areas of quality control and quality assurance. They need to take a more responsible stance on the type of claims they put on their products. Finally, it's imperative that the herb industry fund more clinical research.

At the same time, the government needs to look carefully at the regulation of herbal supplements. Is it fair to place accepted medicines in Europe such as ginkgo, saw palmetto, horse chestnut, kava, and St. John's wort into a regulatory category that serves only to muddle the real use of these clinically proven herbal medicines? Should companies that invest in clinical research proving the effectiveness and safety of their herbal product be constrained in what they can tell consumers and health care professionals?

Thanks to you, the herbal consumer, the past decade has been a wild ride. Let's hope that the next decade brings the clarity and credibility we all want for herbal medicine. Thanks for reading!

part I

How to Choose the Best Herbal Supplement

The best attitude with which to approach the herbal marketplace is open-minded skepticism.

ROB MCCALEB, EVELYN LEIGH, AND KRISTA MORIEN,
THE ENCYCLOPEDIA OF POPULAR HERBS

"GUARANTEED Potency!" "Organically Grown!" "Standardized Full-Spectrum Extracts!" "Clinically Proven by Doctors!"

As you scan the huge selection of herbal supplements on the shelves these days, label claims such as these bombard your senses. Gone are the days when your doctor recommended an herbal remedy that was dispensed by your friendly neighborhood pharmacists. Today's herbal consumer is faced with the daunting task of trying to make heads or tails of label claims, promotional literature, and even store clerks guiding them toward the herbal supplement that's supposedly the best choice. Winning the Power Ball lottery often seems easier.

I wish I had an easy answer for you. Unfortunately, herbal regulations in the United States leave most of the work up to you, the herbal consumer. While I do see positive trends in quality control and quality assurance as well as increased education of health care professionals, it's important that you do your homework before purchasing an herbal supplement. In addition to the obvious considerations such as proper labeling of ingredients and responsible claims, this education may help you more effectively address a health concern successfully. Equally important is knowledge about safety issues such as side effects or potential drug interactions associated with the herbal supplement you are considering.

THE SELF-ACTUALIZATION MODEL
AND HERBAL SUPPLEMENTS

During both undergraduate and postgraduate studies in psychology, I was impressed with Dr. Abraham H. Maslow's theory of self-actualization. Maslow argued that each person has a hierarchy of needs that must be satisfied, ranging from basic physiological requirements to love, esteem, and, finally, self-actualization. As each need is met, the next higher level in the emotional ladder dominates our conscious functioning. Therefore, people who lack food or shelter or who cannot feel safe are unable to move up the ladder and express higher needs. Maslow believed that persons who satisfied the highest level of psychological needs were able to fully integrate all components of their personality, or self.

While baldness, an expanding waistline, and teenagers reminding me of my shortcomings have provided a challenge to my sense of self in the past few years, I've often thought Maslow's model has some application to herbal supplements. Not implying that herbs have a sense of self, the theory provides a framework for us to look at what steps are necessary for an herbal supplement to reach the status of "best."

Figure 1.1 is an attempt to place these criteria in a hierarchy that starts at the bottom as basic requirements and ends with those factors that would elevate an herbal supplement above its peers.

While my hierarchy clearly reflects my bias toward clinically proven herbal products, considering some or all of these requirements in the order presented should help guide your attempt to select the "best" herbal supplement. Let's expand our look at what goes into making an herbal supplement the best in its class.

FIGURE 1.1. HERB QUALITY, SAFETY, AND EFFICACY HIERARCHY

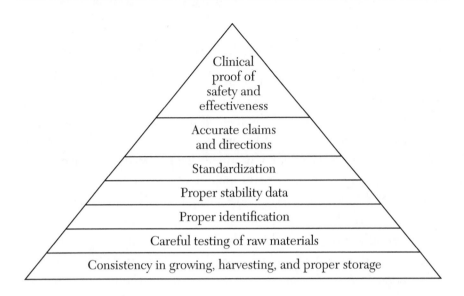

GROWING, HARVESTING, AND STORAGE

When looking at an herbal supplement, our primary concerns are normally whether it is high quality, actually works, and is safe. However, our self-actualization model has to start with the time the seed is planted to time of harvest. The level of certain active constituents in plants can vary depending on the type of soil in which they're grown, the local climate, and harvesting time. Perhaps equally important is how the herbs are stored. Improper storage can lead to contamination and poor-quality raw materials going into the tincture bottle, capsule, or tablet on the shelf.

As the production of herbal products has become more sophisticated, so has the business of growing them. Be sure the company you are buying your herbs from has full knowledge of the source of their herbs.

One other note of importance here is the issue of sustainability. As the herb industry has exploded, the demand of increased sources of certain plants has followed. While wild crafting is a popular concept, it is often unrealistic in these times. American ginseng, goldenseal, and even echinacea have all been threatened by overzealous harvesting in the wild.

Controlled cultivation of herbs on farms helps decrease the risk of certain plant species becoming extinct and is also good for the economy.

GOOD MANUFACTURING PRACTICES

As we work up our hierarchy, numbers 2 through 4 are among the key considerations in deciding the quality of an herbal product. *Good manufacturing practices* (GMPs) is the blanket term used to cover the steps a company must take to ensure the quality of its product. While not fail-safe, GMPs reduce the risk of poor quality leading to safety concerns and lack of effectiveness in the herbal supplement you are buying.

Companies following GMPs will usually have laboratory facilities either in-house or through a reputable contract laboratory that allows for proper identification of the herb. The first question by an herbal manufacturer should always be "Do we have the right herb?" While an experienced botanist may be able to take the first steps of plant identification based on leaf shape, type of flowers, or root configuration, chemical profiling using sophisticated procedures such as high-performance liquid chromatography (HPLC) allows for more accurate identification. This is particularly applicable to standardized extracts with known chemical markers that allow for the development of a common "fingerprint" for an herb.

Next in our GMPs comes the issue of purity. It's important for herb manufacturers to test herbs for contaminants (sometimes called *adulterants*). These could be something as simple as weeds or some other plant that have made their way into the bulk herbal product. More important, purity testing also is a checkpoint for contaminants such as pesticides, heavy metals, bacteria, mold, and even animal or insect contamination.

Next we reach the issue of potency. In many traditional practices of herbal medicine, this quality was determined by the senses: taste, smell, and sight. How the herb tasted, smelled, or looked was often the key to whether an herbalist would choose the plant for medical use. As noted earlier, the development of laboratory analyses, including HPLC, often make this part of our GMP journey easier and more reliable. It is important to keep in mind that determining potency is much easier for those plants with identified active constituents that can be measured. Examples include bilberry, kava, ginkgo, and milk thistle.

Finally, a frequently overlooked issue related to potency is stability. While more related to a finished product that is already in a capsule or tablet, the issue of shelf life is critical to its effectiveness. Some companies automatically slap a three- or four-year expiration date on their products without performing the necessary tests to accurately determine stability. It's important to buy herbal supplements from suppliers that actually perform stability testing to see how long the potency of their product survives on the shelf. The Food and Drug Administration helped this process a bit in 1999 by passing a ruling that requires manufacturers labels to be 100 percent accurate when it comes to potency claims.

STANDARDIZATION

The past two decades have seen an explosion of standardized herbal extracts. This movement has primarily been driven by the influx of standardized extracts from Europe such as bilberry, feverfew, ginkgo, horse chestnut, and St. John's wort. Typically sold in capsule or tablet form, standardized extracts, as we'll note in Part 2, typically guarantee a consistent range of certain constituents from batch to batch in the finished product. This is typically expressed on the label as a percentage of the total weight of the extract.

Standardized extracts have become popular among health care professionals because they allow for more consistency in dosing. Based on the concentration of certain active constituents, these products often have an advantage of delivering a more powerful and efficient medicinal punch. Bilberry extract is a classic example. While you can eat several bowls of blueberries daily to equal the effect you might get with a couple of capsules of bilberry extract, you might be using your improved vision to read magazines on the toilet! Due to the proprietary nature of some of these extracts in Europe, they often have clinical studies supporting their safety and effectiveness. These factors have placed standardized extracts somewhere between our traditional perceptions of herbal remedies and modern pharmaceutical drugs.

It's important to remember that the term *standardization* has become a marketing hook with some products. Standardization implies consistency in a product, and not strength. Although many extracts are standardized to constituents that are medically active in the body (e.g., silymarin in mild thistle and kava lactones in kava), the term may also be extended to *marker* compounds that are used for quality control purposes only. Examples include valerenic acid in valerian and echinacosides in echinacea. This means it's best to consider standardization on an herb-by-herb basis and not buy into a blanket concept that encompasses all herbs.

Standardized extracts are a relatively new development in the long history of herbal medicine and represent only a small minority of what's currently available among herbal products.

PACKAGE CLAIMS AND DIRECTIONS

An herbal manufacturer that you can depend on for quality herbal supplements should be one that gives an accurate depiction of what's inside the bottle or package. Ingredient lists should not only include such issues as accurate identification, potency, and stability—as already discussed—but also encompass full disclosure of what else is in the product. Companies should disclose all additives and excipients used in their products.

Also critical are the instructions for use on the label. Ideally these should be based on clinical research experience with the product in question. Lacking clinical studies to support dosing, herbal pharmacopoeias and textbooks from Europe are the next best bet. Guidelines established by organizations such as the British Herbal Pharmacopoeia, German Commission E, and the European Scientific Cooperative on Phytotherapy often provide dosage guidelines that are based on clinical and historical use of the herb in question.

Full disclosure regarding safety issues is also important to a quality herbal supplement. What are common side effects? Can pregnant or lactating women use the herb safely? Is it safe for children? Are there any drug interactions to be concerned about? All of these are important questions that should be considered when creating an herbal supplement label or package insert.

Finally, are the structure and function claims on the label accurate? We discussed DSHEA and structure and function claims in the foreword. So you know the FDA expects companies to base these claims on valid scientific evidence supporting them. The ideal win-win situation is if these claims are based on research done on the actual product in the package. As we'll note later, *clinically proven* takes us to the top of our self-actualization ladder. Lacking actual clinical studies, companies should at least be aware of the clinical data on related products and create their claims accordingly. While I'm not a fan of this fallback position, it at least provides some guidelines for companies to follow in creating responsible claims.

Use books such as this one to educate yourself about what the scientific literature says about an herbal supplement. Match this up with the claims on the label. If there are notable discrepancies, then move on down the shelf!

Clinically Proven

The pinnacle of our self-actualization is clinical proof of safety and effectiveness. While I don't downplay historical evidence of safety and effectiveness, modern clinical studies give us added focus and assurance of these important considerations. It helps us have a more accurate sense of what dosage to use and for how long. You're likely to have a greater sense of what side effects or potential drug interactions may occur. Finally, the claims on the package are based on firsthand experience, not borrowed information.

That's why my gold standard is those products that have been tested in modern clinical studies. If you look at most clinically proven herbal supplements currently available in the United States (please see Part 3 for a listing of some of these products), you'll note that all of our other requirements to reach the status of "best" have been addressed.

I encourage you to support companies that have gone to the trouble to manufacture products that have reached the top of our self-actualization model. This is your assurance that they are more likely to offer products of the highest quality and are willing to answer questions accurately about their products.

SELF-ACTUALIZATION AND THE HERBAL CONSUMER

OK, so now that the checklist for the herbs is complete, here are a few more pointers to help your herbal self-actualization. These will be echoed throughout the book and should be a conscious part of your choice to use herbal supplements.

1. Read, read, read! As is the case with anything we use medicinally, information on herbs changes rapidly. Try to keep up with your reading of quality books on herbs and databases such as those mentioned in the Resources section at the back of the book.
2. Follow label directions. As we'll note in Part 2, just because you think it's safe because it comes from a plant doesn't mean there's no potential for side effects. Carefully follow dosage recommendations, and don't decide on your own that more is better than less.
3. If you want to use an herbal supplement to treat an ailment or disease, talk to a qualified health care professional first. This is particularly critical if you're taking medication.
4. Be wary of using herbs together with prescription or over-the-counter medications. Again, your doctor or pharmacists may help guide you here.
5. Buy from stores that are committed to educating their employees. Educated employees are more likely to give you accurate information based on quality material provided by credible manufacturers and their own reading. Avoid those stores that try to steer you toward a product because of profit margins or self-interest.

6. You usually get what you pay for. Standardized herbal products that have reached the level of "best" in their class are often more expensive than those that haven't. So, be prepared to pay a little more for quality, clinically proven herbal products. Don't reach for ground-up saw palmetto berries, for example, when a standardized liposterolic extract is what's been clinically proven to treat prostate enlargement.

Watch out, herbal manufactures and retailers—we're self-actualized and comin' to get you!

part 2

QUESTIONS COMMONLY ASKED
ABOUT HERBAL SUPPLEMENTS

ALTHOUGH access to good information on herbs is at an all-time high, Americans still have a lot to learn about herbal medicines—particularly their use in health care. The following questions about herbs are commonly asked by consumers, retailers, and health care professionals. They run the gamut from use of herbs with prescription or over-the-counter medications to questions about different herbal preparations. In Part 1, I've addressed the big question, "How do I choose the best herbal supplement?" Some of the issues regarding quality control are covered again in this section.

I'm a medical professional, not an herb grower or manufacturer. As such, I urge you to call companies selling herbal supplements with your questions. Most of them have customer service departments to serve you. Also, resources such as the American Botanical Council and the Herb Research Foundation may offer assistance.

And remember: The purpose of this book is to help you choose herbal medicines with a sound résumé of clinical research and real-life use for different conditions. These criteria should play a major role in your choice of herbal medicines.

Do herbs really work?

Eighty percent of the world's population can't all be wrong! That's the estimated number of people worldwide who use herbal medicines to stay well.[1] While cultural use of herbs has existed throughout history, many countries have taken this knowledge and applied it to modern medicinal applications. Countries such as Germany, France, China, and Japan have successfully incorporated herbal medicine into their health care systems. Why? Because they work!

These countries have created a model for the effective use of herbal medicine. Thanks to their efforts, we need no longer refer to herbal medicine as "folk medicine." Folklore gave us clues to the medical use of herbs, but the modern research conducted in these countries has provided us with scientific support for their use in modern medical systems. In Part 3, we'll take a detailed look at European phytotherapy as a role model for what herbal medicine could become in this country.

If herbs are so effective, why don't more doctors regularly recommend them in the United States?

There's been a huge increase in doctor's interest in herbal supplements in the past decade. Fueled by published reports that more and more of their patients are taking herbs,[2] doctors are trying to sort through the maze of herbal education for three reasons. The first is to be able to address patient questions. The second is to become more knowledgeable about the safety of herbs. Finally, some, but not all, want to find out whether some of these herbal medicines do have a place in their clinical practice.

The biggest gap for doctors has been lack of education about herbs. This situation is changing rapidly. Current estimates have about two-thirds of the U.S. medical schools either currently teaching or planning to incorporate classes on complementary medicines such as herbs.[3] Also, some companies selling herbal supplements with clinical research support have begun to realize the value of educating doctors.

In the meantime, don't be afraid to talk to your doctor about herbs. It's important for them to know that herbs are part of your treatment program, as some herbs may interact with medications you might be taking.

Educate your doctor—share books like this and those listed in "Herbal Medicine Resources." Also, the references in the book can provide doctors with answers to some of their technical questions.

Don't forget that many health care professionals have been educated in herbal medicines and are licensed to recommend them in certain states. If you are in a state that licenses naturopathic physicians, you're at an advantage. See the resources listed at the back of the book to see whether you live in a state that licenses naturopaths and who's in your area. Remember to use those naturopathic physicians who have a degree from a recognized four-year, postgraduate institution (these school are listed in the resources section).

Can I combine mainstream medical care with alternative therapies such as herbal medicine?

A hot topic in medicine these days is the issue of integrating alternative and complementary medicines. While mainstream doctors and pharmacists are scrambling to catch up in this area, many managed health care systems, insurance companies, and hospitals are beginning to offer alternative medicine practitioners as part of their services.

It doesn't take a rocket scientist to figure out why this is happening. Alternative medicine is big business. In 1998, it was estimated that Americans spent an estimated $27.2 billion on alternative medicine care.[4] Mainstream providers are realizing that the way to keep patients is to offer these services.

So, the answer to this question is an enthusiastic yes! Creating a health care team that includes your medical doctor and alternative practitioners such as a naturopathic physician, chiropractor, or acupuncturist is an ideal way to create a truly holistic approach to your health care.

Why aren't herbs labeled as to what conditions they treat?

Actually, herbal supplement labels can say more now than in the past. The passage of the Dietary Supplement and Health Education Act (DSHEA) in late 1994 (see comments about DSHEA in the foreword) marked a significant change in what can be said on herbal supplement labels. DSHEA allows for supplement manufacturers to explain how an herb or herb constituent influences a structure or function in the body. This is why you'll sometimes encounter the term *structure and function claims* used for these statements.

While these statements about herbs have greatly improved the quality of information for consumers, the law does not allow for specific disease treatment or prevention claims to be made. So, men buying saw palmetto won't see a label telling them that the product can treat benign prostatic hyperplasia; they will see claims that promise support for normal urinary flow and prostate health.

While a new ruling by the Food and Drug Administration at the beginning of 2000 gives a little more scope to herbal supplement claims to include normal events associated with different stages of life (e.g., acne during adolescence, hot flashes during menopause), disease claims are still taboo for herbal manufacturers. This places greater emphasis on finding a health care professional to help in your selection of an herb(s) for treating a condition. This leap also requires greater self-education using books such as this one and those listed in the resources section in the back of the book.

Where do herbs fit into my health care program?

Herbal medicines are often more gentle in their action than commonly prescribed drugs. They may take longer to act and often work to support or influence balance in a body system, instead of doing its job for it. This sometimes makes them good considerations for treatment of the early stages of chronic conditions (e.g., ginkgo for age-related cognitive decline, intermittent claudication) or prevention of illness. Herbs may also play a role in your everyday wellness program.

For some individuals, they also offer means of recovery from illnesses such as anxiety, depression, or insomnia. In these cases, herbal alternatives, while gentler and less likely to cause side effects, do have a notable effect within a reasonable amount of time. In other words, switching over to an herbal alternative such as kava or valerian doesn't mean you're going to have to wait weeks to notice an effect. Herbal medicines may be an option for treatment of some chronic conditions that are not responding to drug therapy. Examples include eczema, rheumatoid arthritis, premenstrual syndrome, and benign enlargement of the prostate. Once improvement occurs, the herbal prescription generally is a safer alternative for continued treatment.

Remember, the best way to decide how herbs fit into your health care program is to find a health care professional trained in herbal medicine to act as your guide (see "Herbal Medicine Resources" at the back of the book).

Can herbs be taken with prescription or over-the-counter drugs?
One of the key friction points for integration of herbs into medical practice has been the issue of potential interaction with drugs. While some herbs have been used safely with mainstream drugs for many years, we are learning more about potential drug–herb interactions. Part of the reason is the large number of people using drugs and herbs together. A survey completed in 1997 estimated that almost 19 percent of people taking herbs and other dietary supplements were using them together with prescription medication.[5]

Drug–herb interactions can take on different faces. The most concerning is if the herb you are taking interacts with a drug to cause potentially dangerous side effects. Examples of this include using garlic with an anticoagulant drug such as warfarin, leading to increased risk of bleeding. Another example would be St. John's wort used with an antidepressant such as Prozac®, leading to a condition known as serotonin syndrome (mental confusion, muscle twitching, sweating).

Some herbs may affect the way the body metabolizes certain drugs. Our old friend St. John's wort has been found to potentially decrease blood levels of certain drugs such as digoxin, cyclosporin, indinavir, theophylline, and warfarin. Dong quai and green tea have been discovered to interfere with the actions of warfarin. The message here is to be sure to discuss what herbs you are taking with your health care professional.

Finally, herbs may counteract the side effects caused by certain drugs. One example is ginkgo counteracting the sexual dysfunction sometimes caused by antidepressant drugs known as selective serotonin reuptake inhibitors or SSRIs (e.g., Prozac, Zoloft). Milk thistle may help prevent potential liver damage caused by some medications.

While discussing the potential for drug–herb interactions with your health care professional is important, some good references on the topic are available in your local bookstore. One that I helped write is the *A–Z Guide to Drug-Herb-Vitamin Interactions* (Prima Health, 1999). Another good resources is Dr. Francis Brinker's book *Herb Contraindications and Drug Interactions* (Eclectic Medical Publications, 1998).

Can herbs act as substitutes for prescription or over-the-counter drugs?
As we'll note in Parts 5 and 6, a number of herbs may be considered alternatives to some drugs. Examples include St. John's wort for mild to moderate depression, kava for mild to moderate anxiety, valerian for insomnia, ginger for motion sickness, and ginkgo for age-related cognitive decline and early-stage Alzheimer's disease. Note that most of these herbal alternative address milder forms of the condition in question. Medical care in the United States stands to improve dramatically if we could start phasing herbal prescriptions into the early treatment of many conditions before they become more serious. We could save precious health care dollars by slowing the progression of conditions that ultimately require expensive medical interventions.

When I begin taking an herb, how do I know what dosage to use and how long to take the product?
Part 5 of this book highlights herbs that have received the scrutiny of modern research. Clinical research has sometimes helped arrive at the "best" dosage for a specific condition. Use this information to select standardized herbal preparations that offer a clear dosing schedule.

However, such standardized products are currently in the minority. Other herbal preparations can be effective when taken at the proper dosage. Use the recommendations in Part 6 as a guide; also, compile a list of quality reference books on herbal medicine (see "Herbal Medicine References").

Like most drugs, herbs affect people in different ways. For instance, men taking saw palmetto report that their nightly trips to the bathroom are notably less within the first week. Others may not notice this effect for three to four weeks. Again, standardized herbal preparations with clinical studies will often give us a little better prediction as to when to expect results.

In the case of more traditional preparations, it may take some experimentation before you determine how long to take a product. The guidance of a qualified health care professional or herbalist can help guide you.

The issue of how long to take an herb varies and, much like many drug therapies, depends a lot on how the person is responding and the nature of the condition being treated. Echinacea is best taken for short periods of seven to ten days for treating the common cold. St. John's wort may do its thing in three to four months for someone dealing with depression due to the death of a loved one. However, someone with more chronic depression may need to be on it for several months, if not longer.

Some herbs used for chronic health conditions are best used on an ongoing, continuous basis. Examples include ginkgo, hawthorn, and saw palmetto.

Note: Seek professional help when deciding on the proper dosage for your child.

Should I take my herbal supplement at mealtimes or between meals?

We don't know for sure with every herbal medicine. Again, this is often based on experience and less frequently on clinical studies. Some herbs probably benefit from mealtime consumption because digestion and assimilation will be at their peak. Oil-based preparations derived from plants such as evening primrose and saw palmetto are usually taken with food.

There are always exceptions to the rule. For example, if you're using bromelain (really not an herb but a proteolytic enzyme from pineapple) to relieve inflammation, take it between meals. Taken during meals, it acts as a digestive enzyme and will offer little anti-inflammatory activity.

I've heard that because herbs are from plants, they're basically safe. Do I have to worry about any side effects?

Most of the herbs covered in this book have few side effects. These are usually mild and affect a small minority of people. Mild gastrointestinal upset is one you'll see mentioned from time to time. Some people may be allergic to an herb or one of its constituents.

Some herbs, however, have the potential to cause significant side effects. If you take an herbal product and have a bad reaction, contact your doctor first. Poison control centers are also expanding their databases to include potential reactions to herbal supplements. Notify herb companies, also. This feedback provides them with important information about their products. Like the drug industry, herb companies should track side effects of their products.

The adage that herbs are safe just because they are from plants is a dangerous one. Herbal laxatives such as senna, aloe, and cascara should be used with the caution afforded any drug. When consumed in large amounts on a regular basis, licorice root products can cause high blood pressure and water retention. Comfrey root may cause damage to the liver when consumed in large amounts.

While the scare tactics employed by the press and some medical publications to make herbs look dangerous are sometimes overblown and often reflect unbalanced reporting, the best rule of thumb is to use the same caution with herbs that you would with any medication. Most of the serious side effects I've been called about over the past five years have stemmed from overuse or misuse of an herbal medicine or an interaction with a prescription drug. Use herbs sensibly and you'll usually avoid trouble. If you're not sure, seek the help of qualified health care professionals or books that address safety issues.

In Part 5, I've tried to give you the breakdown of the most common side effects that have either been seen in clinical studies or reported by people using the herbal supplement.

Can a pregnant or lactating woman take herbal medicines?

As is true with many drugs, the answer is usually "We're not sure." The best rule is to avoid most herbs during pregnancy. Exceptions may be a tea made from red raspberry, ginger capsules to help with nausea, and even an echinacea tincture to help fight a cold.

Herbs that have been found to be potentially dangerous during pregnancy or lactation should bear a warning on the label (I wish I could say this is always the case). Examples include stimulant laxative such as cascara and aloe and may also extend to herbs such as ginseng, kava, and black cohosh.

Many commercial herbal products currently sold don't include information about pregnancy and lactation. If the label of an herbal preparation doesn't say anything, seek the opinion of a health care professional well versed in herbal medicine before taking an herbal supplement.

In Part 5, I address whether an herb is contraindicated during pregnancy and lactation. The great legal two-step is to say "no known contraindications" instead of "safe." So, two-step with your doctor, midwife, or naturopath to decide which is the best choice.

Can children take herbal medicines? Is the dosage the same?

My clinical experience, which is strongly oriented to pediatrics, says that children often respond to treatment with herbal medicine. However, as is the case with herbs during pregnancy, we're often not 100 percent certain of the safety of an herb for children (by the way, this problem is also shared by many prescription and over-the-counter drugs). What's the best dosage and delivery form are frequently asked questions by parents. Taste can often be a major obstacle to even getting an herbal product into a child.

So, I hate to sound like a broken record, but your best bet is to work closely with a health care professional (preferably one with extensive pediatric experience) to decide whether an herb is safe for your child.

DOSAGE

Most pediatricians adjust drug prescriptions for children on the basis of weight. This can be done with some of the standardized herbal preparations we'll discuss in Part 5. However, with many traditional preparations, this approach is difficult, because we often don't know what the optimal dosage is even for an adult. It's sometimes comforting to know that the pediatric dosage of some herbal medicines does not drop significantly; echinacea is a classic example.

Some herbalists use Young's formula, which bases estimated dosage on a child's age. I favor dosage based on weight. While Young's formula is easy to use, the room for error is large. What if your five-year-old weighs the same as most eight-year-olds?

OK, already—I am a broken record: When in doubt, seek professional help!

DELIVERY

This is the hard part—an herbal medicine will benefit children only if you can get it into them. Liquids are the best form of delivery for young children, but they often taste bad and are high in alcohol (a concern for infants less than one year of age). Try mixing these in juice. Glycerin-based liquid preparations are a good-tasting alternative but are often weak in strength (see the later description of tinctures). Powdered herbs can be mixed in applesauce or sweet potatoes.

Be creative and patient. I'm not the best adviser, since my son thinks anything or anyone called "herb" should be avoided!

Are herbal medicines addictive?

The commercial herb industry is not allowed to sell herbal supplements that are addictive. Obviously, many addictive drugs come from the plant kingdom (e.g., opium, heroin, cocaine), but fortunately, they aren't sold in your friendly health food store or natural health section of your pharmacy or grocery store.

One trend that makes me very uneasy is the growing use of herbs high in caffeine (e.g., guarana) for weight loss and energy. Caffeine certainly rates as a mild addiction and has the downside of making people edgy. With time it also runs down your adrenal function (see the section on stress and fatigue under "Endocrine System" in Part 6). Products promising "escalation" or "acceleration" belong on espresso stands and not in health food stores.

Do herbs contain steroids or hormones?

This is a widely held misconception. First, products that are either hormones such as melatonin or hormone precursors such as DHEA are not herbs! Second, some herbs or herb constituents bind hormone receptors in the body. Examples are licorice and ginseng weakly binding estrogen receptors. This action is even more notable for flavonoids known as isoflavones in red clover and soy that are sometime referred to as *phytoestrogens*. Please see the discussion on phytoestrogens in the "Menopause" section in Part 6.

Some herbs actually support glands that produce hormones and steroids. These products will often work on the endocrine system, which includes the hypothalamus, pituitary, thyroid, adrenal glands, and reproductive organs. Examples include vitex, eleuthero (Siberian ginseng), and licorice.

Finally, some herbal products promise the ability to supply precursors to hormones in the body. One of my favorites are the wild yam products that are supposed to increase a woman's progesterone levels naturally. This is false advertising, and women are better off avoiding the "yam scam" and opting instead for an herb such as vitex, which helps the body naturally improve its production of progesterone. What form of herbal medicine is most effective?

This is another question without a clear-cut yes or no answer. Herbal medicines come in many forms. You can have garlic, ginger, or turmeric with your meals. You may choose to have some chamomile tea for your upset stomach. Goldenseal tincture will probably soothe your sore throat better than a capsule. A concentrated extract of ginkgo in tablet form, however, will be far more effective than a tincture in treating poor circulation.

One form of taking herbs that is becoming increasingly popular is in snacks such as potato chips or candy bars as well as some drinks. Popularly known as *nutraceuticals,* most of these preparations contain such small amounts of a particular herb that it is unlikely that you'll get any benefit at all. If you need ginkgo to improve your mental sharpness or kava to manage mild anxiety, don't reach for one of these products. Your best bet is to stick with the product form that has been tested and proven to work in clinical studies.

Commercial herbal preparations are available in many different forms: bulk herbs, teas, tinctures, fluid extracts, powdered herbs in capsules and tablets, and solid extracts. Let's consider each of these.

Herbal Powders

Usually available in capsules or tablets, herbal powders typically have minimal processing and are reasonably priced.

Teas

Herbs are often prepared as medicinal teas. Practitioners of traditional Chinese medicine often use a form of medicinal tea called a *decoction*. A decoction is made by combining bulk herbs in water and boiling them together. The mixture is then strained and the liquid consumed. Decoctions make stronger, more concentrated medicinal teas.

Note: Remember that the development of the modern tea bag has little to do with the traditional preparation of herbal teas as medicines. These preparations typically used very large amounts of the herb to make a very concentrated tea.

Infusions

To make an infusion, pour boiling water over the herb and let it steep. Chamomile is commonly prepared in this manner. Tea bags are the most common form of infusion used in the United States.

Note: Many plants have active constituents that are not soluble in water. You're better off taking a liquid or solid extract in such cases.

Tinctures

Tinctures are an extremely popular form of herbal preparation in the United States. You make a tincture by letting an herb soak in a solvent (usually alcohol or water) for several hours, days, or even weeks, depending on the herb. Tinctures are most commonly made with alcohol.

Over the past few years, glycerin has been used to make "alcohol-free" tinctures. While far more tasty than grain alcohol, glycerin is not as good a carrier as alcohol and results in somewhat weaker preparations. If you're concerned about alcohol in tinctures, try placing the alcohol-based tincture in a tea, and take it that way. This will dilute and even evaporate some of the alcohol.

Tinctures are typically a 1:5 or 1:10 concentration. This means that one part of the herbal material is prepared with five to ten parts (by weight) of the liquid. A tincture is therefore usually considered a more diluted herbal preparation.

FLUID EXTRACTS

Fluid extracts are more concentrated than tinctures. Like tinctures, they are often made with either water or alcohol, but sometimes other solvents may be used in an extraction. The final product is concentrated by distilling some of the solvent and thus increasing the herbal concentration. Fluid extracts are typically a 1:1 concentration.

SOLID EXTRACTS

A solid extract represents the most concentrated form of an herbal product. It results when *all* of the solvent is evaporated off, leaving a solid residue. These residues are usually available in powdered form. An exception would be oil-based preparations containing fatty acids, such as saw palmetto extracts. Solid extracts are typically 2:1 to 8:1 concentrations.

STANDARDIZED EXTRACTS

Many of the herbal medicines discussed in this book have taken the extraction process one step further. *Standardization* means guaranteed levels of a certain constituent or group of constituents in the final product. This quality is usually expressed as a percentage of the total weight of the extract. Standardization allows for accurate dosing based on a measured amount of the proven, active constituents. For example, milk thistle extracts typically contain 80 percent silymarin. The recommended daily dose of silymarin is 420 milligrams. Thus, 525 milligrams of the extract will provide the recommended dose. Other examples of standardized herbal medicines are bilberry, ginkgo, and kava.

Remember that the term *standardization* does not necessarily mean "more active." While some herbs such as milk thistle, ginkgo, and kava are standardized to constituents that have medicinal activity in the body, other herbs, such as valerian and echinacea, may be standardized to constituents that are used as markers for quality control and may have nothing to do with medicinal activity. It's best to take herbal standardization on a case-by-case basis.

Questions Commonly Asked About Herbal Supplements

A FINAL TIP

There's a lot of overlap among the categories. Ask fifteen herbalists or doctors about which preparations they prefer, and you'll probably hear fifteen different opinions. Standardized liquid or solid extracts offer the most reliable dosing forms. Medical professionals looking for measured and often quicker results will usually opt for this form of herbal medicine. You may also want to start here if you're treating a specific health condition.

Tinctures and powdered herbs, while weaker in their effect, do offer a cost-effective alternative for treatment of minor ailments. They can also be employed as part of your daily supplement program.

If I choose to use a tincture or fluid extract, how can I compare dosage with a solid extract?

One gram of a 10:1 solid extract equals 10 milliliters of a 1:1 fluid extract and 100 milliliters of a 1:10 tincture. Remember that some standardized extracts can have very high concentrations. A 50:1 extract of ginkgo leaves would require 50 milliliters of a 1:1 fluid extract and 500 milliliters of a 1:10 tincture to be in the ballpark!

Please keep in mind that these are rough comparisons. A standardized extract has a carefully measured amount of active constituent(s) also. Just because you produce an equal amount of fluid extract or tincture doesn't mean you're guaranteed a proper amount of these active constituents.

Are single herbs or herbal combinations better?

Once again, the answer is an unequivocal "It all depends." If you're taking herbs to help round out your optimal diet and supplement program, then herbal combinations are often an ideal way to go. There's less concern here with therapeutic dosages.

My scientific mind and impatient nature have biased me in favor of using single-herb preparations or combinations with clinical proof for the treatment of health conditions. Most of the herbal medicines discussed in Part 5 are effective therapeutic agents on their own merits without being combined with other herbs. When we start combining herbs, we sometimes lose some of our assurance about the way an individual herb will work in the body. The bottom line is, when you know it works a certain way by itself, use it by itself. Again, the exception to the rule is herbal combinations that have been clinically studied. This doesn't mean that I oppose using herbal combinations. I find these valuable when a condition presents a combination of symptoms. I may choose to combine echinacea with goldenseal for a cold with a sore throat. A person with high cholesterol and intermittent claudication may benefit more if he or she combines red yeast rice and ginkgo.

A key concern about combinations is whether they deliver sufficient dosages of the recommended herbs. If you've got a product with everything but the kitchen sink in it, you're probably looking at a rather weak cumulative effect.

In addition to having sufficient amounts of the featured herbs, an herbal combination should have a rationale for the combination. Combining *Drosera* and thyme for a dry, spasmodic cough makes sense. So does gentian and yellow dock to help with digestion. But putting vitex, black cohosh, and dong quai in a formula for women with PMS doesn't make sense. Here again, a health care professional can be a useful guide. Also, finding a retail outlet with an educated staff will make your decision easier.

What do the designations "organically grown" or "wild-crafted" mean?
An herbal product that bears the designation "organically grown" means that no pesticides, herbicides, chemical fertilizers, or irradiation were used to produce, grow, or preserve the plant. Most herb companies strive to buy organically grown herbs whenever possible.

"Wild-crafted" usually means that the herb is not grown in a controlled setting, such as a farm. Wild-crafted herbs are usually picked in the wild by an experienced herbalist. While this is often romantically perceived as being the best way to harvest herbs, it is fraught with potential problems. The first problem is the environmental impact. If every herb company depended on wild-crafting, our natural supply of wild plants would be so greatly diminished that many herbs would face possible extinction.

The second problem is consistency in wild-crafted herbs. Different growing conditions can significantly change the concentration of medically active constituents.

Large herb companies in the United States and Europe rely primarily on herbs that have been grown under controlled situations. This method means less impact on our wild plants, as well as better quality control. Many U.S., European, and Asian herb companies have developed plant strains and optimal growing conditions that guarantee a higher plant yield and greater concentration of important medical constituents in the herbs.

Where can I obtain accurate and reliable information on herbal medicine?
See the list of resources listed in the back of the book. In addition, health food stores, pharmacies, and other retail outlets can provide you with educational materials.

Be a critical reader!

part 3

PHYTOTHERAPY: A RATIONAL MODEL FOR HERBAL MEDICINE IN THE UNITED STATES

We see the position which medicinal plants should hold in modern medicine: before the major chemotherapeutic agents, and indeed before surgery, in any case in their own position and in their own right. The sequence also establishes the degree of seriousness and danger of the different interventions, being a progression from the least invasive to the most invasive.

RUDOLF FRITZ WEISS, M.D.

WHAT'S A "PHYTO"?

When searching for a model to spur the further development of herbal medicine in this country, one need go no further than the herbal system employed by European countries such as Germany and France. Certainly, the herbal products that have been developed in these countries meet the requirements for clinical effectiveness and safety stated in the Dietary Supplement Health and Education Act of 1994 (DSHEA; see the foreword). The system of herbal regulation in these countries (particularly Germany) offers the most rational approach to the integration of safe and effective herbal medicines into our health care system.

The term used to describe the modern clinical use of herbs in many European countries is *phytotherapy*. Phytotherapy is the science of using plant medicines to treat illness. Efforts in this field have successfully combined modern medical practice with herbal medicine. As a result, countries such as France, Germany, Switzerland, and Italy have adopted a regulatory climate that nurtures clinical research on herbs and encourages acceptance of their use in their health care systems.

PHYTOTHERAPY: HISTORICAL PERSPECTIVE

The French physician Henri Leclerc (1870–1955) is often credited with being the "father of phytotherapy." He published numerous papers on the use of herbal medicines in the clinical setting. His works are summed up in his textbook, *Précis de Phytothérapie*, which continues to be a primary reference in modern phytotherapy.

The real mover and shaker, however, was the German physician Rudolf Fritz Weiss (1898–1991). He inspired the organization of a group of professionals dedicated to phytotherapy and also published the highly influential textbook *Lehrbuch der Phytotherapie* (Textbook of Phytotherapy). This has become one of the leading reference books on the use of herbs in medical practice. Now in its seventh edition in Europe, the sixth edition is available in the United States under the title *Herbal Medicine*. Dr. Weiss also founded the *Zeitschrift für Phytotherapie* (Journal of Phytotherapy), devoted to research on applications of herbal medicines in the health care setting.

While these two figures played an important role in medical acceptance of herbal therapies, the influence of phytomedicinal companies has been huge, both in Europe and now in the United States. Companies such as Madaus, Bionorica, Schwabe, Lichtwer Pharma, Schaper and Bruemmer, and Indena not only have led the charge in the development of quality herbal extracts but have financed important clinical studies that have elevated herbs such as ginkgo, saw palmetto, and St. John's wort to their current level of popularity.

INFLUENCE OF HERBAL MEDICINE
ON EUROPEAN HEALTH CARE

Like pharmaceutical drugs in the United States, herbal medicines used in European phytotherapy undergo extensive laboratory testing and clinical trials prior to approval for use by humans. Known as *phytomedicines*, these herbal products have become an important part of the health care delivery system in many European countries.

Phytomedicines are used largely as supportive therapies for chronic illness or as treatment of minor ailments that do not require drug therapy. Many phytomedicines are also used to prevent disease. Subsequently, health care costs in areas such as geriatric medicine and gynecology have fallen.

The "mainstreaming" of phytotherapy into clinical practice in Germany and France has led to significant numbers of physicians and pharmacists recommending phytomedicines to their patients. More than 70 percent of general practitioners in Germany prescribe phytopharmaceuticals, and many of these are covered by national health care insurance.[1] Approximately 40 percent of the drugs listed in the German *Rote List* (their version of our *Physicians Desk Reference*) are derived from plants.[2] Currently, about 60,000 phytomedicinal products appear on the German market.

COMMISSION E AND ESCOP MONOGRAPHS

We would be wise to look to Germany for a successful model of how to regulate herbal medicine. For example, herbal medicines in Germany have been reviewed by a commission of professionals from a variety of health care disciplines. They have been responsible for the creation of the Commission E monographs on plant medicines. Similar to official summaries used to regulate drugs in the United States, these herbal monographs describe the plant medicine, its health care applications, appropriate dosage, and safety information. Through 1995, more than 300 monographs have been published by this group. These materials currently represent the most comprehensive information available on the use of herbs in the modern health care setting.

The past few years have seen an English translation of the Commission E Monographs completed by the American Botanical Council. An expanded version of the monographs with clinical research became available at the beginning of 2000 and is essential reading for any health care professional interested in herbal medicine.

Since 1995, Commission E has not issued any new monographs. Instead, the group has acted as an expert advisory board to the German Federal Institute for Drugs and Medical Devices and has directed focus to the development of monographs for the entire European Union (EU).[3] With the formation of the EU, the 1990s saw work of the development of monographs that apply to all countries in the EU. Led by the European Scientific Cooperative on Phytotherapy (ESCOP), 50 herbal monographs have been published to date; the monographs are available from the American Botanical Council (see the resources in the back of the book).

The development of herbal monographs has not been limited just to Europe in the past few years. As of June 1999, the World Health Organization (WHO) had published 28 monographs and plans to publish another 29 in 2000.

PHYTOMEDICINES IN THE UNITED STATES

The past decade has seen a huge influx of European phytomedicines into the U.S. herb market. Table 3.1 lists some commonly recommended and researched phytomedicine brands in Europe and who's selling them in the United States. Beginning with popular herbs such as ginkgo, milk thistle, saw palmetto, and St. John's wort, phytomedicines not only have set a higher standard of excellence for the U.S. herb market but also have had a huge economic impact. In 1998, ginkgo, St. John's wort, garlic, saw palmetto, kava, and valerian all ranked among the ten top-selling herbs in the United States.[4]

Table 3.1
COMMONLY RECOMMENDED AND RESEARCHED PHYTOMEDICINES IN EUROPE AND CORRESPONDING U.S. BRANDS

Single Herb Products	European Brand Name/ Manufacturer	U.S. Brand Name/ Manufacturer
Black Cohosh	Remifemin®/Schaper & Brümmer	Remifemin®/ Enzymatic Therapy
Echinacea	Echinacin®/Madaus	Echinaguard®/ Nature's Way
Garlic	Kwai®/Lichtwer Pharma	Kwai®/Lichtwer Pharma
Ginkgo	Tebonin® (EGb 761)/ Schwabe	Ginkgold®/ Nature's Way Ginkoba®/ Pharmaton Quanterra™ Mental Sharpness/ Warner-Lambert (Pfizer)
Hawthorn	Crataegutt® forte/Schwabe	HeartCare®/ Nature's Way
Horse Chestnut	Venostasin®/Klinge Pharma	Venastat®/ Pharmaton
Milk Thistle	Legalon®/Madaus	Thisilyn®/ Nature's Way
Saw Palmetto	Permixon®/Prostate/ Pierre Fabre	Elusan®/Plantes & Médicines, Inc.
St. John's wort	Jarsin® (LI 160)/ Lichtwer Pharma	Kira®/Lichtwer Pharma

continued

Phytotherapy: A Rational Model for Herbal Medicine in the U.S.

Table 3.1 (continued)

Single Herb Products	European Brand Name/ Manufacturer	U.S. Brand Name/ Manufacturer
Vitex	Agnolyt®/Madaus	Femaprin®/ Nature's Way

Combination Products

Echinacea, Wild Indigo, Thuja	Esberitox®/Schaper & Brümmer	Esberitox®/ Enzymatic Therapy
Gentian Root, Elder Flower, European Vervain (aerial parts), Primrose Flower, Sorrel (aerial parts)	Sinupret®/Bionorica	Quanterra™ Sinus Defense/Warner-Lambert (Pfizer)

With an impressive resume of clinical studies and safety data, these products have raised the bar for herbal products in the United States. One of the real windfalls resulting from their introduction is the huge influx of clinical information on herbal medicines from Europe. Along with the Commission E monographs, these textbooks and clinical studies have brought a new level of credibility to herbal medicine in the United States. It has also given health care practitioners an expanded repertoire to treat many common conditions, and consumers reliable products and good standards of quality control.

Last but not least, these herbs are creating a surge in clinical studies on herbs in the United States. The completion of these important studies will add focus to the role that these phytomedicines will play in the U.S. health care delivery system.

Phytotherapy: A Rational Model for Herbal Medicine in the U.S.

32

part 4

CATEGORIES OF
HERBAL MEDICINES

BEFORE diving into some of the most commonly prescribed herbal medicines in Part 5 and herbal recommendations for common health conditions in Part 6, let's take a look at some general categories of herbal medicines to describe their actions in the body. Some of these actions will be familiar (astringents and laxatives) and some less familiar (carminatives and demulcents). Herbs in the adaptogen and antioxidant categories affect a broad spectrum of actions in the body.

These categories give you a framework for the way groups of herbal medicines act in the body. For example, if you're having trouble properly digesting food and suffer a lot of bloating after a meal, you may want to consider a digestive bitter such as yellow dock. If you're run down from stress and overwork, adaptogenic herbs such as eleuthero (Siberian ginseng) or astragalus are extremely useful. These categories are widely accepted and used by health care professionals who prescribe herbal medicines.

Remember that herbs like to defy labels. Some will end up in more than one category. For a more thorough review of herbal categories (including those applicable to traditional herbalism), I highly recommend Chapter 3 in David Hoffman's *The Herbal Handbook: A User's Guide to Medical Herbalism* (Healing Arts Press, 1998).

ADAPTOGENS

It's fitting to begin a discussion of herbal categories with a term that embodies herbal medicine's amazing diversity. An *adaptogen* is a substance that increases the body's resistance to stress and exerts a balancing effect on various systems of the body, including the immune, nervous, and cardiovascular systems.

Adaptogens can trace their descent from the herbal tonics commonly used in the traditional herbal healing systems of China and India. A prime example is Asian ginseng (*Panax ginseng*), which we'll cover in Part 5. Two Russian scientists, I. I. Brekhman and I. V. Dardymov, first applied the term *adaptogen* to Asian ginseng and later to its Russian relative eleuthero (*Eleutherococcus senticous*, Siberian ginseng).[1] Their expanded definition of an adaptogen includes the following three criteria:

- An adaptogen must show a nonspecific effect and raise the powers of resistance to toxins of a physical, chemical, or biological nature.
- An adaptogen effects a normalizing or balancing action independent of the type of pathological condition.
- An adaptogen must be harmless and must not influence normal body functions more than necessary.

The following herbal medicines qualify as adaptogens:

Asian ginseng	Schizandra
Eleuthero (Siberian ginseng)	Ashwagandha
Astragalus	Codonopsis ("Dangshen")

While most of these herbs have an illustrious career in traditional herbal medicine, they may be even more applicable in today's stress-filled world than they were hundreds of years of ago. Adaptogens enhance health by performing the following actions:

- Stress reduction (support normal function of the hypothalamic–pituitary–adrenal [HPA] axis)
- Enhancement of brain and central nervous system activity
- Immunomodulation

- Antioxidant activity
- Liver protection and antitoxin activity
- Improved blood sugar metabolism
- Increased stamina and endurance

The core of an adaptogen's diverse actions is its ability to help the body deal more effectively with stress.[2] The key here is support for the HPA axis. This rather ominous-sounding name is really the part of our endocrine system that is responsible for regulating the body's response to stress. Proper function of the HPA axis depends on healthy communication between the three control centers. When overly large amounts of stress—mental or physical—override this normal communication, we begin to see symptoms of fatigue, anxiety, and even soft-tissue pain. The burden of this dysregulation appears to fall on the adrenal glands. We'll discuss this further in Part 6 under chronic fatigue immunodeficiency syndrome and stress and fatigue.

The adrenals, which sit atop the kidneys, are responsible for helping us respond to stress. They also help us rebound from stress. When the adrenals become overwhelmed, we lose this edge, and different systems in the body begin to break down.

If you're experiencing chronic stress, the number one condition you'll probably notice is fatigue. You may also experience problems with blood sugar metabolism, sluggish immune function, and even general aches and pains in the muscles and joints. Chronic fatigue immuodeficiency syndrome may be the end result of exhausted adrenals.

Adaptogens serve to help reinstate normal HPA axis communications and recharge exhausted adrenal glands. When this task is completed, they continue to support normal HPA axis function and optimize our ability to deal with stress in its many forms.

I'll let the chapters on eleuthero and Asian ginseng in Part 5 serve as an introduction to some of the potential health care applications for adaptogenic herbal medicines. The actions of adaptogens also make them ideal for resisting illness. They should be an important consideration for any supplement regimen aimed at optimizing health.

ANTIOXIDANTS

A popular topic in health care today is the role that free radicals play in many diseases. Particular attention has been focused on age-related conditions such as atherosclerosis, Alzheimer's disease, and macular degeneration. Free radicals may also play a role in other diseases that afflict our society, including cancer.

Free radicals are highly reactive groups of atoms that repeatedly undergo chemical reactions without change to themselves. We all produce them and have substances in the body known as *antioxidants* to keep them in check. When free radicals form in excess, naturally occurring antioxidant substances produced by the body (e.g., glutathione, superoxide dismutase) can be overwhelmed. Damage to cells ensues.

Modern society produces a lot of contributors to free radical formation. These include pesticides, environmental pollution, and secondhand cigarette smoke. Free radicals also rise with overexposure to ultraviolet rays produced by the sun. Stress can raise the level of free radicals, as can chronic illnesses, such as human immunodeficiency virus (HIV) infection. Also, as we get older, our defense systems become less aggressive and free radicals have more opportunity to cause harm.[3]

Unless you've been living in seclusion on some deserted island (although the *New York Times* probably has delivery there), you know that antioxidant nutrients can help counter free radical production in the body. Vitamin C, vitamin E, selenium, and a variety of carotene-like substances provide this antioxidant support.[4]

Many herbal medicines also offer antioxidant support. The herbal constituents that shine in this area are the *bioflavonoids* (usually referred to as *flavonoids*). Occurring in a wide variety of edible plants (including herbs) and common foods, flavonoids are one of nature's most potent antioxidants. In fact, some flavonoids are several times more potent in this regard than vitamin E.[5,6]

Start adding flavonoids to your free radical defense program by way of your diet. Apples, green tea, onions, cherries, and blueberries are excellent sources of flavonoids. High consumption of flavonoids in the diet is associated with lowering the risk of cardiovascular disease.[7] New data

Table 4.1
TISSUE-SPECIFIC BIOFLAVONOIDS

Herbal Medicine	Bioflavonoids	Body System
Bilberry	Anthocyanosides	Eyes, circulatory system
Hawthorn	Oligomeric procyanidins	Heart, circulatory system
Ginkgo biloba	Ginkgo flavone glycosides	Brain, nervous system, cardiovascular system
Milk thistle	Silymarin	Liver and gallbladder

have extended this to cancer prevention as well, an area in which the flavonoids in green tea really shine.[8] As we'll note in Part 6 in our discussion of menopause, foods and herbs high in isoflavones (sometimes called *phytoestrogens*) such as soy and red clover, exert health benefits that may hold an eventual key to offering women an alternative to hormone replacement therapy after menopause.

The health-promoting benefits of flavonoids have been known to herbal medicine for years. Many herbal medicines have complex flavonoid structures as medically active constituents. Examples discussed in Part 5 include bilberry, chamomile, hawthorn, ginkgo, and milk thistle. Owing to research on the way these particular flavonoids work in the body, we've also been able to establish a "tissue-specific" effect for many of them. Table 4.1 lists herbal medicines, their active flavonoids, and the body systems they support. All of these are discussed in greater detail in Part 5.

Flavonoids have become a priority of mainstream medical research. These important dietary and herbal constituents promise to lead the way in further unlocking the preventive and therapeutic potential for antioxidants, particularly in the prevention of cardiovascular disease and cancer.

ASTRINGENTS

If you drink straight black tea, you'll notice a tightening sensation inside your mouth. This is because of substances known as *tannins* in the black

Table 4.2
HEALTH CARE APPLICATIONS FOR ASTRINGENTS

Herbal Astringent	Application
Horse chestnut	Varicose veins, hemorrhoids, leg ulcers, postoperative swelling, and hematomas
Witch hazel	Eczema, hemorrhoids, and varicose veins
Tormentil	Diarrhea

tea. In fact, milk is commonly added to tea to counteract the activity of tannins.

Tannins are the primary component of herbal medicines commonly labeled "astringents." Tannins actually get their name from their use in tanning hides (animal, not human!). When tissue comes in contact with tannins, proteins coagulate, causing a tightening effect. This creates a protective barrier and also helps add "tone" to the tissue.

Tannin-containing herbs are useful in treating inflammation of the skin and mucous membrane (another name for the lining inside the respiratory and gastrointestinal tracts). Inflammation occurs in topical conditions such as eczema and leg ulcers. Topically, tannins are also useful to speed wound healing. Internally, tannins add tone to the gastrointestinal (GI) tract, helping stop diarrhea and soothing irritated tissue. They've also been employed in traditional herbal medicine to help stop bleeding in the GI tract.

Commonly used astringent herbs include witch hazel leaves, oak bark, American cranesbill, and English walnut leaves (see Table 4.2 for some of the health care applications of these herbs).

Note: Internal use of astringents is contraindicated during pregnancy.

CARMINATIVES

Carminative (from the Latin *carminare,* to cleanse) herbs soothe and tone the digestive system. Typically high in volatile oils, these herbs are used in cases of GI upset, irritation, and cramping. They help relieve excess gas and bloating.

Two classic examples of carminative herbs are peppermint and chamomile. As we will note in Part 5, chamomile is revered in Europe and is one of the most commonly prescribed herbs for digestive tract problems. Health care applications for these herbs include indigestion, heartburn, infant colic, and sometimes irritable bowel syndrome. Other carminative herbs include anise, caraway, and fennel. On the basis of our discussion in Part 5, ginger may also be considered a carminative.

The key to the gastrointestinal actions of carminatives is their volatile oil content. Since volatile oils are not water soluble, the typical teacup of peppermint or chamomile is medicinally weak. Unless you're brewing a highly concentrated tea of dried chamomile flowers or fresh peppermint leaves, you're better off using concentrated fluid extracts or alcohol-based tinctures. These will offer a more reliable source of medically active volatile oils.[9]

Cholagogues

An area that has long been the focus of natural medicine is healthy liver function. The liver, as we will note in the chapter on milk thistle in Part 5, is the primary organ of detoxification in the body. In addition, it works with the gallbladder to digest and assimilate fats. One key to proper fat digestion is *bile:* When bile production in the gallbladder and flow from the liver become impaired, many people experience a sense of fullness or bloating following the consumption of fats in the meal.

Herbs classified as *cholagogues* have two primary actions. The first is to stimulate the production of bile. The second is to stimulate the proper flow of bile. Some herbal texts refer to the second action as *choleretic*. By improving bile production and flow, these herbs also reduce the risk of gallstone formation. They are also associated with improving fat digestion and promoting healthy liver function.[10]

Listed here are commonly prescribed cholagogues:

Dandelion root	Milk thistle
Turmeric	Artichoke
Goldenseal root	Chelidonium

Note again the overlap of categories. Many digestive bitters (see the section "Digestive Bitters") can also be classified as cholagogues.

DEMULCENTS

Demulcents are herbs that are high in *mucilage* (a slimy, soothing substance). These herbs are noted for their ability to soothe or protect irritated mucous membranes inside the body. When applied topically to the skin, a demulcent herb is commonly referred to as an *emollient*. These herbs have demulcent properties:

Marshmallow root	Slippery elm
Mullein flowers	Aloe leaves (only the mucilaginous part)
Plantain leaves	Fenugreek seeds

The slimy mucilage in these herbs produces remarkable effects on the body. A demulcent[11]

- eases irritation in the bronchioles secondary to a cough;
- reduces irritation in the GI tract secondary to diarrhea;
- relaxes and eases urinary tract irritation; and
- soothes skin irritation and inflammation, speeding wound healing.

Traditional herbalists and some naturopaths prescribe demulcent herbs to ease the following conditions:

- Sore throats/coughs
- Diarrhea
- Irritable bowel syndrome
- Inflammatory bowel conditions
- Urinary tract irritation (e.g., following an infection)
- Burns

Note that some herbal texts list comfrey and coltsfoot as commonly prescribed demulcents. These herbs contain a group of constituents known as pyrrolizidine alkaloids, which are potentially harmful to the liver.[12,13] Internal consumption of comfrey and coltsfoot is not recommended.

DIGESTIVE BITTERS

My son would argue that all herbs are bitter and taste like something intended to poison him. His perspective is clouded by the fact that his dear old dad used to try out different vile-tasting herbal tinctures on him during naturopathic training.

The bitter taste associated with many herbs (particularly the root or rhizome portion) is the basis for using them to stimulate digestion. When a bitter substance hits your tongue, taste buds tell the brain to signal the mouth to produce more saliva and the stomach to release more acid to help break down food. Some research on bitters also suggests a stimulating effect on the pancreas and increased production of digestive enzymes. As mentioned previously (see "Cholagogues"), these herbal bitters also stimulate bile flow. The bottom line is that one feels hungrier and digests better after consuming an herbal bitter.

If your digestion is sluggish due to poor production of stomach acid, you'll find bitters particularly useful. If you notice a lot of bloating and gas after eating a meal high in protein, try taking an herbal bitter immediately before eating. Stomach acid production also has a tendency to decrease as we age. Herbal bitters are frequently prescribed for elderly persons who produce less stomach acid and experience sluggish digestion.

Commonly prescribed herbal digestive bitters include the following:

Gentian root and rhizome	Dandelion root
Yellow dock	Blessed thistle
Centaury	Wormwood
Rue	Boldo

IMMUNOMODULATORS

More attention is being paid to the effect that many herbs have on the immune system. Examples covered in Part 5 include echinacea, eleuthero (Siberian ginseng), and Asian ginseng.

Immunomodulation describes the ability of an herb, nutrient, or other substance to promote healthy immune function. The immune system is a complex interplay of cells that dictate the body's resistance to infections. These include macrophages, lymphocytes (B and T), and other factors known as cytokines (e.g., interleukin, interferon, and tumor necrosis factor). Lymphocytes, the body's primary defense against viral infections, have been a primary area of focus with regard to HIV infection.

A common denominator among immunomodulating herbs is the presence of complex sugar molecules known as *polysaccharides*. Polysaccharides improve the activity of lymphocytes and other cells of the immune system, thus strengthening the overall immune response.[14]

Perhaps the most well-known example of an immunomodulating herb is echinacea. As we will note in Part 5, echinacea is thought to increase the immune response, which makes it valuable for strengthening a potentially healthy immune system to fight infections such as colds and flu more efficiently. It may also speed the body's recovery from infections and reduce the recurrence of bacterial and yeast infections. Echinacea is the perfect short-term boost that many immune systems require from time to time.

However, a "get busy" immune stimulant like echinacea is not for everybody. If your immune system is already overactive, as is the case in people with autoimmune diseases, echinacea may not be your first choice. It's also not recommended for progressive diseases such as multiple sclerosis. Finally, the jury is still out on whether echinacea should be used by persons with HIV infection.

In my opinion, these conditions are the domain of the adaptogenic herbs listed earlier. Adaptogens such as astragalus and eleuthero (Siberian ginseng) tend to enhance the immune system by way of a balancing approach, as opposed to the more nonspecific approach taken by echinacea. This means adaptogens can be used as potentially supportive therapy in conditions in which the immune system is either depressed or overactive. The following is a list of immune-related conditions for which herbal adaptogens might be considered:

- HIV infection
- Chronic fatigue immunodeficiency syndrome
- Chronic hepatitis
- Cancer recovery from radiation or chemotherapy

Keep in mind that with most of these conditions, immune-enhancing actions represent only one aspect of a complete health care program.

Some mushrooms, including shiitake, reishi, and maitake, contain a high concentration of polysaccharides. These polysaccharides, like those of immunomodulating herbs, affect the immune system. Traditionally employed as tonics, these mushrooms have many of the same applications as the herbal adaptogens.

LAXATIVES

By the time you finish this book, you may be thinking laxative. From prunes to good ol' Ex-Lax, laxatives are among the most commonly sold over-the-counter remedies in both the United States and Europe. Herbal laxatives are sold most often.

Herbal laxatives are usually placed into two categories: stimulant or bulk-forming. Table 4.3 gives common examples of the two categories.

Table 4.3
HERBAL LAXATIVES

Bulk-Forming	Stimulant
Psyllium seed	Senna leaves
	Cascara bark
	Aloe (latex from the leaves)

BULK-FORMING LAXATIVES

Bulk-forming laxatives, which are high in fiber as well as mucilage, expand when they come in contact with water (try leaving some psyllium seeds in a bowl of water for a couple of days). As they increase in volume in the bowel, they stimulate a reflex contraction of the walls of the bowel, followed by emptying. This class of laxatives exerts a milder effect than stimulant laxatives and are most suitable for long-term use.

Since they are high in fiber, bulk-forming laxatives also contribute to keeping cholesterol in check. Research also suggests that diabetics can benefit from the dietary fiber in guar gum, psyllium, and fenugreek. The dietary fiber helps lower blood sugar in people with non-insulin-dependent diabetes (also known as *adult-onset* or *type 2 diabetes*).[15]

STIMULANT LAXATIVES

Stimulant laxatives increase bowel movements, owing to the presence of active constituents known as *anthraquinones*. Anthraquinones increase the contraction of the muscles of the bowel wall primarily by acting as mild irritants. This reaction is not dissimilar to a cough in response to a throat irritant.

Stimulant laxatives are wonderful short-term cures for constipation. However, long-term use is not recommended without medical supervision. Long-term overuse of stimulant laxatives can cause dehydration and also create a dependence on laxatives for a normal bowel movement. Stimulant laxatives are normally not recommended for pregnant or lactating women (senna is the exception). These laxatives should be avoided if you have an inflammatory bowel disease such as ulcerative colitis or Crohn's disease.

The best researched and most widely used stimulant laxative is senna. One of the best products for treatment of chronic constipation in elderly people is a combination of senna (18 percent) and psyllium (82 percent). In a study of seventy-seven elderly patients in a nursing care home, the use of this combination was found to be far more effective and cost-efficient than a synthetic laxative (lactulose) in the treatment of chronic constipation.[16]

Cascara, another laxative, is milder in action than senna. Aloe is an extremely potent laxative and is usually employed only when senna or cascara are not effective.

part 5

Commonly Prescribed
Herbal Medicines

PICKING herbal medicines that meet my criteria for excellence was easy. Keeping the list to a manageable size, however, was not. It reminded me of the time someone asked me to name my favorite jazz albums of all time. Unfortunately, I was only given five choices!

The herbal medicines presented here won primarily on the strength of clinical research, history of clinical use, safety, and a lot of personal bias. Many of them fill gaps not currently addressed by our medical system. As I look them over, I'm struck by how easily they would fit into the U.S. health care system. Wouldn't it be great to have urologists recommending saw palmetto as a therapeutic starting point in the treatment of benign prostatic hyperplasia? How about hawthorn extracts being recommended by cardiologists for early stages of congestive heart failure and angina?

The herb chapters that follow are formatted with a quick-reference introduction that summarizes the particulars on each herb, including common uses, notes on recommended use and proper dosage, and safety issues including potential drug interactions. The text that follows tells the story behind each herb, with a focus on how it might fit into your health care choices.

Also, please remember the following guidelines before deciding to use any of the following herbal medicines:

- Do not self-diagnose. Many of the herbal medicines are recommended for conditions that require proper medical diagnosis and close monitoring by your physician. Once this part of the picture is clear, discuss your desire to use herbal medicines with your doctor. A naturopathic physician or medical doctor, osteopath, or chiropractor trained in natural health care is an optimal choice.
- Don't discontinue any prescription medications without first discussing it with your doctor.
- Don't be afraid to share your herbal education with your doctor. Most physicians are concerned that you may be self-medicating with something that may potentially harm you. Share books like this one and those recommended in "Herbal Medicine Resources" with them. Once they become familiar with the fact that most of these herbs are approved for medical use in other countries and have clinical research, they may choose to become students of herbal medicine also!
- Herbal recommendations, like drugs, don't stand alone in our approach to health. Try to integrate them into a comprehensive health care program that focuses on diet and lifestyle factors.

Bilberry

Vaccinium myrtillus

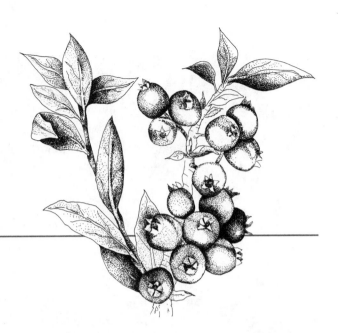

Part Used
The ripe berries

Common/Potential Uses
- Poor night vision
- Prevention and treatment of diabetic retinopathy
- Prevention and treatment of macular degeneration
- Prevention of cataracts
- Easy bruising

Active Constituents
Anthocyanosides (a bioflavonoid complex)

How It Works
Like other bioflavonoids (flavonoids), anthocyanosides are potent antioxidants. In addition, they assist with normal formation of collagen in connective tissue and help strengthen capillaries in the body. Anthocyanosides are also associated with improving capillary and venous blood flow.

Recommended Use

Standardized extract containing 25 percent anthocyanosides—120 to 240 milligrams (prevention) or 480 to 600 milligrams (treatment of early-stage macular degeneration or diabetic retinopathy). Take in two to three divided dosages daily.

Side Effects

At dosages listed above, there are no known side effects with bilberry extracts.

Safety Issues/Drug Interactions

There are no known interactions with commonly prescribed drugs. There are no known contraindications to the use of bilberry during pregnancy or lactation.

LIKE other plants high in complex flavonoids (e.g., pine bark, grape seeds), bilberry has received much attention in medical circles over the past few years. Flavonoids are extremely efficient antioxidants and assist the body in counteracting the effect of potentially harmful free radicals. Many plants high in flavonoids target different tissues and organs of the body (see Part 4). Examples include milk thistle for the liver as well as hawthorn for the cardiovascular system.

Bilberry, with its high content of a flavonoid complex known as anthocyanosides, exerts positive effects on the eyes and vision. It is commonly used for a wide array of eye conditions ranging from night blindness to diabetic retinopathy. Bilberry extract may also be a useful supplement to promote healthy circulation throughout the body and improve the strength and health of the walls of blood vessels.

Plant Facts

A close relative of the American blueberry, bilberry grows in the woods and forest meadows of northern Europe and in sandy areas of Canada and the United States. A member of the Ericaceae family, it is a shrublike perennial that grows to about 1 foot in height. The plant flowers in May or June and the ripe fruits are normally collected between July and September.[1] Although there are historical uses of the leaves, modern medicinal extracts use only the ripe fruit of the plant.

History

As a food, bilberries and blueberries have a long history of use that extends to the present. Medically, dried berry and leaf preparations have been used to treat everything under the sun. Bilberry was recommended to treat scurvy, urinary tract infections, kidney stones, and diabetes and to stop milk flow in a nursing mother.

Perhaps the most sound historical recommendation for bilberries and blueberries is for the treatment of diarrhea. The dried berries were crushed and boiled in water, then strained; the patient was then given the tea to drink. The *astringent* effect (see Part 4) speeded recovery and soothed the irritated intestinal tract following diarrhea.[2]

Modern medical research on the use of bilberry began after World War II. During the war, bombers didn't have the computerized screens in use today; if you wanted to bomb something, you had to *see* it. British Royal Air Force (RAF) pilots noted that their night vision improved when they consumed bilberry jam prior to night bombing raids. These anecdotal reports of improved night vision led to French and Italian research on the medical use of bilberry for a variety of visual disturbances.

Medically Active Constituents

Research over the past three decades has pointed very clearly to the flavonoids in bilberry as the medically active constituents. In particular, the anthocyanosides have received attention.[3] Bilberry contains more than fifteen types of naturally occurring anthocyanosides. Closely related plants, such as blueberries, black currants, and grapes, also contain these flavonoid complexes.

Research into the medical potential of anthocyanosides has led to the development of a standardized bilberry extract with a highly concentrated amount of anthocyanosides. The most frequently prescribed form has 25 percent anthocyanoside content.[4] The magnitude of this concentration is perhaps best reflected in the fact that the fresh fruit contains only 0.1 to 0.25 percent anthocyanoside content! So remember, you might improve your vision with six to ten bowls of blueberries daily, but you'd be using it for reading magazines on the toilet!

Bilberry is a classic example of the advantage of a modern herbal extract compared to more traditional preparations like tea. First, extracts allow a greater dosage of the medically active component. Also, the measured amount of anthocyanosides in an extract allows more consistent dosing and therapeutic activity.[5]

It's interesting to note the introduction of other types of extract high in anthocyanoside-like flavonoid complexes known as *proanthocyanidins* (sometimes called *oligomeric proanthocyanidins*). These include standardized extracts from grape seeds as well as pine bark. Preliminary research on grape seed extract proanthocyanidins suggests there may be some overlap in the effectiveness of these products, particularly in the eyes and cardiovascular system.[6] We'll revisit oligomeric proanthocyanidins in the chapter on hawthorn.

How Bilberry Works

Support for Normal Vision

Following the reports of those wild and crazy RAF pilots, initial research centered on bilberry's effects on the eyes and vision. Studies performed in animals revealed that the anthocyanosides actually speeded the regeneration of rhodopsin (visual purple) in the retina of the eye.[7]

The retina, which lies at the back of the eye, is the part of your eye that "sees"—that is, responds to light. It does so by way of specialized cells called *cones* and *rods*. The cones are used for detailed vision (e.g., reading) and color perception. The rods are involved in night vision and adaptation to light.[8] Rhodopsin is a purple pigment that is critical for the proper functioning of the rods. By speeding up the regeneration of rhodopsin, bilberry may support better adaptation to both dark and light.

SUPPORT FOR NORMAL CIRCULATION

Anthocyanosides strengthen the body's small blood vessels, known as *capillaries*. When capillaries become fragile (a condition that is not uncommon with aging), bruising occurs more often. Capillary fragility can also have harmful effects on other areas of the body. In the eyes, it can lead to areas of microhemorrhaging known as *retinopathy*. This is a common complication of diabetes. Weak capillaries also lead to poor blood supply to connective tissues in the body, which can hinder healing of tissue in cases of trauma and inflammatory conditions such as arthritis.

Anthocyanosides help strengthen capillaries. Owing to their antioxidant capabilities, they protect the capillary from free radical damage.[9] Anthocyanosides also help build stronger capillaries by stimulating the formation of healthy connective tissue.[10] Finally, anthocyanosides are also associated with the formation of new, healthy capillaries.[11]

Anthocyanosides also improve circulation through larger blood vessels. Studies indicate that blood vessel tone is improved in both arteries and veins after exposure to anthocyanosides.[12] Anthocyanosides have been shown to reduce the stickiness of platelets (also known as platelet aggregation)—an effect that is associated with a reduction the risk of atherosclerosis.[13] These combined effects have made anthocyanosides popular in the management of such circulatory conditions as varicose veins and hemorrhoids. It also points to these and other bioflavonoids as valuable aids in the long-term maintenance of a healthy circulatory system.

SUPPORT FOR NORMAL CONNECTIVE TISSUE

As is the case with many bioflavonoids, anthocyanosides also enhance the formation of normal connective tissue throughout the body. They do this by promoting the normal cross-linking of collagen—the backbone of healthy connective tissue.[14]

Anthocyanosides are particularly useful for the protection of connective tissue from damage secondary to inflammation.[15] They also assist in the regeneration of healthy connective tissue following injury.

HEALTH CARE APPLICATIONS

EYE CONDITIONS

Bilberry extract has become a leading herbal recommendation for the maintenance of healthy vision and for the treatment of some early-stage eye diseases. In the 1960s, French researchers discovered that bilberry extracts improved night vision and a person's ability to adjust visually to bright light.[16] This led to the use of bilberry extracts for persons with night blindness and/or poor ability to visually adapt to bright light.[17]

A newer study, however, has cast some doubt on bilberry's ability to improve night vision.[18] Young men given 480 milligrams of bilberry extract daily showed no improvement in their night vision.

In my clinical experience, persons with poor night vision (not you healthy youngsters) will sometimes note improvement using bilberry. It's safe, and two to three weeks of use should tell you whether it's going to work.

I sometimes recommend bilberry for eye strain—particularly for those of us sitting behind a computer for long stretches of time! Long-term use may also help improve the vision of near-sighted people.[19]

Bilberry may help diabetics diagnosed with retinopathy. Diabetic retinopathy is the leading cause of blindness among diabetics and is characterized by damage to the capillaries in the retina. One uncontrolled study (this means there was no placebo group) indicates that daily use of 600 milligrams of bilberry extract leads to a reduction in capillary fragility and hemorrhaging.[20] Note, however, that the results of this study are based on the reactions of only a small number of patients. Another placebo-controlled study with persons with diabetic retinopathy and hypertensive retinopathy also showed benefit of treatment with a bilberry extract.[21] Long-term use is optimal for treatment and possibly prevention of retinopathy.

Many herbal prescriptions—including gingko and evening primrose oil—help reduce the risk of some of the complications of diabetes, including retinopathy and neuropathy. Perhaps most notable is the fact that these herbal preparations also address healthy circulation in the diabetic patient and are not associated with causing problems with regulation of blood sugar control (see the discussion on diabetes in Part 6, "Endocrine System").

The small uncontrolled study on capillary fragility mentioned earlier (note 18) also indicated that bilberry may be of use for persons with early-stage macular degeneration—a form of retinopathy that primarily affects the elderly. Again, use of bilberry for preventing this condition makes most sense. While there are only small clinical observations with cataracts,[22] bilberry's antioxidant actions in the eyes also make it a logical choice for reduction of cataract risk. Clearly, more research is needed to understand the potential for bilberry in the prevention and treatment of these chronic eye diseases.

CIRCULATION PROBLEMS

Because bilberry extract improves large vessel and small vessel circulation, it may help elderly people with poor circulation to the extremities.[23] Although unlikely to be as effective as horse chestnut seed extract, it is sometimes recommended for conditions associated with the veins— namely, chronic venous insufficiency varicose veins. It should also be considered useful for improving circulation and subsequent healing in persons who have had surgery.

One notable area of use for bilberry extracts is in the prevention and treatment of varicose veins and hemorrhoids during pregnancy. These occur frequently among women in their third trimester, when the weight of the fetus and gravity combine to pull blood toward the point of least resistance. Using bilberry extract both during and after pregnancy may reduce symptoms and even the possible onset of these conditions.[24] The study noting these effects marks bilberry extract as an herbal prescription that deserves the "safe during pregnancy" seal of approval.

The anthocyanosides in bilberry have also been shown to decrease the basement membrane thickness of capillaries in persons with diabetes.[25] The possible reduction in the risk of blood vessel disease is another benefit of bilberry for persons with diabetes.

Finally, owing to bilberry's ability to strengthen capillaries, it is also a practical recommendation for people who bruise easily. I frequently recommend it with vitamin C. This combination also benefits children with frequent nosebleeds.

HOW TO USE BILBERRY

For use in diagnosed eye conditions, such as early-stage diabetic retinopathy and macular degeneration as well as circulatory disorders, bilberry extract standardized to 25 percent anthocyanoside content is recommended at a daily dose of 480 to 600 milligrams in two to three divided dosages. Following improvement, this may be reduced to a maintenance dose of 120 to 240 milligrams daily. The lower dose may be used by persons interested in the prevention of eye or circulation disorders.

There are no known side effects to bilberry at the therapeutic or maintenance dosages listed here. Bilberry is not known to interact with drugs commonly prescribed for the eyes or circulation. There are no contraindications to the use of bilberry during pregnancy and lactation. Night bombing raids, with or without bilberry, are contraindicated for the health of the planet!

RELATED CONDITIONS DISCUSSED IN PART 6

- Atherosclerosis
- Bruising
- Cataracts
- Diabetic retinopathy
- Macular degeneration
- Poor night vision

Black Cohosh

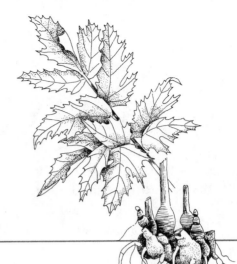

Cimicifuga racemosa

Part Used
The dried root and rhizome

Common/Potential Uses
- Hot flashes and other symptoms of menopause
- Dysmenorrhea (painful menstruation)

Active Constituents
Although the exact constituents that give black cohosh its activity are not clear, some studies have suggested that the triterpenoid glycosides and isoflavones in the root and rhizome are responsible.

How It Works
The exact mechanism of action is unknown. Previous belief that black cohosh has estrogen-like actions has been disproven in recent years.

Recommended Use

Standardized ethanolic extract of the rhizome (1 milligram of deoxyactein per 20 milligrams of extract), 20 milligrams twice daily.

Side Effects

Mild gastrointestinal upset has been reported at the doses listed above. At very high doses (several grams per day), the herb may cause abdominal pain, nausea, headaches, and dizziness.

Safety Issues/Drug Interactions

Black cohosh should not be used by pregnant or lactating women. While it may treat symptoms of menopause, it is not a substitute for estrogen replacement therapy with regard to bone and cardiovascular health.

I FOUND myself in the midst of a near-riot 5 years ago during a lecture in Fort Lauderdale, Florida. Speaking to a group of senior citizens in a large health food store, I was asked to recommend treatment for hot flashes associated with menopause. Before I had a chance to answer, a loud voice from the other side of the room boomed, "They're not flashes, dahling, they're flushes." Within seconds, the flashes and flushes had squared off in a battle reminiscent of the Yooks (butter side up) and Zooks (butter side down) in the *Butter Battle Book* by Dr. Seuss.

Two weeks later I finally discovered the truth. While I was relating the story of the flashes versus the flushes, a woman calmly raised her hand and set us all straight. "Dr. Brown, they're simply power surges."

Anyway, whatever your description for those uncomfortable temperature changes that suddenly occur at the onset and often throughout menopause, black cohosh has been the leading source of symptom relief in many European countries for the past two decades.[1] While new studies have dispelled previous beliefs that black cohosh is a phytoestrogen, the standardized extract continues to offer safe and effective treatment of acute symptoms associated with menopause. It's also the focus of current studies to determine its effectiveness for treating hot flashes in women who have been treated for estrogen-receptor-positive breast cancer—a group for whom estrogen-replacement therapy is not an option for treating hot flashes.

PLANT FACTS

Black cohosh (*Cimicifuga racemosa*) is a shrublike plant native to the deciduous forests of eastern North America, ranging from southern Ontario to Georgia, north Wisconsin, and west to Arkansas.[2] A member of the buttercup family, it is also known by the common names black snakeroot and bugbane. Black cohosh is a perennial and grows to about 3 feet tall without flowers and as high as 8 feet tall when flowering. An upright stalk grows out of the thick rootstock. The leaves are deeply serrated, and the plant produces small white flowers in late May. While the dried root and rhizome have been used in traditional herbal preparations, most modern extracts use only the rhizome (a rootlike stem growing along or under the ground and sending out both roots and shoots).

HISTORY

Black cohosh was valued by Native Americans and used for many conditions, ranging from gynecological problems to rattlesnake bites. Medical use of black cohosh dates back to the early nineteenth century in the United States.[3] American physicians at the time used the herb for rheumatism, smallpox, and fevers. During the nineteenth century, use of the plant began to focus on use for gynecological complaints with special focus on "uterine disorders." By the late 1800s, the use of black cohosh in this country had largely disappeared from medical circles.

As is the case with other medicinal herbs native to the United States such as echinacea and saw palmetto, black cohosh was introduced to Europe. It was introduced to Germany in the late nineteenth century and used primarily as a homeopathic remedy until the 1930s, when it became a therapeutic phytomedicine for treatment of gynecological disorders. To date, all of the key clinical studies on black cohosh for menopausal complaints have been completed in Germany. While the German Commission E monograph continues to cite premenstrual syndrome and dysmenorrhea (painful menstruation) as potential uses, these indications are largely based on historical use of the herb.[4] Modern use of black cohosh is primarily focused on relief of those "power surges" during menopause.

MEDICALLY ACTIVE CONSTITUENTS

As we'll note a little later when we discuss how black cohosh works, there's been a bit of recent uncertainty about which constituents in black cohosh make it work. The root and rhizome are rich in compounds known as triterpene glycosides such as cimicifugoside and actein.[5] These are the constituents to which many European extracts are standardized. In fact, the leading extract in Germany, Remifemin® (Schaper and Bruemmer, Salzgitter, Germany), is standardized to contain 1 milligram of the triterpene glycoside deoxyactein per 20 milligrams of the extract. While we're not exactly sure how these compounds work in the body, they are thought to be the most important in black cohosh.

The root and rhizome also contain isoflavones such as formononetin. While these were originally thought to provide phytoestrogenic actions, current research (cited later) appears to minimize their contribution to the actions of black cohosh.

HOW BLACK COHOSH WORKS

In herbal medicine, there's a humbling process that comes with trying to make definite statement about an herb's specific mechanism of action. Nowhere has this been more apparent than in the case of black cohosh.

As a woman approaches menopause, the signals between the ovaries and pituitary gland begin to diminish, slowing down estrogen production and increasing secretion of luteinizing hormone (LH). Hot flashes and other acute symptoms of menopause are usually attributed to these changes. Earlier studies with rats (I get power surges when I think of rats!) suggested a hormone-like action for black cohosh. One study found that constituents in black cohosh bound estrogen receptor sites in the rat uterus.[6] Another found it caused a reduction in blood concentrations of LH.[7] This latter finding was also shown in a study with menopausal women taking a standardized extract of black cohosh rhizome.[8] The conclusion was that black cohosh had mild estrogenic actions and also reduced the amount of LH—both effects expected to reduce hot flashes in menopausal women.

In the last 5 years, however, both animal and human research has indicated that the above findings are not accurate. One study with mice (did Minnie have hot flashes?) and rats found that black cohosh had no estrogenic effect at all.[9] The final blow to the estrogenic theory of black cohosh came when a study looked at the effect of the black cohosh extract Remifemin in menopausal women ages 43 to 60 years.[10] Women were given either 40 or 127 milligrams of the extract daily for three months. While their symptoms such as hot flashes improved equally at both doses, no estrogen-like effect was noted at all.

The bottom line is that, contrary to previous belief, black cohosh is not a phytoestrogen. On one hand, this means menopausal women should not consider it a substitute for estrogen-replacement. While we're several studies away, isoflavone extracts from soy and red clover may fill this bill. However, as we'll note later, black cohosh continues to be the most studied alternative for relief of hot flashes and doesn't possess the side effects or potentially harmful health effects (e.g., increased risk of cancer) associated with estrogen replacement therapy.

HEALTH CARE APPLICATIONS

A review of eight German clinical trials on the use of black cohosh for treatment of symptoms of menopause published in the *Journal of Women's Health* concluded that the herb is both safe and effective and a suitable alternative to estrogen replacement therapy in those women for whom estrogen therapy is either refused or potentially harmful.[11] Remember, when we say, "alternative to estrogen replacement therapy," we're referring to symptom relief only. Black cohosh has not been found to reduce risk of osteoporosis or cardiovascular disease.

Small clinical studies completed in the 1980s in Germany using the Remifemin extract suggest that black cohosh not only reduces hot flashes effectively but also compares favorably to hormone replacement therapy and anti-anxiety medications (e.g., Valium) for symptom relief.[12] One study compared black cohosh extract (80 milligrams per day) with conjugated estrogens (0.625 milligrams per day) or placebo in eighty menopausal women.[13] After 12 weeks, women taking black cohosh had a significantly greater reduction in scores on a standard measure of menopausal symptoms known as the Kupperman Index. The Kupperman Index rates severity of hot flashes, outbreaks of sweating, sleep disorders, nervousness/irritability, dizziness, difficulty in concentrating, joint pains, headaches, and heart palpitations. Side effects were virtually absent in the black cohosh group.

Another study compared black cohosh (similar dose but liquid preparation) with conjugated estrogens (same dose as noted earlier) or Valium (2 milligrams per day) in 100 menopausal women.[14] Again, after 12 weeks of treatment, hot flashes and other symptoms on the Kupperman Index were more effectively reduced in the black cohosh group. It should be noted that women taking black cohosh also had a greater reduction in depression and anxiety. These effects have also been seen in younger women experiencing hot flashes following a hysterectomy.[15]

The best study to date on black cohosh not only supports its effectiveness in treating hot flashes but also suggests that a rather low daily dose is effective.[16] Partially summarized above during our discussion of how black cohosh works, the study compared 40 and 127 milligrams of black cohosh extract in 152 women ages 43 to 60 years. After three months of treatment, both dosages of black cohosh were found to be equal in reducing symptoms on the Kupperman Index. Self-rating scales and physician evaluation supported these results. No serious side effects were noted at either dose. This study confirms that the 40-milligram dose is as effective as higher doses of black cohosh for successful treatment of hot flashes—a finding good for the power surges and the wallet.

How to Use Black Cohosh

The gold standard for black cohosh extracts is the Remifemin product. Take 20 milligrams (one tablet) of the extract twice daily. More traditional preparations (tinctures, dried root in capsules) do not have the research support of the standardized extract. Remember that black cohosh probably won't work immediately. Most women notice results after about two to four weeks of use. The German Commission E monograph recommends limiting continuous use of black cohosh to six months.[17]

Side effects are rare with use of black cohosh. In clinical studies, there were rare reports of mild gastrointestinal upset, headaches, and heaviness in the lower legs. Earlier reports suggesting that black cohosh may interact with estrogen replacement therapy have been disproved by the recent findings showing no estrogenic effect for the herb. This conclusion also seems to contradict earlier concerns that black cohosh may be harmful to women with estrogen-receptor-positive breast cancer. Pregnant or lactating women should not use black cohosh.

Product update: The Remifemin extract is available in the United States under the same name from Enzymatic Therapy (Green Bay, Wisconsin).

Related Condition Discussed in Part 6

- Hot flashes (associated with menopause)

Chamomile

German chamomile
Matricaria recutita

Part Used
  Dried flowers

Common/Potential Uses
Internal Uses

- Infant colic
- Peptic ulcers
- Indigestion and heartburn
- Irritable bowel syndrome
- Mouthwash for canker sores and other irritations of the mouth and gums
- Restlessness or sleeplessness in infants (especially with teething) and young children

External Use

- Inflammatory skin conditions (such as eczema)

Active Constituents

Volatile oil components: α-bisabolol, α-bisabolol oxides A and B, and matricin, as well as flavonoids, including apigenin and luteolin

How It Works

Chamomile exerts both an anti-inflammatory and an antispasmodic effect in the gastrointestinal tract. Topically, it also has anti-inflammatory properties. It promotes wound healing and has mild antibacterial properties.

Recommended Use

Chamomile is typically taken in tea form. Boiling water is poured over a heaping tablespoon of dried flowers and covered. After 5 to 10 minutes, the water is passed through a tea strainer. A cup of freshly brewed tea is drunk three to four times daily, between meals.

Alternatively, you could mix a dried, encapsulated product or alcohol-based tincture with hot water. The dosage should be 2 to 3 grams of the encapsulated product or 1/2 to 1 teaspoon of the tincture three times daily, between meals.

Use chamomile as a mouthwash for irritations and minor infections in the mouth. Topical preparations for use on the skin are usually in the form of creams or ointments that contain 3 to 10 percent chamomile. Medicinal baths containing chamomile can also be used for inflammatory skin conditions.

Side Effects

Although rare, allergic reactions to chamomile have been reported. These reactions include bronchial constriction with internal use and allergic skin reactions following topical use. While such side effects are extremely uncommon, people with allergies to plants of the Asteraceae family (e.g., ragweed, asters, and chrysanthemums) should avoid using chamomile.

*I am sorry to say that Peter was not very well during the evening. His mother
put him to bed and made some chamomile tea; and she gave a dose to Peter!
One tablespoon to be taken at bedtime.*

BEATRIX POTTER, *THE TALE OF PETER RABBIT*

CHAMOMILE is as popular in German herbal medicine as ginseng is in
Chinese herbal medicine. Used historically as a folk remedy for digestive
complaints and inflammatory skin conditions, chamomile continues to be
a cornerstone of European and American herbal medicine today. With
4,000 tons of chamomile produced annually, the herb has become important worldwide both medically and economically.[1]

PLANT FACTS

Since the intent of this book is to transform you into a responsible herbal
consumer, not a botanist, I won't burden you with the confusion surrounding different forms of chamomile. Two major forms are used worldwide—German and Roman chamomile. With the exception of Great
Britain, where Roman chamomile is preferred, German chamomile (previously referred to in older literature as *Matricaria chamomilla*) is the
most commonly used and best researched form of chamomile.[2] Since it's
also the most frequently used in the United States, we'll limit our discussion in this chapter to the German form.

Chamomile is a member of the daisy family and is native to Europe
and western Asia. An annual, it grows from 1 to 2 feet high and forms dis-

tinctive yellow flowers with white rays. The flowers typically bloom in late July or early August.[3] Traditional and modern medical preparations of chamomile use the flower heads just prior to blooming.

HISTORY

German and Roman chamomile have been used for centuries as medicinal plants. The Egyptians believed the plant was a treatment for "ague," or malarial fever. The origin of the name *chamomile* comes from the Greek *kamai* (on the ground) and *melon* (an apple). This name referred to the freshly harvested plant, which carries the scent of apples. During the Middle Ages, the plant was cultivated for use as an aromatic stewing herb.[4]

In Europe, the herb became something of a cure-all. Germans use the phrase *alles zutraut* (capable of anything) to describe chamomile. The plant reached its pinnacle of popularity in 1987, when the Germans named it "plant of the year" (a kind of Academy Award of plants, I guess).[5]

Today, the chamomile industry is huge in Europe. Chamomile is found in liquid and dried preparations for internal use, ointments, creams, bath products, cosmetics, and even hair dyes. In Germany alone, more than ninety licensed products contain chamomile.

MEDICALLY ACTIVE CONSTITUENTS

The flowers of chamomile contain volatile oil, anywhere from 1 to 2 percent. Key constituents in the volatile oil are α-bisabolol, α-bisabolol oxides A and B, and matricin. Matricin is usually converted to chamazulene during the extraction process. German chamomile extracts are often produced to contain an established amount of chamazulene and α-bisabolol.

Also among chamomile's active constituents are bioflavonoids. These include apigenin, luteolin, and quercetin.[6]

The medical benefits of chamomile result from a complex interplay of these two groups. The primary anti-inflammatory activity was originally attributed to the essential oil constituents;[7,8] however, more recent studies with flavonoids indicate that they also possess significant anti-inflammatory activity.[9]

Both components also contribute to the antispasmodic, or muscle-relaxing, effect of chamomile. This effect is particularly noteworthy in the smooth muscles of the gastrointestinal tract.[10]

Recently, apigenin (as well as other flavonoids) was found to inhibit the growth of *Helicobacter pylori* in test tubes,[11] a bacteria thought to contribute to peptic ulcer disease. This may point to wider use of chamomile in the long-term management of peptic ulcer disease.

HEALTH CARE APPLICATIONS

Americans have relegated chamomile to the status of a "calming" herb. This is largely because of its use in commercial teas suggesting a calming or sleep-inducing effect. But the clinical applications of chamomile are more wide-ranging than this. For example, homeopathic chamomile products are available for teething and colic in young children. Rudolf Fritz Weiss (see Part 3) advocates the use of chamomile for intestinal ailments and skin conditions. He suggests chamomile as a gentle, long-term alternative to aggressive, short-term therapies such as atropine and cortisone.[12]

Varo Tyler, a respected advocate for the rational use of herbal medicine in the United States, gets right to the point when he calls chamomile "perhaps the best example of the wide chasm separating medicinal practice in Western Europe and the United States."[13] However, despite European enthusiasm for chamomile, well-controlled clinical trials would help focus the use of this popular herb.

GASTROINTESTINAL TRACT SPASMS AND IRRITATION

Peter Rabbit's mother was an insightful herbalist. Along with peppermint, chamomile is probably the perfect embodiment of the term *carminative* (see "Carminatives" in Part 4). The major advantage of chamomile is its noted anti-inflammatory action. This makes it valuable for a wide range of gastrointestinal (GI) tract disorders.

While I'm attempting to be specific here, keep in mind that chamomile's broad-spectrum approach to the GI tract leaves room for you to use it to treat a variety of conditions and even for mild, soothing effects. It should be considered whenever the GI tract is either cramping or irritated due to anxiety or stress. Chamomile also heals and calms the GI tract following a bout of diarrhea.

Use chamomile as a supportive treatment in the following conditions:[14]

- Irritable bowel syndrome
- Indigestion
- Infant colic
- Gastritis
- Peptic ulcer disease
- Cramping secondary to diarrhea
- Spastic colon

One study found that a tea that combined chamomile, vervain, licorice, fennel, and lemon balm was effective in relieving colic in infants more effectively than a placebo tea.[15] The dose of tea used in the study was approximately 1/2 cup (150 milliliters) given during each colic episode for a maximum of three times per day.

Remember that inflammatory conditions of the GI tract, such as ulcers, Crohn's disease, and ulcerative colitis, can also lead to bleeding and possible anemia. While chamomile may help in the long-term management of these serious conditions, it should not be thought of as a substitute for proper medical monitoring and more aggressive short-term therapies.

Chamomile can be used as part of a program to keep your GI tract well. In addition to helping maintain normal GI tone, it also stimulates normal digestion.[16]

MOUTH IRRITATIONS AND GUM DISEASE

Because of its soothing effect on mucous membranes (the area lining the inside of your mouth and GI tract) and healing properties, chamomile is also useful for the treatment of canker sores and other irritations or sores inside the mouth.[17]

The added benefit of antibacterial activity by the essential oil constituents makes it potentially valuable in the treatment and prevention of gum diseases such as gingivitis.[18] The best approach here is to gargle with a strong tea several times daily.

Topical application to the gums is also useful for infants during teething. I usually recommend that parents apply a strong tea or liquid extract directly to the gums every 2 to 3 hours. Chamomile will help your child's gums feel better and may also exert a calming effect that will help them sleep.

SKIN IRRITATIONS AND ECZEMA

Chamomile is widely used in Europe for the treatment of skin irritations.[19] Topical chamomile creams and ointments are used to treat eczema, insect bites, and poison ivy or poison oak rashes. I find it useful in combination with calendula (marigold) ointment or cream for the treatment of diaper rash in infants.

Owing to the aforementioned wound-healing and antibacterial effects, Europeans often apply chamomile in wound dressings. Topical use of chamomile ointment was also found to successfully treat mild stasis ulcers in elderly bed-ridden patients.[20]

Note: Please use chamomile as a wound-healing treatment only under the supervision of a health care professional.

Topically, chamomile may also work well for eczema. Remember, it's not the knockout punch some people are looking for. One study found chamomile to be about 60 percent as strong as 0.25 percent hydrocortisone when applied topically.[21] In a study with eczema patients previously treated with a topical anti-inflammatory (difluocotolone valerate), a topical chamomile cream was found to be about as effective as 0.25% hydrocortisone in alleviating symptoms.[22]

HOW TO USE CHAMOMILE

The German Commission E monograph[23] gives the following instructions for the preparation and use of chamomile tea for medicinal purposes:

> Pour hot water (150 ml) over a heaped tablespoonful of matricaria flowers (approx. 3 grams), covered, and after 5–10 minutes, pass through a tea strainer. Unless otherwise prescribed, for gastrointestinal complaints a cup of the freshly prepared tea is drunk three or four times a day between meals. For inflammation of the mucous

membranes of the mouth and throat, the freshly prepared tea is used as a wash or gargle.

If you don't want to prepare your own chamomile tea, take a short-cut: use either a powdered, encapsulated herb preparation or an alcohol-based tincture. The dosage of the powdered herb is 2 to 3 grams, two to three times daily between meals. Tinctures are usually dosed at ½ to 1 teaspoon three times daily. I'm a big proponent of placing these delivery forms in hot water and drinking them like a tea. European extracts, which are usually liquid based, are much stronger than U.S. commercial chamomile products. They would be a welcome addition to herbal product offerings in the United States.

For infants and young children, I recommend one-half the adult dosage. Chamomile tea is unique among the many herbs discussed in this book because it actually tastes good. This makes it a bit easier to give directly to infants.

Topically, European creams and ointments are usually made with a 3 to 10 percent concentration of chamomile. A similar concentration is also used for medicinal baths and poultices.

Side effects are extremely rare with either internal or external use of chamomile tea. The big red flag that's been waved in the faces of herb users is the risk of an allergic reaction. Bronchial tightness and shortness of breath, as well as a skin rash, have been reported. How common has this been? Between the years 1887 and 1982, fifty allergic reactions resulting from chamomile use have been reported. Only five could be attributed to German chamomile![24]

Concern about allergies is primarily limited to those with allergies to members of the Asteraceae family. If you're allergic to ragweed, asters, or chrysanthemums, you're probably better off avoiding chamomile.

European monographs list no contraindication to the use of chamomile during pregnancy and lactation. One tragic case has been reported of a woman using a chamomile-containing enema during labor, leading to the death of her newborn.[25] However, this should not dissuade women from using it orally. No interactions with commonly prescribed medications have been reported.

Related Conditions Discussed in Part 6

- Blocked tear duct
- Canker sores
- Colic
- Diarrhea
- Eczema
- Heartburn
- Insomnia
- Irritable bowel syndrome

Cranberry

Vaccinium macrocarpon

Part Used
  The ripe fruit

Common/Potential Uses
  - Recurrent urinary tract infections
  - Prevention of urinary tract infections

How It Works
  Cranberry inhibits the adherence of *Escherichia coli* (*E. coli*) bacteria to the cells lining the wall of the bladder. These bacteria are responsible for the large majority of recurrent urinary tract infections.

Recommended Use
  Take one capsule (400 milligrams) of a concentrated cranberry juice extract in the morning and one capsule in the evening. Ample intake of fluids throughout the day is also recommended. Several glasses of a high-quality cranberry juice daily will approximate the effect of the encapsulated concentrate.

Side Effects
None known

Safety Issues/Drug Interactions
There are no known contraindications to the use of cranberry during pregnancy or lactation. There are no known interactions with antibiotics. However, cranberry should not be used as a substitute for antibiotics during an acute urinary tract infection. Omeprazole, a drug used to treat ulcers, interferes with absorption of vitamin B_{12}. Cranberry may increase vitamin B_{12} absorption in persons taking the drug.

CRANBERRY is the perfect example of the Hippocrates adage, "Let your food be your medicine." Regularly recommended by health care professionals and widely used by consumers for the prevention of urinary tract infections, cranberry is one of those herbal medicines that has enjoyed acceptance in modern medical circles for quite some time. New research is clarifying the way cranberry works to protect the urinary tract. This work has served to validate its historical use and to expand the use of this common food in the future.

PLANT FACTS

A close relative of American blueberry and European bilberry, cranberry has been used for centuries in cooking and as a garnish. More recently, it has become a major cash crop due to the commercial sales of cranberry juice cocktail. Cranberry is cultivated extensively in natural and artificial bogs throughout the United States, especially in Massachusetts and Washington.

HISTORY

The Pilgrims learned about cranberries from American Indians. Use of the berry spread, both as a food and in some medical applications. Historically, cranberry was used to prevent kidney stones and "bladder gravel." It was also believed to remove blood "toxins" from the body.

Since the early part of the twentieth century, however, most of the focus on cranberry has been related to the urinary tract, especially for the prevention of urinary tract infections. In 1923, American scientists showed that the urine of individuals consuming large amounts of cranberries became more acidic.[1]

Part of this acidifying process included an increase in hippuric acid, a chemical that can have a potent antibiotic effect in the urinary tract.[2] Because the bacteria (*Escherichia coli*) causing most urinary tract infections (UTIs) prefer an alkaline pH, cranberry became a common recommendation among physicians for prevention of UTIs and treatment of women with recurrent UTIs.[3,4]

FACTS ABOUT URINARY TRACT INFECTIONS

Women suffering from UTIs account for approximately 5.2 million visits to physicians' offices each year. One of five women in the United States will suffer a UTI at some time in their lives. If you've been treated for an acute urinary tract infection, your risk of recurrence is 20 percent! Recurring UTIs increase the risk of kidney infections and may result in scarring of the bladder wall.[5]

That nasty bug *E. coli* causes 90 percent of first-time UTIs in women (by the way, they don't contract it by eating hamburgers). Among women it is also the leading cause of recurrent UTIs. *Escherichia coli* causes UTIs by adhering to the wall of the bladder and causing inflammation. It is interesting to note that among women with recurrent UTIs, *E. coli* seems to adhere more easily to the cells lining the bladder. Thus, their risk of recurrent UTIs goes up dramatically.[6]

How Cranberry Works

In 1984, A. E. Sobota of Youngstown State University (Ohio), disproved the acidifying theory of cranberry.[7] He demonstrated that cranberry does not acidify the urine sufficiently to produce an antibacterial effect. Instead, he showed that cranberry prevented *E. coli* from adhering to the cells lining the bladder wall.[8] If *E. coli* can't adhere, it can't cause an infection. His work altered thinking about the way cranberry prevents UTIs and has actually strengthened the rationale for using it to prevent recurrent UTIs—especially when long-term antibiotic therapy has failed.

Sobota's work has been expanded by a group of researchers in Israel. Their work has focused on the most virulent strains of *E. coli* and shows that cranberry powerfully deters the adhesion of these strains in the bladder.[9] Their work also indicates that other members of the *Vaccinium* genus (e.g., blueberry and bilberry) also possess anti-adherence properties.[10]

Recently, researchers at Rutgers University discovered that the anti-adherence activity of cranberry lies primarily with the proanthocyanidins in the fruit.[11] This conclusion will hopefully lead to the development of a standardized cranberry extract with more predictable anti-adherence activity.

Health Care Applications

Recurrent Urinary Tract Infections

As noted earlier, the primary group suffering from recurrent UTIs is younger women. To date only one small clinical study has looked at the effectiveness of cranberry in this group. Women ages 18 to 45 years with a history of recurrent urinary tract infections were given either a concentrated cranberry extract in a capsule (400 milligrams twice daily) or a placebo for 3 months and then were switched to placebo or cranberry for another 3 months.[12] Only ten of nineteen women completed the study. However, while these women were taking cranberry, only six UTIs occurred compared to fifteen while taking placebo. This study will hopefully inspire larger studies in the future.

PREVENTION OF URINARY TRACT INFECTIONS

Two studies suggest that cranberry may also protect elderly individuals from *E. coli* in the urinary tract. The first study, involving 153 women (average age, 78.5 years), found that cranberry juice (300 milliliters daily) reduced the amount of bacteria in their urine.[13] While the study used a very weak cranberry preparation (they sweetened it with saccharin!), it does demonstrate the ability to lower the risk of UTI in this population. The importance of this study lies in the reduction of bacteria in the urinary tract. People over the age of 65 years are more likely to have higher urinary levels of *E. coli*. It's important to note that these higher levels, presaging a UTI, may not produce any noticeable signs or symptoms, but such people are nevertheless at greater risk of a UTI. A higher risk of kidney infection is also a possibility.

The second, smaller study found that 4 to 6 ounces of cranberry juice administered daily to twenty-eight nursing home patients resulted in an absence of UTIs in nineteen of the patients.[14] The same researchers later administered an encapsulated cranberry juice extract to twenty-one patients for varying lengths of time. Although the results were observational, twenty of these patients reported no UTIs while taking cranberry.

OTHER POTENTIAL USES

An article in a nursing journal suggests expanding the list of uses for cranberry when it comes to the urinary tract.[15] In addition to prevention of UTIs, the author suggests using cranberry to prevent some types of kidney stones and to reduce urine odor and other complications in persons with urostomies and enterocystoplasties (bladder reconstruction).

HOW TO USE CRANBERRY

Take one capsule (400 milligrams of concentrated, cranberry juice extract) in the morning and one capsule in the evening. Make sure you drink plenty of water throughout the day. Several glasses of a good-quality cranberry juice can be used as an alternative to the capsules. Don't rely on commercial cranberry cocktail, which usually contains sweeteners and only a small amount of actual cranberry juice.

Encapsulated cranberry juice extract seems to offer more consistent anti-adherence activity and is certainly lower in sugar than cranberry juice cocktail. It's a good alternative for people who don't like the taste of cranberry and aren't willing to drink several glasses daily.

For those of you with recurrent UTIs, proper medical diagnosis is essential. Remember, improperly treated UTIs can lead to serious kidney infections. Cranberry is not a substitute for antibiotics in the treatment of UTIs!

Finally, the drug omeprazole (Prilosec®), used to treat ulcers and reflux, may reduce absorption of vitamin B_{12} in some persons. One study found that drinking cranberry juice with your omeprazole may increase absorption of vitamin B_{12}.[16] It doesn't take a rocket scientist to know that vitamin B_{12} absorption relies to a large extent on stomach acid. Cranberry's mild acidifying effect is the likely cause in the improved vitamin B_{12} absorption reported in this study.

Product update: The encapsulated form of cranberry used in the study cited in note 12 is Cranactin® from Solaray. The juice used in the other study, cited in note 13, was good ol' Ocean Spray Cranberry Juice Cocktail.

RELATED CONDITION DISCUSSED IN PART 6

- Urinary tract infections (recurrent)

Echinacea

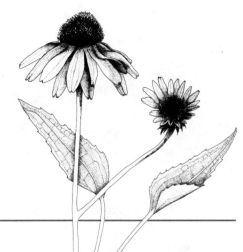

Purple coneflower
Echinacea purpurea, Echinacea angustifolia, Echinacea pallida

Parts Used

The most-researched form of echinacea is a juice made from the aboveground portion (aerial parts) of *E. purpurea* (including leaves and flowers). Herbal preparations made from the aerial parts and roots of *E. purpurea* and *E. angustifolia* have also been studied and used in herbal medicine.

Common/Potential Uses

- Treatment of colds and flu
- Supportive treatment of recurrent infections of the ears, respiratory tract, and urinary tract
- Recurrent vaginal yeast infections

How It Works

Stimulates the immune system

Recommended Use

Use the expressed (i.e., squeezed) juice of the *E. purpurea* herb. For short-term use, take 20 to 40 drops of the juice initially; then

20 to 40 drops of the juice every 2 hours throughout the day for 48 hours or until symptom relief is noted. Alternatively, 900 to 1,200 milligrams of dried herb or root of either *E. purpurea* or *E. angustifolia* or 3 to 5 milliliters of tincture daily may replace the expressed juice product. Limit use to 7 to 10 days.

Side Effects

Rare reports of allergic reactions

Safety Issues/Drug Interactions

The German Commission E monograph says that persons with autoimmune illness such as lupus or other progressive systemic diseases such as tuberculosis, multiple sclerosis, and HIV infection/ AIDS should avoid echinacea. Although I agree, this recommendation is controversial and not based on clinical evidence. There are no known contraindications to use of echinacea during pregnancy and lactation. Persons with allergies to plants of the Asteraceae family (e.g., ragweed, asters, and chrysanthemums) should use echinacea cautiously. There are no known drug interactions with echinacea.

HERBAL preparations of echinacea are among the most popular in both Europe and the United States. On the German market, more than 300 echinacea products are available. In 1994, German doctors and pharmacists prescribed echinacea more than 2.5 million times![1] It is continually among the top-selling herbal supplements in the U.S. dietary supplement market.[2] The primary use has been for prevention or treatment of colds and flu.

To date, medicinal preparations of *E. purpurea* and other echinacea species (e.g., *E. angustifolia* and *E. pallida*) have 200 journal articles to their credit.[3] In addition to its general use for colds and flu, echinacea has also been applied to treat recurrent vaginal yeast infections, chronic prostate inflammation (prostatitis), and bronchitis. In Europe, both injectible and oral forms are used.

PLANT FACTS

Echinacea is a native American wildflower belonging to the sunflower family. It is commonly referred to as "purple coneflower" because of the flower's distinctive shape and color. Of the nine species native to the United States and Canada, three are used medicinally: *E. purpurea, E. angustifolia,* and *E. pallida.* Although echinacea can be found growing in the wild, almost all current commercial preparations are harvested from cultivated plants in either the United States or Europe.[4]

HISTORY

The history of echinacea's medicinal use begins in American and Western herbal lore. It was used by Native Americans for a variety of ailments, including treatment of venomous bites and external wounds. Echinacea was first introduced into U.S. medical practice by John King in 1887. Also recommended by John Uri Lloyd (a pharmacist of Cincinnati, Ohio), echinacea was very popular among medical professionals in the late nineteenth century. By the early part of the twentieth century, however, echinacea had largely disappeared from U.S. medicine.[5]

Echinacea was "rediscovered" in the 1930s by Dr. Gerhard Madaus of Germany. Madaus, the founder of the pharmaceutical manufacturing firm Madaus AG of Cologne, Germany, came to the United States in search of *E. angustifolia* seeds. This species of echinacea was the most widely used medicinally at that time. Perhaps fooled by some tricky U.S. herbalist, Madaus returned to Germany with seeds of *E. purpurea* instead of *E. angustifolia.* By default, *E. purpurea* became the subject of Madaus's pharmacological studies. The result was the development of a product called Echinacin®, an expressed juice prepared from the above-ground part of the plant. This preparation has become the most extensively researched and frequently prescribed echinacea monoprepa-ration worldwide.

MEDICALLY ACTIVE CONSTITUENTS

Studies suggest that echinacea boosts the activity of the immune system. Most of echinacea's immunostimulating properties are probably due to three major groups of constituents: the alkylamides/polyacetylenes, caf-feic acid derivatives, and polysaccharides.[6,7] One of echinacea's polysac-charides, arabinogalactan, has shown significant ability to stimulate the cells of the immune system in test tube studies.[8]

HOW ECHINACEA WORKS

Echinacea is thought to stimulate the immune system making it more ef-fective in fighting off infections. Echinacea appears to increase the pro-duction of and activity of white blood cells, including those known as natural killer cells (no relation to the "natural born killers" in the movie!). It also increases production of interferon, an important part of the body's response to viral infections such as colds and the flu.[9,10,11] Besides sup-porting a healthy immune system, echinacea may also help strengthen the immune response to reduce the incidence of recurrent infections. Significantly more research needs to be completed to more clearly define how echinacea works in the body.

HEALTH CARE APPLICATIONS

COMMON COLD AND THE FLU
The past decade has been a real roller-coaster ride for echinacea. Previously thought to be the ideal product for both prevention and treat-ment of colds and flu, echinacea has been shown recently to be best used at the very beginning of a cold or flu to help shorten the duration and get you back to your normal routine quicker. On the other hand, it looks like

taking it on a daily basis to help defer colds and flu is probably not going to help much. So keep some in the medicine cabinet as part of your cold and flu medication armament.

Let's start with the good news on echinacea for colds. Two studies using *E. pupurea* products have clearly shown the ability to reduce the duration of the common cold. In the first, a product made from the expressed juice of the aerial parts of *E. purpurea* (Echinacin) reduced the duration of the common cold in a group of Swedish furniture factory employees by 50 percent.[12] It's important to note that participants in this study started on their echinacea at the first sign of a cold and took it every 2 hours during the first day of treatment. Boy, talk about a result that corporations everywhere should be looking at!

The second study used a Swiss echinacea product known as Echinaforce® (a combination of 95 percent aerial parts and 5 percent root) that is delivered in tablet form.[13] Persons taking the regular Echinaforce and a more concentrated version had a significantly greater reduction in cold symptom complaints and got better quicker than persons taking a product with just the root of the plant or a placebo.

Finally, similar results have been shown using other types of echinacea preparations. One study found that *E. pallida* root tincture significantly decreased cold symptom severity and duration.[14] Another product, Esberitox®, which combines *E. purpurea* and *E. pallida* root with wild indigo root and thuja in a chewable tablet, has also shown the ability to help shorten the severity and duration of the common cold.[15]

OK, now the bad news. Two published studies and an unpublished third have suggested no benefit in taking echinacea to prevent colds. The first compared *E. purpurea* and *E. angustifolia* root tinctures with placebo in a group of 289 adults susceptible to getting colds frequently.[16] There were no differences between echinacea and placebo in the prevention of colds. It was interesting that those taking echinacea did report thinking they had a benefit significantly more than those taking placebo.

The second study used a liquid expressed juice product (Echinacin) in 108 adults.[17] Again, the results found that the average number of colds suffered was the same for both the echinacea and placebo groups. One criticism of this study is the fact that it was actually a reanalysis of research data from 1991, and not a new study.

Bastyr University in Seattle completed a large prevention study with the same preparation of echinacea as used in this second study just described.[18] It also showed no benefit for using echinacea to prevent colds in persons with a history of frequent upper respiratory tract infections. While this herb is not as widely studied for its impact on the flu, one study did look at the effect of an echinacea preparation (*E. pupurea* root) on people afflicted by the flu.[19] One hundred eighty volunteers (age range, 18 to 60 years) with the flu were assigned to one of three groups: (1) placebo; (2) 450 milligrams of echinacea daily; and (3) 900 milligrams of echinacea daily. Those receiving 900 milligrams daily showed a significant reduction in flu symptoms, such as weakness/low energy, chills/sweating, sore throat, muscle/joint aches, and headaches. Results were not favorable at the lower dosage of 450 milligrams daily.

RECURRENT INFECTIONS

Echinacea can also be a supportive therapy for people with recurring infections. I commonly recommend echinacea for my pediatric patients with recurring ear infections. It's particularly useful when antibiotic therapy is failing. While echinacea should not be considered a substitute for antibiotics, it may stimulate a sluggish immune system to resist infection more effectively.

Others likely to benefit from echinacea are women with recurring vaginal yeast infections. Recurrence even with topical antifungal medications exceeds 60 percent! This is another indication that killing the bug doesn't address the underlying problem: an immune system that's not mounting a strong enough defense.

The positive effect of *E. purpurea* was illustrated in a study of 203 women suffering from recurrent vaginal yeast infections.[20] All of these women were being treated with a topical econazole nitrate cream (a commonly prescribed antifungal/antiyeast medication). Women using the econazole nitrate alone experienced a 60.5 percent recurrence rate. Those taking echinacea orally lowered this recurrence rate to 16.7 percent!

Researchers also noted a normalization of immune function (as measured by skin test) in all of the women receiving echinacea.

HOW TO USE ECHINACEA

Take echinacea at the onset of a cold or flu for a period of 7 to 10 days, without interruption. Remember, it's probably more effective if you take it every 2 hours during the first day and then three to four times daily thereafter. I'm currently recommending that even persons using it for recurrent infections not exceed 14 days of continuous use. The emphasis is on a quick burst of immune function and not pounding the immune system over the head for weeks or months.

Use the expressed (i.e., squeezed) juice of the *E. purpurea* herb. For short-term use, take 20 to 40 drops of the juice initially; then 20 to 40 drops of the juice every 2 hours throughout the day for 48 hours or until symptom relief is noted. Alternatively, 900 to 1,200 milligrams of dried herb or root of either *E. purpurea* or *E. angustifolia* or 3 to 5 milliliters of tincture daily may replace the expressed juice product. Children ages 6 to 12 years can take half to three-fourths of the adult dose; children below 6 years may take one-fourth to half the adult dose. I'm not a big fan of using alcohol-based preparations in young children, so opt for either a alcohol-free liquid preparation or a chewable tablet. The Esberitox combination of echinacea, wild indigo, and thuja comes in chewable tablets. The adult dose is three tablets three times daily (follow label instructions for children).

The current German Commission E monograph suggests that persons with an autoimmune illness such as lupus or other progressive systemic diseases such as tuberculosis, multiple sclerosis, and HIV infection/AIDS avoid use of echinacea.[21] The monograph lists no contraindications to the use of the expressed juice of *E. purpurea* herb during pregnancy and lactation. Persons with allergies to plants of the Asteraceae family (e.g., ragweed, asters, and chrysanthemums) should use echinacea cautiously. There are no known drug interactions with echinacea.

Product update: The Echinacin expressed juice product is sold in the United States by Nature's Way. The product name is Echinaguard®.

Echinaforce is sold in the United States by Bioforce. The Esberitox tablet product is sold in the United States by Enzymatic Therapy.

RELATED CONDITIONS DISCUSSED IN PART 6

- Canker sores
- Colds and flu
- Cold sores
- Recurrent ear infections
- Periodontal disease
- Recurrent sinus infections
- Sore throat
- Recurrent urinary tract infections
- Vaginal yeast infections

Eleuthero

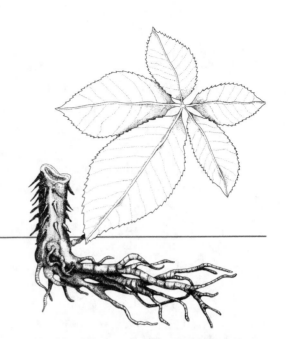

Eleutherococcus senticosus,
Acanthopanax senticosus
Siberian ginseng, ci-wu-jia

Part Used
The root and rhizomes

Common/Potential Uses
- Fatigue and declining work ability
- Support during exercise and physical exertion
- Support for the body during times of stress
- Prevention of colds and flu
- Supportive use following radiation or chemotherapy
- Chronic fatigue immunodeficiency syndrome
- Human immunodeficiency virus (HIV) infection

Active Constituents
A complex group of glycosides known as eleutherosides as well as polysaccharides

How It Works

Eleuthero is notable for its ability to support and enhance adrenal function. Optimal adrenal function is associated with greater energy and better reaction to stress. Eleuthero also supports and strengthens the immune system. In addition, it maximizes the utilization of oxygen by working muscles, keeping them in an aerobic state for a longer period of time.

Recommended Use

Dry extract of the root, 2 to 3 grams daily in two or three divided dosages; concentrated solid extract standardized for eleutherosides B and E, 300 to 400 milligrams daily; alcohol-based extract, 8 to 10 milliliters in two to three divided dosages. Historically, eleuthero is taken continuously for 6 to 8 weeks, followed by a 1- to 2-week break before resuming.

Side Effects

Eleuthero has few reported side effects. Mild, transient diarrhea has been reported by a small number of users. Eleuthero may cause insomnia in some people if taken too close to bedtime. It should be used cautiously by persons with uncontrolled high blood pressure.

Safety Issues/Drug Interactions

There are no known contraindications to use of eleuthero during pregnancy or lactation. However, pregnant or lactating women using eleuthero should avoid products that have been adulterated with *Panax ginseng* or other related species that are contraindicated. One case report suggests that eleuthero may increase serum levels of digoxin.

ELEUTHERO, often referred to as Siberian ginseng, is a frequently prescribed herbal tonic. Used for hundreds of years in Asian and Eastern European countries, eleuthero is an *adaptogen*—a substance that can increase our resistance to a wide variety of negative influences (see "Adaptogens" in Part 4).

Today, eleuthero is used to enhance recovery following exercise. It is a major ally in stress management because it supports the normal functioning of the adrenal glands. Clinical research also points to eleuthero as a promising supplement in the long-term management of conditions such as chronic fatigue immunodeficiency syndrome. It may also be a useful tool for persons recovering after chemotherapy.

PLANT FACTS

Eleuthero belongs to the Araliaceae family and is a distant relative of Asian ginseng (*Panax ginseng*). Also known commonly as touch-me-not, ci-wu-jia, and devil's shrub, eleuthero has been most frequently nicknamed Siberian ginseng in the United States. The common botanical name for the plant is *Eleutherococcus senticosus*, although some oriental textbooks also refer to it as *Acanthopanax senticosus*.

Eleutherococcus senticosus is a slender, thorny shrub that grows to a height of 3 to 15 feet. It is native to the taiga forests of the Far East (southeastern part of Russia, northern China, Korea, and Japan). Medicinal preparations of the plant are made largely from the root. The largest share of raw herb used for extracts in the United States comes from Russia.[1]

HISTORY

Although not as popular as *Panax ginseng*, eleuthero dates back 2,000 years in the records of Chinese medicine. Referred to as *ci-wu-jia* in Chinese medicine, it was used to prevent respiratory tract infections, as well as colds and flu. The Chinese also believed eleuthero provided energy and vitality.[2]

In Russia, eleuthero was originally used by people in the Siberian taiga to increase performance and quality of life and decrease infections. In 1856, the Russian botanists Franz J. Ruprecht and Karl Johann Maximowicz named the plant *Hedra sentocosa*. Maximowicz later changed the name to *Eleutherococcus senticosus*.

Modern Development

The modern history of eleuthero began with I. I. Brekhman and colleagues in the 1940s. During a search for a more economical herbal alternative to Asian (Chinese or Korean) ginseng, Brekhman discovered that eleuthero offered many of the same benefits as the famous Asian tonic. Having already investigated the actions of *Panax ginseng* (and coining the term *adaptogen* to describe them), Brekhman shifted his attention to eleuthero.[3] Eleuthero became the center of extensive clinical research over the next 3 decades.

In Russia, eleuthero's ability to increase stamina and endurance was so well regarded that the cosmonauts used it instead of the amphetamines taken by American astronauts. Soviet Olympic athletes used it to enhance their training and then went on to dominate many of the endurance sports. Explorers, divers, sailors, and miners used eleuthero to prevent stress-related illness.[4] After the Chernobyl accident, many Russian and Ukrainian citizens were given eleuthero to counteract the effects of radiation.

Medically Active Constituents

The constituents in eleuthero that have received the most attention are the *eleutherosides*. Predominantly glycosides, these constituents are thought to contribute to the adaptogenic actions of eleuthero.[5] Seven primary eleutherosides have been identified, with the most research focusing on eleutherosides B and E.[6] These substances are not the same as ginseng's active constituents, known as *ginsenosides*.

Eleuthero also contains complex polysaccharides (a kind of supersugar molecule).[7] These constituents play a critical role in eleuthero's ability to support immune function.

HOW ELEUTHERO WORKS

Together with Asian ginseng, I can't think of an herbal medicine that better fits the definition of an adaptogen. Acting on a wide range of body functions, eleuthero has a remarkable ability to increase the body's resistance to stress and provide an impetus to move toward a state of balance.

STRESS REDUCTION

Stress takes its toll on our bodies daily. Psychological stress due to deadlines, emotional distress, and existential dilemmas has been shown to affect the body. More easily measured are the physical stresses such as physical labor, strenuous exercise, poor diets, and environmental pollution. While stress can eventually wreak havoc on a number of body systems, its initial target is the adrenal glands. Chronic stress can overwhelm the adrenals and lead to chronic fatigue, poor immune function, and improper blood sugar metabolism.[8]

As an adaptogen, eleuthero helps us adapt to stress by providing fuel to the adrenal glands, allowing them to function optimally when challenged by stress.[9] This means eleuthero should be considered as a daily supplement for anyone experiencing stress on a regular basis. I firmly believe that many of the chronic conditions unique to our modern society could be reduced significantly with stress reduction and better care for our adrenal glands.

ENHANCED MENTAL PERFORMANCE

The most common response to mental fatigue in our society is to grab a cup of coffee. You can even buy herbal supplements that are high in caffeine to increase mental alertness. Eleuthero has been shown to enhance mental acuity without the letdown that comes with caffeinated products.[10]

This effect again is due to eleuthero's ability to support adrenal function as well as the optimal functioning of the hypothalamic pituitary adrenal axis (HPA axis). My Chinese medical colleagues continually remind me that it's a cooperation of the three and to quit focusing on just the adrenals.[11]

ENHANCED PHYSICAL PERFORMANCE

Owing to the extensive use of eleuthero by Russian and East German athletes, research has accumulated on its ability to enhance physical performance. However, the results are mixed.

A 1986 study[12] conducted at the Institute of Health and Sport Sciences at the University of Tsukba in Japan demonstrated that eleuthero improves the use of oxygen by the exercising muscle. Twelve male athletes were given either eleuthero or a placebo. Athletes taking eleuthero showed a 23.3 percent increase in total exercise duration and stamina compared to only 7.5 percent in those taking the placebo.

While eleuthero may help your muscles use oxygen more efficiently and improve recovery following exercise, it's unlikely to make your marathon times significantly better or, for that matter, your dash for the door when the kids are stressing you out that much quicker. One study giving eleuthero to athletes found minimal effect on performance.[13]

Another study completed at Old Dominion University found no improvement in the running time of twenty highly trained college distance runners taking 60 drops of a liquid eleuthero preparation (Maxim-L®) daily for 6 weeks.[14]

The ability of eleuthero to enhance physical performance may extend beyond the boundaries of athletics. Research also indicates eleuthero enhances the stamina of airline personnel and people engaged in physical labor.[15]

My personal feeling is you're less likely to see an improvement in performance using eleuthero if you're an elite athlete. If you're a weekend warrior like me, you're likely to note less muscle aches and fatigue on Monday morning. For you athletes, remember—one of the biggest problems with the stress of those hard workouts is the stress on the adrenals and immune system. Eleuthero might be a good choice to counteract these negative effects of exercise.

ANTITOXIN ACTIONS

Eleuthero also reduces bodily stress by combating harmful toxins. In animal studies, the herb has exerted a protective effect against such chemicals as ethanol, sodium barbital, tetanus toxoid, and chemotherapeutic agents.[16] Eleuthero may also reduce the side effects of radiation exposure.[17]

These actions have led to the specific use of eleuthero in alcohol rehabilitation centers. It is also used extensively as a supportive treatment for cancer patients receiving radiation or chemotherapy.

IMMUNE SYSTEM ENHANCING ACTIONS

Evidence is also mounting that eleuthero enhances and supports the immune response. Russian studies have found eleuthero useful as a preventive measure during cold and flu season. Recent evidence suggests that eleuthero may prove valuable in the long-term management of various diseases of the immune system, including HIV infection, chronic fatigue immunodeficiency syndrome, and autoimmune illnesses such as lupus.

Research in Germany shows that eleuthero increases important components of the immune system known as lymphocytes.[18] Lymphocytes act as one of the body's primary defenses against viral infection and have become the target of study, particularly with regard to HIV infection. Research has focused on agents that possess the ability to enhance certain subsets of lymphocytes. These agents have been coined *immunomodulators* (see the discussion of herbal immunomodulators in Part 4).

According to the German study, eleuthero increases the activity and number of T lymphocytes. The most significant increase is in the subset of T lymphocytes known as *helper/inducer* or *CD4 cells*. Without proper CD4 cell activity, the rest of the immune system cannot function properly. CD4 cells are a major target of HIV and decrease in number significantly following HIV infection and the progression to AIDS (acquired immunodeficiency syndrome).

HEALTH CARE APPLICATIONS

OPTIMIZING WELLNESS

Unlike the situation with ginkgo or milk thistle, it's difficult to zero in on conditions specifically requiring eleuthero. Many of its actions fall into the preventive category; hence, the use of eleuthero should address the goal of optimizing wellness. Eleuthero often forms the centerpiece of my daily supplement recommendations for many patients.

I highly recommend it for patients under stress, as it helps by optimizing the ability of the HPA axis (the stress modulator of the body) to deal with stress more optimally. Eleuthero often becomes a cornerstone of treatment for patients dealing with chronic viral illnesses and autoimmune conditions.

PREVENTION OF COLDS AND FLU

I like to think of eleuthero as long-term insurance against colds and flu, whereas echinacea takes care of short-term needs. Several studies in Russia suggest that it greatly reduces the incidence of influenza, colds, and pharyngitis.

A Russian auto plant gave each of more than 13,000 employees 2 milliliters of eleuthero daily during November and December. Colds, flu, and other infections dropped an average of 40 percent compared to previous winters. In another study, 1,000 employees of a mining/smelting plant enjoyed a more than twofold reduction in acute respiratory diseases and influenza with daily use of eleuthero.[19]

M. P. Zykov and S. F. Protasova of the Research Institute of Influenza in Leningrad have suggested that eleuthero be used either in combination with influenza vaccinations or by itself in the prevention of influenza—particularly in high-risk populations.[20] Their research indicates that it protects against postvaccination reactions.

SUPPORTIVE USE FOR CANCER PATIENTS

Eleuthero may be a valuable supplement for persons receiving treatment for cancer. Oncology clinics in Russia and Germany have reported success in improving the general health of cancer patients by adding eleuthero to their treatment regimen; immune function also improved.[21] Also noted was a reduction in the number and intensity of side effects commonly encountered with radiation and chemotherapy.

The Institute of Oncology (Georgia, Russia) examined the effects of daily supplementation of 2 milliliters of a liquid eleuthero extract in women being treated for breast cancer.[22] A group of eighty patients was chosen, all of whom had gone through surgery for cancer and were receiving both chemotherapy and radiation treatment.

Half of the women were given eleuthero, while the other group received no additional treatment. The patients in the eleuthero group showed a significant reduction in side effects caused by radiation and chemotherapeutic treatment (i.e., nausea, dizziness, and loss of appetite).

Adaptogens such as eleuthero and astragalus have been shown to help the bone marrow bounce back more quickly following chemotherapy. This means that patients can begin producing infection-fighting white blood cells (i.e., lymphocytes and macrophages) more quickly. Eleuthero also appears to improve appetite, promote weight gain, and increase lymphocyte activity in cancer patients.[23] Clearly, more studies need to be done to clearly identify what role eleuthero may play in improving the quality of life in cancer patients.

OTHER POTENTIAL USES

Potential health care applications for eleuthero include the following:

HIV infection	Chronic fatigue immunodeficiency syndrome
Chronic hepatitis	Lupus
Recovering alcoholics	Recovery following long-term steroid use

Eleuthero, in combination with a polypeptide extract from spleen tissue, has been studied in the United States and Africa for potential use against HIV infection. Preliminary results indicate that this combination may slow the progression of the disease. It has also shown some promise in reversing some of the weight loss noticed in AIDS patients with wasting syndrome.[24]

Chronic fatigue immunodeficiency syndrome (CFIDS) is emerging both as a disease of the immune system and as the outward manifestation of dysregulation of the HPA axis. Eleuthero has become a cornerstone of my long-term treatment recommendations for CFIDS.

HOW TO USE ELEUTHERO

The most extensively researched form of eleuthero is an alcohol extract made from the root. The recommended daily dosage is 8 to 10 milliliters in two to three divided dosages. Encapsulated, dried root supplements are recommended at a dosage of 2 to 3 grams daily in two or three divided dosages. Concentrated solid extracts, standardized for eleutherosides B and E, have recently been introduced. The dosage of this form is 300 to 400 milligrams daily. Eleuthero should be taken continuously for 6 to 8 weeks followed by a 1- to 2-week break before resuming.

Reported side effects have been minimal. Mild, transient diarrhea has been reported by a very small number of users. Eleuthero is less likely to cause the overstimulation reported by some individuals taking Asian ginseng. However, the final dose of the day should not be taken too close to bedtime, or it may keep you up beyond the *Late Show*. Eleuthero is not associated with any masculinizing effect in women and will not interfere with a normal menstrual cycle (these effects have been reported anecdotally by women using Asian ginseng).

Current European monographs list no contraindications during pregnancy or lactation. However, pregnant or lactating women should avoid products that may be adulterated with Asian ginseng or other related species. Eleuthero has been reported in one case study to possibly interact with digoxin.[25] In this case, a man taking digoxin and eleuthero together developed dangerously high serum digoxin levels. Although a clear relationship could not be established, it is wise to talk with your doctor before using the two together.

RELATED CONDITIONS DISCUSSED IN PART 6

- Alcohol-related liver disease
- Chronic fatigue immunodeficiency syndrome
- Diabetes
- HIV infection/AIDS
- Stress and fatigue

Evening Primrose

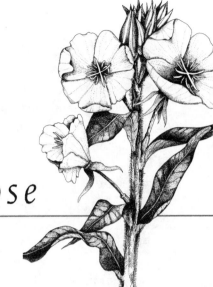

Oenothera biennis

Part Used
  Oil extracted from the seed

Common/Potential Uses
  • Eczema
  • Diabetic neuropathy
  • Rheumatoid arthritis
  • Breast pain and tenderness associated with menstrual cycle

Active Constituents
  The essential fatty acid gamma-linolenic acid (GLA) and the
  triglyceride structure to which it is attached (also known as
  enotherol)

How It Works
  Evening primrose oil provides a highly available source of GLA to
  the body. This is particularly useful for persons with conditions that
  are associated with a poor conversion of dietary oils to GLA and

other important essential fatty acid metabolites. Providing GLA allows for more efficient incorporation of important essential fatty acids into the membranes of cells. Higher levels of GLA in the body also tend to decrease inflammation and smooth muscle cramping.

Recommended Use
Oil of evening primrose—3 to 6 grams daily taken with meals

Side Effects
Side effects are rare with the use of a high-quality, extracted evening primrose oil (EPO). At the recommended dosages, vague abdominal discomfort, nausea, and headache have been reported by less than 2 percent of people taking EPO long-term.

Safety Issues/Drug Interactions
Evening primrose oil is not known to interact with commonly prescribed medications. There are no known contraindications to the use of EPO during pregnancy or lactation. There are no known drug interactions with EPO.

DIETARY fats have become a rallying point for nutritional educators in our country. We know that consuming diets high in saturated fats from animal sources (e.g., beef, cow's milk, cheese) and fried foods is associated with an increased risk of cardiovascular disease. High saturated fat consumption is also linked to increased risk of cancer of the prostate, breast, and colon.[1]

The public health message has been to urge reduction of these fats in the diet and increase the "good" fats—largely those coming under the heading of polyunsaturated. Vegetable and fish oils have received most of the good press and are being consumed in greater quantities by health-conscious individuals. In the case of vegetables, the combination of healthy oils, fiber, and antioxidant nutrients make these one of nature's most powerful deterrents to many diseases common in American culture.

While diet should be the cornerstone of any plan for optimal health, three decades of research also indicate that concentrated amounts of beneficial oils are useful in the treatment of certain diseases. Use of fish oil to lower cholesterol and treat psoriasis is one example. In this chapter, we'll look at the use of oil extracted from the seeds of evening primrose and its use in the treatment of conditions such as eczema, premenstrual syndrome (PMS), and diabetic neuropathy. Before exploring medical applications for evening primrose oil (EPO), let's take a little detour and discuss essential fatty acids (EFAs).

ESSENTIAL FATTY ACIDS: HOW YOUR BODY USES THEM

Fatty acids are the building blocks that make up the fats and oils we consume in our diet. Adding the designation "essential" implies that the fatty acid is required by our body but can't be produced by it. Essential fatty acids can be obtained only from our diets. Note also that EFAs are polyunsaturated (although not all polyunsaturated fats are EFAs). Polyunsaturated fats (PUFAs) contain two or more special double bonds, described as "cis," between carbon atoms. Polyunsaturated fats can readily become saturated; that is, the healthy cis bonds can be converted to unhealthy "trans" bonds, by heat, rancidity, and food processing.

The two primary categories of EFAs are the omega-6 EFAs and the omega-3 EFAs. The "6" and "3" designations refer to the position of the first carbon double bond (there will be a chemistry quiz at the end of the chapter!) when counting from a designated end of the fatty acid.[2] Seed oils such as flax, sunflower, pumpkin, and walnut contain both omega-6 and omega-3 EFAs, with one category often predominant (e.g., flax seed oil is 58 percent omega-3, and safflower is 65 percent omega-6).

When we consume EFAs, our bodies go through a complex series of steps to convert an EFA to a form that can be used by the body. This is accomplished largely through the actions of enzymes. One of these

FIGURE 5.1. OUTLINE OF THE PATHWAYS OF OMEGA 6 (*n*-6) AND OMEGA-3 (*n*-3) ESSENTIAL FATTY ACID METABOLISM

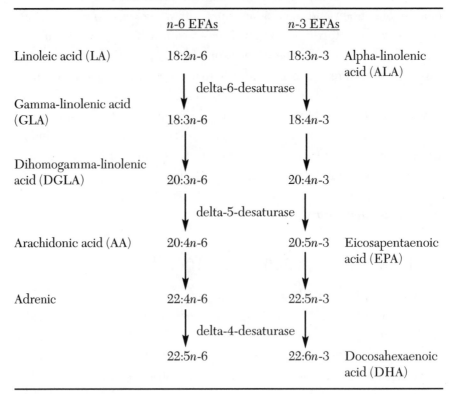

enzymes is delta-6-desaturase (see Figure 5.1, which outlines the steps in the metabolism of EFAs). Delta-6-desaturase performs the first step in the metabolism of dietary EFAs.

Dietary oils such as flaxseed oil and safflower oil contribute linoleic acid (an omega-6 EFA) and alpha-linolenic acid (an omega-3 EFA), which enter at the beginning of this cascade of steps. Other oils, such as fish oil and evening primrose oil, provide the body with omega-6 and omega-3 EFAs that actually bypass some of the initial steps of metabolism (including delta-6-desaturase). This quality has made these oils valuable for persons who have difficulty converting the more common dietary oils into the important EFA metabolites so essential to the health of the body.

Essential fatty acids contribute to a variety of mechanisms essential to the normal, healthy functioning of the body.[3] Major roles of EFAs in the body include the following:

- EFAs are required for the normal structure of all cell membranes in the body. They confer a fluid and flexible property on cell membranes and allow for normal passage of important nutrients to the operating centers of the cells.
- EFAs are essential for the formation of prostaglandins. These hormone-like substances orchestrate a number of actions in the body, including smooth muscle contraction and inflammation. Buildup (i.e., an excess) of certain types of prostaglandins can be detrimental to the health. Essential fatty acids can modulate the production of prostaglandins so as to reduce inflammation and smooth muscle cramping.
- EFAs are involved in the transport and metabolism of cholesterol in the body. They are associated with lowering cholesterol levels in the bloodstream.
- EFAs are required to keep the skin healthy.

DISEASES AND CONDITIONS ASSOCIATED WITH IMPROPER ESSENTIAL FATTY ACID METABOLISM

On the basis of this information, what to do seems perfectly simple: Change the types of fats in your diet by eating more vegetables, vegetable oils, and fish, and be healthier. If you were taking odds, you'd be right most of the time. However, some people don't seem able to convert EFAs properly at the step involving the enzyme delta-6-desaturase. What results is a buildup of dietary EFAs such as linoleic acid and alpha-linoleic acid without conversion to a form that is useful to the body (see Figure 5.1). This seems to apply particularly to the production of gamma-linolenic acid (GLA) from linoleic acid.[4]

Certain conditions are associated with improper conversion of EFAs at the delta-6-desaturase step:

- Nutritional deficiencies (e.g., zinc, magnesium, vitamin B_6)
- Aging
- Diabetes
- Alcoholism
- Viral infections
- Cancer
- Eczema
- Premenstrual syndrome
- Cyclical breast pain

Most research has linked these conditions to a defect in the normal activity of delta-6-desaturase. In the case of diabetics, there also appears to be some malfunctioning in the activity of delta-5-desaturase.[5]

You should know that EFAs such as GLA, dihomogamma-linoleic acid (DGLA), and arachidonic acid are important components of human breast milk.[6] These preformed omega-6 metabolites are used by infants for the development of many body tissues—most notably the brain. Infant formulas, which are high in linoleic acid, don't provide the same levels of these metabolites. This point creates obvious concerns for the developing nervous system in very young infants. Later, we'll explore the use of supplemental GLA, in the form of EPO, in the nurturing of both formula-fed infants and infants whose mothers may be producing low amounts of breast milk GLA.

EVENING PRIMROSE OIL: A THERAPEUTIC ESSENTIAL FATTY ACID

Science has pointed to the therapeutic use of EFAs that bypass the delta-6-desaturase step. As mentioned earlier, fish oil is one common example. Fish oil from cold-water species such as salmon is a source of the omega-3 EFAs eicosapentaenoic acid (EPA) and docosahexaenoic acid (DHA) (see Figure 5.1). Fish oil supplements high in these two metabolites are frequently recommended for the treatment of psoriasis and ulcerative colitis.

The most widely researched plant source of omega-6 EFAs is the evening primrose. Evening primrose is noted for its large and delicate flower, which blooms and lasts for only one evening. The small seeds of the plant are high in GLA as well as linoleic acid. Cross-breeding has led to the cultivation of plants whose seeds consistently yield 7 to 10 percent GLA.[7]

Years of research have pointed to EPO as the most reliable source of GLA. This is due to its very simple structure, which allows for greater absorption of GLA without interference from other fats. More complex plant sources of GLA, including borage oil and black currant oil, contain higher concentrations of GLA compared to EPO, but they also have a number of competing fatty acids (including saturated fats in the case of borage oil). This leads to inferior GLA absorption and utilization in the body. Borage and black currant oils, being less researched, may also contain other, toxic substances. In fact, the long-term use of either of these oils may be associated with an increased risk of overaggregation of platelets in the bloodstream—an event associated with an increased risk of atherosclerosis.[8,9]

What this means is that a person taking EPO will be assured of a balanced increase in omega-6 metabolites such as DGLA and also (to a lesser extent) arachidonic acid. This leads to a more efficient production of prostaglandins of the "1" series (see the previous discussion on prostaglandins). These prostaglandins (along with those of the "3" series produced from omega-3 EFA metabolites) have a tendency to discourage inflammation, smooth muscle cramping, and even overaggregation of platelets in the bloodstream.[10]

A remarkable body of medical research on EPO has led to EPO becoming one of the most widely prescribed plant-derived medicines in the world. Let's take a look at some of these applications next.

HEALTH CARE APPLICATIONS

ECZEMA

Eczema is an allergy-based skin disease with a clear hereditary link. One of the things that seems to be inherited in children with eczema is a difficulty in converting EFAs such as linoleic and alpha-linolenic acids to GLA.[11] This has led to the use of EPO, alone or in combination with fish oil, in the treatment of children and adults with eczema.

Before jumping into a review of some of the clinical results concerning EPO treatment for eczema, let's look a little more closely at young children with the condition. First, we know that breast-feeding lowers the risk of eczema, whereas early introduction of cow's milk formulas boosts the risk.[12] Breast milk is high in preformed GLA and DGLA, whereas formula is not.

However, another variable comes into play when Mom also has eczema. Research shows that mothers with a history of eczema, or who have children with recently developed eczema, have higher levels of linoleic acid and lower levels of GLA and DGLA in their breast milk.[13] This means that they are not properly converting EFAs. As a result, their breast milk does not transfer any protection from eczema to their infant.

One solution that has proven helpful to both mother and child is dietary EPO supplementation. Studies have indicated that maternal consumption of EPO is effective in raising breast milk levels of omega-6 EFA metabolites.[14] In Japan, many infant formulas actually contain added GLA.

So, what about using EPO to treat eczema? This has become a leading area for use of EPO in the clinical setting. In fact, EPO (sold under the trade name Epogam®) is recognized by the governments of Great Britain, Germany, Denmark, Ireland, Spain, Greece, South Africa, Australia, and New Zealand as a treatment for eczema. The typical dosage for adults is 4 to 6 grams daily; for children, 2 to 4 grams daily. Remember that evening primrose oil is a long-term therapy—immediate results should not be expected.

Studies on EPO as a treatment for eczema indicate that, when successful, patients benefit after 3 to 4 months of use. The most notable benefit: relief from itching.[15] This result is significant, because it means patients can decrease and sometimes stop using topical steroid creams. Patients have also noted a decrease in skin roughness.

Studies indicate that the best candidates for EPO treatment are younger children with eczema.[16] Adult patients with severe eczema who have been on steroids for long periods of time will probably see only minor results.[17,18] One study with adults suffering from chronic hand dermatitis (not necessarily eczema) found that 6 grams of EPO daily for 16 weeks led to no improvement in their condition.[19] Evening primrose oil is clearly best when started before eczema becomes too serious. Even then, remember that clinical results have not been overwhelmingly positive, and other treatments are likely to be needed along with EPO.

How about just good ol' dry skin? One study using a cream containing 12.5% EPO in adults with dry skin and a tendency toward eczema found that twice daily applications improved skin smoothness.[20]

DIABETIC NEUROPATHY

Evening primrose oil, like other herbal medicines and nutritional supplements (e.g., *Ginkgo biloba* and bilberry), offers a safe and nontoxic way to possibly slow many of the complications of diabetes. It has emerged as a promising long-term therapy to delay the onset and help slow the progression of diabetic neuropathy.[21]

As we will note in our discussion of diabetes in Part 6, neuropathy is an extremely common complication that affects approximately 30 percent of all diabetics. This progressive disorder of the nerves leads to an initial "pins and needles" sensation in the soles of the feet and palms of the hands. Later, it advances to such a point that the ability to differentiate temperature and pressure changes in the extremities is impaired.

A 1990 study conducted over 6 months at the University of Glasgow in Scotland[22] examined the effect of 4 grams of EPO daily versus placebo in diabetic patients with confirmed diabetic neuropathy. Researchers found that patients taking EPO experienced an improvement in sensing cold, heat, and pain. Numbness and weakness also were diminished with EPO. A key finding was the fact that EPO supplementation did not disrupt control of blood sugar.

A follow-up study[23] of 111 diabetic patients with mild neuropathy confirmed the results of the Glasgow study. In a comparison of EPO and placebo (6 grams of EPO daily or placebo for 1 year), seven different medical centers found that administration of EPO resulted in an improvement in nerve conduction, sensation in the extremities, and other signs and symptoms associated with neuropathy. The authors noted that clinical outcomes were better in those patients with better blood sugar control. As in the Glasgow study, EPO did not result in any loss of control of blood sugar.

Again, early intervention is preferable when considering EPO as a treatment for diabetic neuropathy. Finally, news flash to the medical community: As of early in the year 2000, no follow-up studies have been done. Why?

PMS AND BREAST PAIN

One of the most popular uses for EPO has been for PMS and for breast pain—particularly pain associated with a woman's period. Research indicates that EFA metabolism is often impaired in women with PMS and cyclical breast pain.[24,25] Correcting EFA metabolism may benefit women with these conditions.

Clinical studies of EPO treatments for these conditions (which often appear together) indicate that the most notable relief provided by EPO is for breast pain and tenderness. Using EPO at a dosage of 3 grams daily for 4 to 6 months has resulted in a notable reduction in cyclical breast pain and cyst formation about 40 to 50 percent of the time.[26]

Perhaps most notable is the fact that EPO compares favorably to commonly used drug therapies for cyclical breast pain. These include bromocriptine and danazol. Two large clinical reports[27,28] indicate that EPO matches symptom relief. What makes EPO superior, particularly as an initial therapeutic choice, is that it has virtually no side effects. The two drugs mentioned earlier result in side effects in almost one-third of the women using them. Evening primrose oil has become a front-line treatment in Great Britain for the initial treatment of cyclical breast pain and fibrocystic breast disease.[29]

The results of clinical trials of EPO for women suffering from PMS are less convincing.[30,31] It is essential with any treatment for PMS that therapy be monitored for at least three to four cycles to determine success. Evening primrose oil appears to be fairly slow in its actions and probably requires at least four to six cycles before an accurate assessment of results can be made. Even then, herbs such as vitex (see that chapter in this book) and nutrients such as vitamin B_6 and magnesium are more likely to give relief for PMS.

Evening primrose oil should be considered as one part of a comprehensive treatment approach to PMS. See the section on PMS in "Female Health Conditions" in Part 6.

OTHER CLINICAL APPLICATIONS

Other conditions that may be helped by EPO include the following:

- Rheumatoid arthritis
- Dry eyes associated with Sjögren's syndrome
- Endometriosis
- Raynaud's disease

Notable among these conditions is rheumatoid arthritis and dry eyes associated with Sjögren's syndrome (an autoimmune illness). Rheumatoid arthritis may respond best to a combination of EPO and fish oil.

HOW TO USE EVENING PRIMROSE OIL

The recommended daily dose of EPO varies according to the condition. If you're using EPO for eczema, diabetic neuropathy, or rheumatoid arthritis, take 4 to 6 grams daily. Women with PMS and cyclical breast pain can use 3 grams daily. Children with eczema should take 2 to 4 grams daily. Because it is an oil, EPO should be taken with meals for proper absorption.

I highly recommend taking any EFA supplement with some vitamin E. The amount contained in most good-quality multivitamin–mineral supplements is probably fine. Vitamin E is a natural antioxidant for EFAs and will protect them from free radical damage. Taking a good daily multiple also provides nutritional cofactors (e.g., zinc, vitamin B_6, biotin, magnesium) needed for proper EFA metabolism.

Evening primrose oil is virtually devoid of side effects. In clinical studies, a handful of people (less than 2 percent) sometimes experienced bloating and mild abdominal discomfort. Mild headache was also reported, but the frequency of occurrence of this side effect was about the same as for the people taking placebo.

There are no known contraindications to the use of EPO with prescription medications. Some have speculated that steroids and nonsteroidal anti-inflammatory medicines may interfere with proper metabolism of GLA.[32] Research has yet to test this theory. There are no known contraindications to the use of EPO during pregnancy or lactation.

RELATED CONDITIONS DISCUSSED IN PART 6

- Atherosclerosis
- Chronic fatigue immunodeficiency syndrome
- Diabetic neuropathy
- Dry eyes associated with Sjögren's syndrome (sicca syndrome)
- Eczema
- Fibrocystic breast disease
- Premenstrual syndrome
- Rheumatoid arthritis
- Raynaud's disease

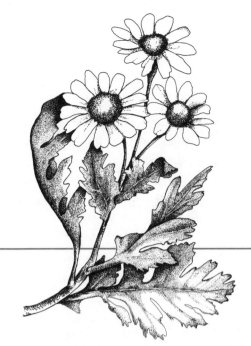

Feverfew

Tanacetum parthenium

Part Used
Dried leaves

Common/Potential Use
- Long-term treatment and prevention of migraine headaches

Active Constituents
Some think it is the sesquiterpene lactones—particularly parthenolide

How It Works
Feverfew blocks the overaggregation of platelets as well as the release of serotonin from platelets. It also blocks the formation and action of pro-inflammatory mediators released from cells.

Recommended Use
Feverfew dried leaf extract with a standardized parthenolide content of at least 250 micrograms per daily dose; continuous use is recommended for the treatment and prevention of migraine headaches.

Side Effects

No studies have been conducted on the long-term toxicity of feverfew. Studies using standardized feverfew tablets have demonstrated minimal side effects; these have been minor (i.e., nervousness and mild gastrointestinal upset). Chewing the leaves of feverfew has resulted in mouth ulceration and swelling of the tongue and mouth in about 10 percent of cases.

Safety Issues/Drug Interactions

Feverfew is not recommended during pregnancy or lactation. Children under the age of 2 years should not use feverfew. There are no known drug interactions with feverfew.

FEVERFEW'S recognition as an effective treatment for migraine headaches is due to a group of outspoken health care consumers. Some British citizens who had successfully used feverfew leaves for treatment of their migraines were not shy about sharing their success stories. Thanks to their efforts, feverfew is recognized today by both the British and Canadian governments as a long-term treatment and preventive measure for migraines.

PLANT FACTS

Feverfew is a member of the daisy family. It is a short, bushy perennial that grows along fields and roadsides all over Europe. Its yellow–green leaves and yellow flowers resemble those of chamomile, with which it is often confused. The flowers bloom from July to October. The leaves are used in medicinal preparations.[1]

History

The name *feverfew* is derived from the Latin for "chase away fevers." Feverfew is mentioned in the ancient Greek medical literature as a remedy for inflammation and menstrual discomfort. It once enjoyed wide use by British herbalists in the treatment of fevers and as a pain reliever but later faded into obscurity. Only in the past two decades has feverfew experienced a revival, owing primarily to its use in the treatment of migraine headaches.[2]

Medically Active Constituents

Feverfew contains compounds known as *sesquiterpene lactones* (STLs). The most important of these compounds is thought to be parthenolide. First identified in 1960, parthenolide represents about 85 percent of the STL content in feverfew and is thought to be the portion of the leaf responsible for feverfew's antimigraine activity.[3]

A critical consideration in commercial feverfew products has been the highly variable content of parthenolide. An analysis of commercial feverfew products in Canada found about half to be virtually devoid of this compound.[4] The Health Protection Branch of the Health and Welfare Department of the Canadian government has proposed that feverfew preparations should contain at least 0.2 percent parthenolide content. If you want to use feverfew to treat your migraines, seek out products that guarantee a stable parthenolide content. I've been recommending an extract that contains 0.7 percent parthenolide and getting great feedback from patients.

Lately, the role of parthenolide in feverfew's antimigraine effects has been questioned by Dr. Dennis Awang, a Canadian herbal expert who was one of the early proponents of using feverfew products with an adequate concentration of parthenolide.[5] This opinion is partly based on the negative results of the Dutch study summarized later that used an alcohol extract instead of the typical dried leaf preparations used in successful studies. While the alcohol-based preparation did have adequate parthenolide, Dr. Awang suggests that other constituents may have been eliminated, making the feverfew less effective. I'm interested in Dr. Awang's about-face but would like a bit more evidence until I steer away from recommending high-quality extracts of feverfew leaf standardized to parthenolide content.

HOW FEVERFEW WORKS

Migraine headaches are, for the most part, a mystery; medical research and drug development are currently focused on the role of platelets and the neurotransmitter serotonin. Platelets, which are a normal part of the blood and are involved in clotting, appear to act abnormally in migraine sufferers. During a migraine attack, platelets not only tend to overcongregate (aggregate) but also to release the substance *serotonin*. Serotonin and inflammatory substances released from platelets are widely believed to be the primary chemical triggers of migraine headaches.[6]

Feverfew, and specifically parthenolide, counters overaggregation of platelets and the release of serotonin.[7,8] This may result in a reduction in the severity, duration, and frequency of migraine headaches and an improvement in blood vessel tone.

Feverfew also discourages the formation of certain inflammatory substances released from platelets and other cells.[9,10] While this is another plus for migraine sufferers, it may also explain its historical use for inflammatory conditions such as arthritis. However, it should be noted that a British clinical study did not show any benefit for rheumatoid arthritis patients using feverfew.[11]

HEALTH CARE APPLICATIONS

Feverfew is the premier herbal therapy for migraine sufferers. By prescribing feverfew along with stress reduction, dietary modifications, and the nutrients magnesium and riboflavin, I have witnessed a major drop in the severity, duration, and frequency of migraine headaches in many of my patients (see my recommendations for migraines in "Nervous System" in Part 6). It's important to remember that feverfew works best when used over several weeks to months. The herb is not designed to give you immediate relief once a migraine is under way.

Modern interest in feverfew arose in Great Britain because of its use by a group of people determined to treat their migraines successfully. Their results, published in *Prevention* magazine in 1978, gained widespread attention. The story related the success of a certain Mrs. Jenkins, who used feverfew for her migraines. A migraine sufferer for more than 50 years, Mrs. Jenkins found relief after self-administering feverfew leaves daily for 10 months. She became an outspoken advocate for feverfew treatment of migraines, and her experience prompted the Migraine Trust of the United Kingdom to start medical studies.

The initial clinical study[12] involved migraine patients who had been using feverfew for several years. Seventeen patients were enrolled and given either feverfew dried leaf extract (50 milligrams per day) or placebo. Eight patients, who had the good fortune to stay on feverfew, experienced continued relief from migraines over a 6-month period. The nine receiving placebo suffered an almost threefold increase in migraines! While this study had too few patients to draw many conclusions, it does suggest that abrupt cessation of feverfew may not be a wise choice. If it's working and you decide you want to try going off it, work closely with your health care provider to develop a closely monitored tapering schedule over 2 to 3 weeks.

A second study[13] enrolled 72 migraine sufferers. They received either 82 milligrams of feverfew dried leaf extract (containing approximately 500 micrograms of parthenolide) daily or placebo. After 4 months with feverfew treatment, fewer migraines occurred, and those that did were less severe. Feverfew also led to fewer vomiting attacks and fewer visual disturbances during migraines. Side effects included mild gastrointestinal upset and nervousness but did not result in discontinuation of treatment or any absences at afternoon tea.

A third study completed in Israel found that 200 milligrams a day of a feverfew dried leaf extract (standardized to 0.2 percent parthenolide) for 60 days had a significant decrease in pain intensity and a decrease in vomiting and sensitivity to light and sound during their migraines.[14] During a second phase of the study, patients were split up into those continuing to take feverfew and others receiving placebo. As was the case in the first study mentioned, persons continuing to take feverfew had fewer symptoms and less pain, while those switching over the to the placebo had the predictable blast from the past.

Finally, a fourth study found no benefit for feverfew in the prophylactic treatment of migraines.[15] In this Dutch study, fifty migraine patients received either a dried alcoholic extract of feverfew leaves (providing 500 micrograms of parthenolide) or placebo for 4 months, and then each group was switched to the other treatment (or lack thereof in the case of placebo). While the study was considered a failure for feverfew, it is interesting to note that, while on feverfew, patients did use fewer drugs to manage their acute migraine attacks than those taking placebo. This study probably points out that the dried leaf extracts and not the alcohol extracts are the ones to use.

HOW TO USE FEVERFEW

As mentioned earlier, I'm still partial to the dried leaf extracts that provide a standardized parthenolide content. Canada's Health Protection Branch recommends a daily dosage of 125 milligrams of a dried feverfew leaf preparation, from authentic *Tanacetum parthenium* containing at least 0.2 percent parthenolide for the treatment and prevention of migraines. This dosage equates to approximately 250 micrograms of parthenolide daily. I've been recently recommending an extract standardized to 0.7 percent parthenolide at a daily dose of 100 milligrams (equivalent to 700 micrograms of parthenolide). The one-a-day dosing has worked great for convenience, and I've been extremely pleased with the positive feedback from patients.

Feverfew is a long-term, prophylactic treatment, not an immediate cure for a migraine attack. My clinical experience suggests that 4 to 6 weeks are usually required to note an initial response. However, average duration of use will vary among migraine patients. Success should be measured by decreased frequency, severity, and duration of migraine attacks.

Don't use feverfew if you are pregnant or lactating. Parents should not give feverfew to children under the age of 2 years. If you're taking prescription medications for migraines, consult a health care professional before using feverfew.

RELATED CONDITION DISCUSSED IN PART 6

- Migraine headache

Garlic

Allium sativum

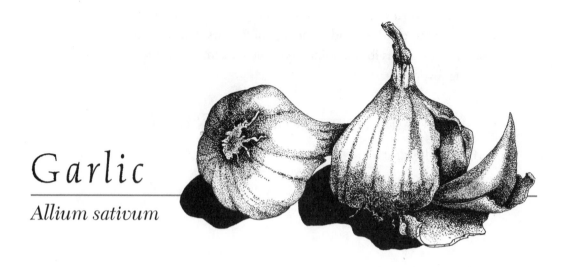

Part Used
The bulb

Common/Potential Uses
- Prevention of atherosclerosis
- Reduction of mildly elevated high cholesterol and triglyceride levels
- Lowering of mildly elevated blood pressure
- Prevention of yeast infections
- Cancer prevention

Active Constituents
The sulfur compound allicin, which is produced with crushing or chewing of the fresh bulb. Allicin in turn produces other sulfur compounds, including allyl sulfides, ajoene, and the vinyldithiins. These compounds are found only in garlic oil products produced by maceration (not in steam-distilled garlic oils).

How It Works

Garlic helps prevent atherosclerosis and improves the health of the arteries. In some persons, it may lower mildly elevated serum cholesterol and triglycerides while raising "good" HDL cholesterol (lipoproteins that help transport cholesterol from various parts of the body to the liver). Garlic also reduces the "stickiness" of platelets, making blood circulation more efficient. It may cause a mild reduction in blood pressure in persons with mild hypertension. Regular dietary consumption of garlic has been associated with lowered risk of stomach and colon cancer in some population studies.

Recommended Use

Standardized garlic powder product containing 1.3 percent alliin and providing 5,000 to 6,000 micrograms of allicin potential daily—600 to 900 milligrams daily in two to three divided doses.

Side Effects

Consumption at these doses rarely poses health risks. Heartburn and flatulence may be experienced by some persons sensitive to garlic. There are rare reports of allergic reactions to garlic.

Safety Issues/Drug Interactions

Because of garlic's anticlotting properties, people undergoing anticoagulant or antiplatelet aggregation drug therapy (e.g., Coumadin®, Ticlid®) or taking aspirin regularly should avoid the use of garlic. There are no known contraindications to the use of garlic during pregnancy and lactation.

The Professor's actions were certainly odd and not to be found in any phar-macopoeia that I ever heard of. First he fastened up the windows and latched them securely; next, taking a handful of the flowers, he rubbed them all over the sashes, as though to ensure that every whiff of air that might get in would be laden with garlic smell.

BRAM STOKER, DRACULA

GARLIC may be the best example of the continuum between plants as food and plants as medicine. One of the most ancient remedies known to humanity, garlic is a staple in the diets of an incredibly diverse number of cultures. Most of these cultures use garlic for medicinal purposes.

But let's not dwell on the past! Garlic has enjoyed a surge in popularity over the last decade. The star of more than numerous research publications (primarily in Europe), garlic is best known for promoting cardiovascular health. Not only obnoxious to vampires, garlic also seems to be the bane of nasty little beasts like bacteria, viruses, and yeast.

While making garlic part of your regular diet, new findings are suggesting that supplementing garlic may be one of the best tools available to stave off atherosclerosis. This places garlic right toward the top of the list of herbal and nutritional considerations for prevention of coronary artery disease.

PLANT FACTS

Garlic is a member of the lily family and belongs to the genus *Allium,* which also includes onions. *Allium* is the Latin name for garlic and derives from a Celtic word meaning "hot" or "burning." The word *sativum* means that the plant is cultivated (i.e., planted). Garlic in its present form is not found in the wild, having evolved to its present form after thousands of years of cultivation.[1]

Garlic bulbs are typically harvested in the early summer. The largest commercial production of garlic is in central California, which harvests about 250 million pounds of garlic every year. (I won't burden you with stories of a young college student hallucinating about pesto while hurtling through the garlic-saturated air of Gilroy, California.) China is also a supplier of commercial garlic.

HISTORY

Talk about stories to tell! Garlic has seen the rise and fall of the pharaohs in Egypt. The Book of Numbers in the Bible reports of dissent among the Israelites as they fled Egypt, owing to a lack of garlic in their travel provisions. Apparently manna without a little babaghanoush really is unacceptable! Even more racy is the fact that the Talmud encourages the consumption of garlic to encourage matrimonial lovemaking![2]

Garlic has been cultivated in the Middle East for more than 5,000 years. It was a common crop and dietary staple in Mesopotamia. It was also a common trade commodity in Babylon.

Greek and Roman physicians such as Hippocrates, Galen, Pliny the Elder, and Dioscorides recommended garlic for a dizzying array of conditions. Among these were parasites, respiratory problems, weight loss, poor digestion, and low energy.

Garlic has also been an important part of traditional Chinese medical history. Known as *da-suan* in China, medicinal use of garlic is first mentioned in Tao Hong-jing's *Ming Yi Bie Lu* (Miscellaneous Records of Famous Physicians), written in 510 A.D. Garlic was administered for digestive difficulties, diarrhea, dysentery, colds, and tuberculosis. It was also used externally in the treatment of pinworms, snake bites, and fungal infections of the skin.[3]

Garlic did not escape the scientific eye of Louis Pasteur. In 1858, the father of pasteurization engaged in studies to confirm the antibacterial activity of garlic. Albert Schweitzer used garlic to treat amebic dysentery during his sojourn in Africa.

MEDICALLY ACTIVE CONSTITUENTS

Garlic's medicinal effects in the body depend on a series of chemical reactions. Figure 5.2 shows what happens when you crush or chew a garlic

FIGURE 5.2. TRANSFORMATION OF GARLIC'S ACTIVE INGREDIENTS

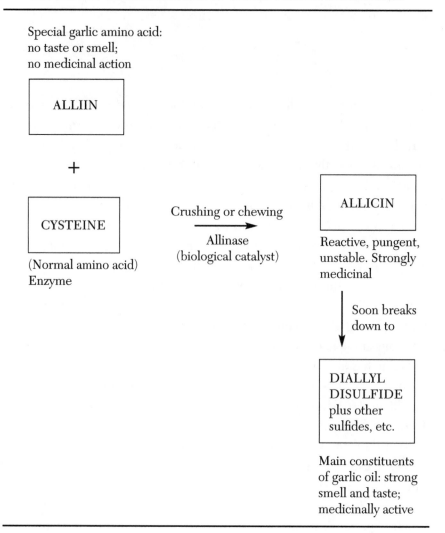

clove. Garlic cloves, before they are crushed or chewed, are high in an odorless, sulfur-containing amino acid known as alliin. With crushing or chewing, alliin comes into contact with the enzyme alliinase. Alliinase very rapidly (in less than 6 seconds) transforms alliin into allicin, which is the source of the familiar garlic odor.

Allicin is not very stable. Depending on the conditions, it breaks down into a number of other sulfur compounds, including ajoene, vinyldithiins, and diallyl disulfide and trisulfide.[4] These compounds are found only in macerated garlic oil products—not in garlic powder supplements.

Allicin and its fellow sulfur compounds fuel many of garlic's actions in the body. Allicin is known to have extensive antimicrobial activity. It inhibits the growth of many bacteria and fungi (including *Candida albicans*). Ajoene also has weak antifungal effects and can reduce the "stickiness" of platelets.[5] Some of the other sulfur compounds have antitumor activity.

All of this rambling about alliin and allicin is based on what happens when you eat *raw* garlic. With chewing, allicin forms quickly in the mouth. Allicin does not form in the stomach, because alliinase is inactivated by stomach acid.[6] Once you've chopped up garlic and dried it or cooked it, a good amount of the allicin is lost. Raw garlic is clearly the best source of allicin.

Research suggests that the best garlic supplements closely approximate the eating of raw garlic. Carefully prepared garlic powder will yield allicin almost as efficiently as raw garlic (only 4 percent less). Aged garlic products don't make the grade, since they yield no allicin and only about 10 percent of the other sulfur compounds present in garlic. Allicin is not present in garlic oil macerates.

Stomach acid inhibits allicin formation. The best way to counter this is to purchase garlic tablets that are enteric coated. Enteric coating allows safe passage through the intensely acidic environment of the stomach and refuge in the more alkaline pH of the small intestine. There the conversion to allicin can safely occur.[7]

How Garlic Works

In the past 40 years, the "stinking rose" (as garlic has been called) has been as busy in the laboratory as in the kitchen. Table 5.1 breaks down the focus of this research.

Table 5.1
GARLIC RESEARCH PUBLICATIONS (1950–1992)

Topic	Number of Publications
Antibiotic effect	171
Cardiovascular (including cholesterol-lowering) effect	258
Anticancer effect	154
Effect on blood sugar level	13
Effectiveness as heavy metal antidote	14
Potential alleviation of intestinal problems	8
Other biological effects	150
Chemical studies	320
Total	1088

Reprinted by permission from L. D. Lawson, *Human Medicinal Agents from Plants*, ACS, Washington, D.C., 1993.

CARDIOVASCULAR EFFECTS

High levels of cholesterol and triglycerides in the blood are major risk factors for the development of coronary artery disease. Concern also arises when platelets in the blood become sticky and clump together in what's known as *platelet aggregation*. Finally, like a hose that becomes hard and brittle after years of use, the walls of the arteries loss their elasticity as we age—a condition known as arteriosclerosis. Together, these conditions lead to poor circulation and even obstruction of blood vessels, which in turn can lead to angina, heart attack, and a host of problems involving blood flow to the extremities, including intermittent claudication.

Garlic is a full-service herbal prescription for cardiovascular system health. More than 250 publications have shown that garlic sometimes lowers mildly elevated cholesterol and triglycerides, reduces oxidation of low-density lipoprotein (LDL) cholesterol, inhibits platelet aggregation, and increases fibrinolysis, which results in a slowing of blood coagulation.[8] It's also been shown to improve the elasticity of the arteries and counteract the age-related arterial stiffness mentioned earlier.[9] Add to this a mild antihypertensive effect as well as antioxidant activity, and garlic emerges as one of nature's most potent weapons against cardiovascular disease.[10,11]

Garlic interferes with the creation of cholesterol in the liver.[12] This means that less cholesterol is released into the bloodstream. Allicin appears to be the sulfur compound in garlic responsible for this action.[13] Garlic, both with allicin potential and aged garlic (which doesn't have allicin potential), has been found to reduce the oxidation of LDL cholesterol.[14,15] Keeping LDL cholesterol free of oxidation is a very important consideration in the prevention of atherosclerosis. Finally, garlic helps package the remaining cholesterol as HDL cholesterol. This form of cholesterol is associated with decreased risk of cardiovascular disease because it's transported to the liver and broken down.[16]

Garlic also reduces platelet stickiness and excessive blood clotting—two factors associated with blockage of blood vessels and sluggish circulation. In one study,[17] ten "healthy" volunteers were given 900 milligrams of garlic powder daily; 2 to 4 hours after garlic ingestion, platelet stickiness was found to be reduced. The *fibrinolytic*, or anticlotting, activity took several days to be noted. Ajoene, which is present only in garlic oil macerates, also appears to help reduce platelet stickiness.[18] I regularly tell people to consider switching their daily aspirin for garlic. The overall cardiovascular benefits are far more convincing for garlic, and you don't have to worry about stomach problems.

By the way, the anticlotting effect of garlic won't cause you to bleed excessively if you're cut. It keeps *excess* clotting in check, a benefit for persons at risk for cardiovascular disease. *Note:* This is not meant to suggest that garlic can effectively replace stronger anticlotting drugs; its primary value is as a preventive.

ANTIMICROBIAL ACTIONS

Another potential benefit of garlic is the creation of an environment that is inhospitable to a wide variety of micro-organisms bent on wreaking havoc in our bodies. In test tube studies and some preliminary human research, garlic exerts antibacterial, antiviral, and antifungal activity. It has even been shown to chase away intestinal worms!

As mentioned earlier, garlic's antibacterial effect was first noted by Louis Pasteur in 1858. The strength of garlic appears to be about 1 percent that of penicillin in killing certain types of bacteria. This means it's not a substitute for antibiotics but may potentially serve as a defense against bacterial infections—particularly by those of you with recurrent infections.[19]

One of the more intriguing potential uses of garlic is for the prevention of tuberculosis (TB). Garlic has noted anti-TB activity and was actually used for this purpose during the 1800s. As described further on, individuals infected with the human immunodeficiency virus (HIV), particularly those with AIDS-related complex (ARC) or acquired immunodeficiency syndrome (AIDS), may find some added benefit by taking garlic to increase resistance to secondary infections from bacteria and yeast. Future research should explore this cost-effective alternative.

In test tube studies, garlic and some of its sulfur compounds are emerging as promising antiviral substances. These studies show that garlic inhibits the herpes simplex virus type 1 (HSV-1), cytomegalovirus (which can cause eye and lung problems in immunocompromised individuals), and also HIV.[20,21,22]

The anti-HIV activity is associated with isolated ajoene and allyl disulfide, which are found only in garlic oil macerates, not garlic powder products. In the case of all three viruses, we don't know whether real-life use of garlic can match these results.

A final area of antimicrobial action for garlic is in the treatment of yeast infections. Growth of *Candida albicans*, the organism most widely responsible for intestinal, vaginal, and oral yeast infections, is inhibited by garlic.[23] Many health care professionals use garlic to prevent recurrent, chronic yeast infections. This approach should be limited to localized yeast infections. Systemic yeast infections can be dangerous and should be treated with stronger drugs.

Once again, I'd like to emphasize that the best protection against a wide variety of micro-organisms is going to come from raw garlic or garlic supplements that approximate the allicin potential of raw garlic. Studies have shown conclusively that allicin exerts the most broad-spectrum antimicrobial activity of any sulfur compound in garlic.[24]

ANTICANCER ACTIONS

Human population studies suggest that regular garlic intake reduces the risk of esophageal, stomach, and colon cancer (discussed later). This is partly due to garlic's ability to reduce the formation of N-nitroso compounds such as nitrosamine.[25] A major source of nitrosamines is the charcoal broiling of fats. You'd be better off getting rid of flame-broiled hamburgers altogether, but if that's the break you need, at least take some garlic along for the ride.

Animal and test tube studies also show that garlic and its sulfur compounds inhibit the growth of different types of cancer. Notable among them are breast cancer and skin tumors.[26,27] More research is needed to determine whether garlic will actually aid persons with cancer. The evidence does argue for a protective/preventive effect of regular garlic intake.

HEALTH CARE APPLICATIONS

ATHEROSCLEROSIS

While the past few years have seen a lot of debate about garlic's ability to lower cholesterol, a new study suggests that we may want to refocus our use of garlic. A landmark study published in the journal *Atherosclerosis* in 1999 suggests that garlic may not only prevent atherosclerosis but, in some cases, actually slow progression and even reverse plaque formation![28]

In this study, volunteers ages 44 to 74 years with diagnosed atherosclerotic plaques were given 300 milligrams of a garlic extract (Kwai®) or placebo three times daily for 4 years. At the end of the study, the placebo group showed a predictable increase in the size of their atherosclerotic plaques, while the garlic group actually showed a slight regression in the size of their plaques! This change was most notable in women who, on average, had a plaque reduction of 4.6 percent. When considering just persons over 50 years old, plaque reduction ranged from 6 to 13 percent.

While this sort of plaque reduction has been shown for some of the newer cholesterol-lowering drugs (e.g., lovastatin), garlic may end up being our first choice for the long-term prevention and perhaps even treatment of atherosclerosis.

Table 5.2

EFFECTS OF GARLIC POWDER WITH STANDARDIZED
ALLICIN POTENTIAL ON ELEVATED CHOLESTEROL AND
TRIGLYCERIDES: THREE POSITIVE HUMAN STUDIES

Number of Patients	Daily Dose	Length of Study	Decrease in Cholesterol	Decrease in Triglycerides	Study
261	800 mg	16 weeks	12%	17%	Mader, 1990 (Ref. 29)
40	900 mg	16 weeks	21%	24%	Vorberg and Schneider, 1990 (Ref. 30)
42	900 mg	12 weeks	6%	11%	Jain et al., 1993 (Ref. 31)

HIGH CHOLESTEROL AND TRIGLYCERIDES

Boy, talk about an abrupt about-face! Look at any article on garlic before the mid-1990s (including the first edition of this book), and the treatment of high cholesterol was featured. Newer research and a closer look at some of the earlier "successful" studies have clouded the picture a bit.

From 1975 to 1998, more than thirty-five human studies have been done on the cholesterol- and triglyceride-lowering (lipid-lowering) effects of garlic. Of these, the majority were performed with Kwai garlic powder tablets standardized to 1.3 percent alliin and 0.6 percent allicin (potential). The dosages ranged from 600 to 900 milligrams daily, and the lengths of the studies ranged from 4 to 16 weeks. Patients with high cholesterol, high triglycerides, or both were studied. Table 5.2 summarizes the results of three of these earlier studies.[29,30,31]

One study[32] compared garlic with bezafibrate (similar to the U.S. drug clofibrate). Ninety-eight patients with high cholesterol and triglycerides received one of two treatments: garlic at 900 milligrams/day or bezafibrate at 600 milligrams/day. At the end of the 12-week study, reduction in cholesterol and LDL ("bad") cholesterol was almost identical for both treatments, as was the rise in HDL ("good") cholesterol. No studies have

Table 5.3
Effects of Garlic Powder with Standardized Allicin Potential on Elevated Cholesterol and Triglycerides: Three Negative Human Studies

Number of Patients	Daily Dose	Length of Study	Decrease in Cholesterol	Decrease in Triglycerides	Study
50	900 mg	12 weeks	not significant	not significant	Isaachson, 1998 (Ref. 35)
115	900 mg	24 weeks	not significant	not significant	Neil, 1996 (Ref. 36)
31	900 mg	12 weeks	not significant	not significant	Simons, 1995 (Ref. 37)

compared garlic directly to the new generation of cholesterol-lowering drugs known as HMG-CoA reductase inhibitors or "statins" (e.g., Lipitor, Mevacor).

Two review articles[33,34] analyzed the results of some of these earlier studies on the cholesterol-/triglyceride-lowering effects of garlic powder. They indicate that over a 1- to 4-month period, the administration of garlic powder tablets (dosage, 600 to 900 milligrams daily) resulted in an average reduction in total serum cholesterol of 9 to 12 percent (range, 6 to 21 percent); triglyceride levels fell from 8 to 27 percent. Both analyses called for better designed and larger studies.

Since 1995, three well-designed studies found no success using garlic for lowering cholesterol.[35,36,37] Table 5.3 summarizes the results of these studies. It should be noted that each of these studies used the Kwai garlic product at a daily dosage of 900 milligrams for 3 to 6 months. All these studies also placed each subject on a uniform diet that carefully controlled the type of food they ingested just prior to and during the study. Two other well-publicized studies also found negative results. These will not be considered, because one dealt with children,[38] and the other used a form of garlic (steam-distilled garlic "oil" bound to β-cyclodextrin) that has no track record of use for this indication.[39]

So, why the discrepancy in the findings? One explanation may be that the earlier studies with garlic did not use a consistent diet for all study participants. It's fairly standard these days to use the American Heart Association Step 1 diet. By more closely controlling intake of certain types of foods (especially those high in fat), the effect of the cholesterol-lowering medication is measured more accurately. Older studies with garlic let people eat a less standardized diet, resulting in the possibility that some of the drops in cholesterol were somewhat exaggerated.

Others have argued that the quality of the garlic products was inconsistent, resulting in different amounts of allicin being released and hence different effects on lowering cholesterol.[40]

The bottom line is this: Garlic should be considered a secondary tool for lowering very mildly elevated cholesterol and triglycerides. This means those of you with the very high levels of cholesterol and triglycerides should see your doctor about using one of the new turbo-charged cholesterol-lowering drugs such as Lipitor® or Mevacor®. Once your cholesterol levels are in check, garlic may be a useful long-term supplement for prevention of coronary artery disease (please see Part 6 for more details on herbal and nutritional considerations for a healthy cardiovascular system).

HIGH BLOOD PRESSURE

Garlic exerts a mild blood pressure lowering effect.[41] This is probably due to its ability to make circulation more efficient (see earlier comments). You should consider garlic as only one part of an overall program for lowering mildly elevated blood pressure, and not as a substitute for stronger blood pressure medications.

INTERMITTENT CLAUDICATION

Most common in the elderly, intermittent claudication involves severe cramping of the muscles in the back of the lower legs during walking or running. It is caused by poor blood flow to the muscles.

While the best herbal prescription for this condition is ginkgo (see the chapter on *Ginkgo biloba*), one study has shown that garlic offers promise.[42] This 12-week study found that garlic powder tablets (800 milligrams daily) led to a significant increase in pain-free walking distance.

INCREASING RESISTANCE TO INFECTION

Garlic may help your body resist infection. As we discussed earlier, this effect may be partly due to garlic's wide-spectrum antimicrobial properties. I heartily endorse using it as a supportive treatment for recurrent yeast infections.

While I don't have any solid clinical research data to back my beliefs, I'm a big proponent of making garlic part of the regular supplement regimen for HIV-infected individuals. Although it probably doesn't have much direct effect on HIV, garlic may deter organisms and viruses that are responsible for secondary (opportunistic) infections that characterize the more advanced stages of the illness. These include cytomegalovirus (CMV), *Mycobacterium avium* (the cause of tuberculosis in AIDS patients), and *Cryptococcus*, the fungus responsible for intestinal infections as well as meningitis in AIDS patients.[43,44]

Again, I'm talking prevention and stronger defenses here. We're a long way from using garlic as a treatment for any of these conditions.

CANCER PREVENTION

The medical establishment has finally gotten smart and realized that diet can be a powerful preventive tool against many forms of cancer. Mainstream research has discovered antioxidants and fiber, and how more of them means less cancer. Garlic should be near the top of the list.

As mentioned previously, garlic appears to have its greatest benefit in the prevention of esophageal, stomach, and colon cancer. An Iowa study[45] examining the diets of women (ranging in age from 55 to 69 years old) found that consumption of garlic was a greater deterrent to colon cancer than dietary fiber and vegetables. The risk of colon cancer dropped by 35 percent with one or more servings of garlic weekly! This reached 50 percent with even greater consumption.

Population studies in China and Italy have shown that consumption of garlic also reduces the risk of esophageal and stomach cancer.[46]

How to Use Garlic

For you bold souls, take about one or two whole cloves of raw garlic daily. If you dislike the smell and the social ramifications, try an odor-controlled, enteric-coated garlic powder tablet with standardized alliin content (approximately 1.3 percent) and allicin potential (approximately 0.6 percent). The daily dose should be 600 to 900 milligrams (about 5,000 to 6,000 micrograms of allicin potential) taken in two or three divided doses. While I constantly get threatening mail from the people who make "odor-free" aged garlic products, I'm still not convinced that their research matches up.

Consumption of garlic at these doses does not pose health risks for most people. Heartburn and flatulence may be experienced by those who are sensitive to garlic. A garlicky taste can sometimes be noticed even with so-called "deodorized" garlic products. There are rare reports of allergic reactions to garlic.

Because of the mild anticlotting properties of garlic, persons undergoing anticoagulant drug therapy—for example, Coumadin®, antiplatelet aggregation drug therapy such as Ticlid®, or the use of aspirin on a regular basis—should avoid the use of garlic. Persons scheduled for surgery should notify their surgeon if they are taking garlic and probably stop it well in advance of the surgery. There are no known contraindications to the use of garlic during pregnancy and lactation.

An interesting study[47] has disproved the popular belief that mothers who consume garlic while nursing cause their infants to shun the garlic-laden breast milk. The study actually found that infants breast-fed longer when mom ate garlic! Of course, pasta with a garlic-laden red sauce was in high demand when solid foods were introduced.

Product update: Kwai garlic products are sold in the United States by Lichtwer Pharma. Other high-quality garlic products include Garlicin® from Nature's Way and Garlitrin® from Enzymatic Therapy.

Related Conditions Discussed in Part 6

- Atherosclerosis
- HIV infection/AIDS
- Hypercholesterolemia (high cholesterol)
- Intermittent claudication
- Interviews with vampires
- Sore throat
- Vaginal yeast infections (recurrent)

Ginger

Zingiber officinale

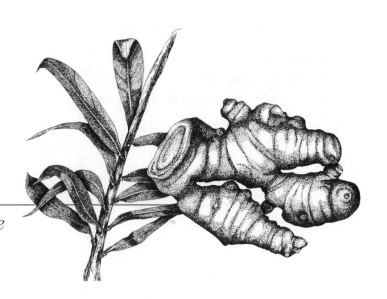

Part Used

The rhizome (the underground stem)

Common/Potential Uses

- Promotes normal digestion
- Alleviates motion sickness
- Reduces nausea associated with pregnancy
- Counteracts postanesthesia nausea following surgery or nausea following chemotherapy

Active Constituents

Volatile oil components, including gingerols and shogaols

How It Works

Ginger acts as a bitter and carminative herb. It helps stimulate digestion and also improves the tone of intestinal muscles. It also soothes upset stomachs. The gingerols and shogaols in the essential oil counter nausea and vomiting. Ginger also reduces platelet "stickiness" in the blood, aiding circulation. It also exerts mild anti-inflammatory actions.

Recommended Use

For prevention/treatment of motion sickness, take 500 milligrams ½ to 1 hour before travel and then 500 milligrams every 2 to 4 hours as needed. Children below the age of 6 years may use half the adult dose. For treatment of nausea of pregnancy, women may use up to 1 gram daily but should only use ginger as needed and not on an ongoing basis. Use of ginger for nausea associated with anesthesia or chemotherapy should only be done under the supervision of a physician.

Side Effects

Some persons sensitive to the taste of ginger may experience heartburn.

Safety Issues/Drug Interactions

The German Commission E monograph suggests persons with a history of gallstones use ginger cautiously. Ginger may interact with anticoagulant drugs (Coumadin®), antiplatelet aggregation drugs (Ticlid®), or aspirin to increase the chance of bleeding. Be sure to inform your doctor if you are taking this type of medication and want to take ginger.

FOLLOWING a chapter on garlic with one on ginger is pure torture! One minute I'm daydreaming about calamari with roasted garlic, and the next it's sushi with pickled ginger. Who said writing a book on herbal medicine is easy?

Like garlic, ginger fits very nicely into the classification of food or spice as medicine. Ginger is commonly used in the cooking of many cultures, particularly in Asia. It is also a common household remedy for digestive disorders, nausea, and coughs. Modern research has established ginger as a safe and effective alternative in the treatment of two conditions: motion sickness and the nausea and vomiting associated with pregnancy.

PLANT FACTS

Ginger is a perennial plant, growing from 1 to 3 feet in height. The underground stem of the plant, known as the *rhizome*, is light brown or tan on the outside and yellow on the inside. Most of the ginger in the U.S. market arrives with its outer, barklike layer scraped off, giving it a pale appearance. The branches off the rhizome are irregularly shaped and are sometimes referred to as hands or fingers.[1]

The annual world production of ginger is estimated at 100,000 tons. Major exporting countries include India, Fiji, Nigeria, Mexico, and China. During the 1980s, the United States imported more than 4,000 metric tons of ginger per year.[2]

HISTORY

Cultivated for thousands of years in China and India, ginger was sold to the ancient Greeks and Romans by Arabian traders. It was actually subject to Roman taxes in the second century A.D. (the money paid for that new luxury stadium). Tariff duties on ginger appear in the records of Barcelona in 1221, Marseilles in 1228, and Paris in 1296. About 1280, Marco Polo reported ginger production in China and India.[3]

Traditional Chinese medicine has recommended ginger for more than 2,500 years. Chinese herbalists prescribe it for abdominal distension, coughing, vomiting, diarrhea, and rheumatism. They view fresh ginger and dried ginger as having different medicinal properties.[4] Ginger is also an important part of the traditional healing systems of Nigeria, the West Indies, and India.

MEDICALLY ACTIVE CONSTITUENTS

The dried rhizome of ginger contains about 1 to 4 percent volatile oils. These oils are responsible for ginger's characteristic odor and taste and contain the medically active constituents. The aromatic principals include the sesquiterpene hydrocarbons zingiberene and bisabolene. The pungent counterparts, known as *gingerols* and *shogaols*, have received most of the research attention in the last few years.[5] They give ginger its characteristic taste and are credited with its antinausea and antivomiting effect.

While most of the clinical research over the past two decades has focused on the powdered rhizome, ginger products produced in the last 5 years have concentrated the volatile oils and established a standardized content of gingerols and shogaols. However, clinical studies have not yet been completed on these "standardized" extracts.

How Ginger Works

DIGESTIVE SYSTEM ACTIONS

Ginger is a classic tonic for the digestive tract. Classified as an "aromatic bitter," it stimulates digestion and benefits those with sluggish digestion. By keeping the intestinal muscles "toned,"[6] ginger also eases the transport of substances through the digestive tract, lessening irritation to the intestinal walls.[7] Ginger improves the production and secretion of bile from the liver and gallbladder. This aids digestion of fats and helps lower the amount of cholesterol in the bloodstream.[8]

Ginger also qualifies as a carminative herb (see Part 4 for more on carminatives). If you're having problems with flatulence, intestinal spasms, or irritation, you'll benefit from the use of ginger.

An animal study conducted in Saudi Arabia[9] showed that ginger protects the stomach from the damaging effects of nonsteroidal anti-inflammatory drugs (e.g., ibuprofen) and alcohol. Another study in Japan found similar results with a bunch of rats that the researchers got all liquored up![10] It is interesting that as opposed to licorice, which worked on the surface of the stomach, ginger increased production of protective mucin in the deeper parts of the stomach lining. This result suggests that ginger may be another plant medicine that offers help against ulcers.

ANTINAUSEA/ANTIVOMITING ACTIONS

Ever wonder what to do when your pet frog starts vomiting? Well, another one of those wonderful animal studies has your answer!

A Japanese study conducted on frogs[11] found that shogaols and gingerols isolated from ginger prevented vomiting induced by chemicals.

What is particularly interesting about their findings is that at least part of ginger's action may occur in the central nervous system (CNS) and not just in the gastrointestinal tract. This observation supports an earlier study in mice indicating that gingerol and shogaol activity was partially centered in the CNS.[12]

A study with dogs given cisplatin, a chemotherapeutic drug, found that ginger significantly reduced vomiting due to the drug.[13]

Studies with humans, on the other hand, have led us to believe that the antinausea and antivomiting actions of ginger are limited to the gastrointestinal tract.[14] But these studies looked only at ginger powder and not at the isolated gingerols and shogaols. Whether ginger extracts with concentrated amounts of these constituents would also exert a CNS effect in humans remains to be proven.

CIRCULATORY EFFECTS

Ginger may also improves the health of the cardiovascular system. Like garlic, ginger makes platelets less "sticky"—that is, less likely to aggregate. This action reduces a major risk factor for atherosclerosis. Ginger does this by raising levels of a substance known as *prostacyclin*. Prostacyclin inhibits the action of thromboxane, a substance associated with increasing platelet aggregation.[15]

A study involving twenty healthy males[16] explored the effect of ginger on platelet aggregation when large amounts of fat were consumed. The men in this study were fed 100 grams of butter daily for 7 days. Not surprisingly, their platelet aggregation went up significantly. However, the addition of 2.5 grams of ginger twice daily led to a significant drop in platelet aggregation. Add ginger to your list of herbs and foods that may reduce the risk of cardiovascular disease.

ANTI-INFLAMMATORY AND ANALGESIC EFFECTS

The Ayurvedic system of medicine offers ginger in the treatment of inflammatory joint diseases, including arthritis. Ginger counters the formation of pro-inflammatory substances such as leukotrienes and certain prostaglandins. The gingerols seem to be the most effective constituents in this activity.[17]

Studies with experimental animals also suggest ginger acts as a mild pain reliever. In fact, the shogaols may act very much like capsaicin, the hot and pungent portion of cayenne pepper.[18] Capsaicin is widely used in topical creams for arthritis and the treatment of pain following a shingles outbreak.

HEALTH CARE APPLICATIONS

MOTION SICKNESS

Ginger has been widely used to treat motion sickness in Europe. However, research results have been mixed, leaving it in a sort of limbo here in the United States. The bottom line appears to be that it probably works best for those "real-life" situations (you know, like those barfing kids on the MTV show) such as seasickness during boat trips or getting sick in the car. It's not likely to reverse the severe motion sickness experienced by astronauts or after a ride on the Kumba roller coaster at Busch Gardens in Tampa.

In 1982, Daniel Mowrey of Brigham Young University (Provo, Utah) and Dennis Clayson of Mount Union College (Alliance, Ohio) found that ginger was superior to dimenhydrinate (Dramamine) for reducing motion sickness (caused by rotating a chair).[19] The dose of ginger was 940 milligrams, consumed 20 to 25 minutes before the test.

A handful of studies since have both agreed and disagreed with Mowrey and Clayson's results. A study that I love because of its subtitle, "A Controlled Trial on the Open Sea," tested ginger against seasickness in eighty Danish naval cadets unaccustomed to sailing in heavy seas.[20] One gram of ginger reduced vomiting and cold sweating. In addition, fewer symptoms of nausea and vertigo were reported. Reduced seasickness allowed them more free time to engage in useful activities, such as watching reruns of *Sea Hunt* or reading *Mutiny on the Bounty*.

A couple of studies that have been hiding in the European herbal archives and recently published show that ginger is comparable to Dramamine® in the prevention/treatment of seasickness in older children and adults and general motion sickness in younger children. In the first study, sixty passengers (ages 10 to 77 years) on a cruise ship were given either a ginger root product (Zintona®) or Dramamine ½ hour before embarking on their trip.[21] The dose of ginger was 500 milligrams; the dose of Dramamine, 100 milligrams. After the trip started, this dose could be repeated every 4 hours as needed for symptoms of motion sickness. Reduction in symptoms of motion sickness was comparable for both groups. However, fewer passengers taking ginger complained of side effects (particularly drowsiness) compared to those taking Dramamine.

The second study is a small one with children ages 4 to 8 years with a history of motion sickness due to car, air, or boat travel.[22] As was the case in the first study, children were given either the ginger rhizome product Zintona® or Dramamine 1/2 hour before travel and then every 4 hours as needed for symptoms during travel. The dose of ginger used in this study were the same for children 6 years or older and 250 milligrams for children younger than 6 years. The dose of Dramamine was 25 milligrams for all age groups. Treatment lasted for 2 days, and this time researchers found that ginger was actually superior to Dramamine for reducing symptoms of motion sickness. Apparently, one nonresponder named Linda Blair had to be kept in the ship's hold until a priest could treat her at the next port.

In another "real-life" study, over 1,700 tourists planning a whale-watching trip in Norway were talked into participating in a study comparing seven different treatments for motion sickness.[23] The Zintona ginger product again matched up favorably to Dramamine as well as some heavy hitters such as scopolamine and meclizine. The whales were particularly grateful at the reduced number of people hurling into their home waters!

A study completed at Louisiana State University (Baton Rouge, Louisiana) and funded by the National Aeronautics and Space Administration (NASA) is more skeptical.[24] Because motion sickness is common among astronauts, the researchers compared the anti–motion sickness activity of ginger and scopolamine (commonly used as a topical patch in the treatment of motion sickness). Using a more sophisticated version of the rotating chair test, they found that scopolamine was effective in reducing motion sickness, whereas 1 gram of either fresh or dried ginger was not.

I have some problems with this study. First, in their discussion of the results, the authors note that the incidence of vomiting and sweating (but not nausea and vertigo) in the ginger group decreased noticeably—so there was some clinical effect!

Second, the comparison substance, scopolamine, is a potent antinausea drug. While astronauts may require the "strong stuff," are we to believe that ginger should be written off for car sickness, sea sickness, and even air sickness in planes? The comparison doesn't seem fair.

I find that ginger works best when taken right before the planned excursion. I instruct patients to take 500 milligrams of ginger root ½ to 1 hour before their trip and then every 2 to 4 hours as needed for nausea. Judging from patient feedback, the results have been on a par with milder anti–motion sickness drugs such as Dramamine, but without drowsiness and other side effects. Ginger is a particularly good alternative for children as well as pet frogs! While I haven't developed a dose for frogs, children below the age of 6 years can use half the adult dose.

NAUSEA AND VOMITING ASSOCIATED WITH PREGNANCY

Ginger is often recommended by practitioners of herbal medicine for the morning sickness that afflicts many women during the first trimester of pregnancy. It is sometimes recommended as a tea, but capsules may work better for some women sensitive to the taste. It should only be used as needed for nausea.

This recommendation is not without controversy. The German Commission E monograph on ginger lists pregnancy as a contraindication for use of ginger.[25] However, a review of the clinical literature could not justify this warning, and there is no evidence that ginger at the low doses recommended could harm a pregnant mother or fetus.[26]

The nausea and vomiting associated with pregnancy can sometimes become much more than just morning sickness. Severe vomiting can lead to hospitalization in some cases. This condition is known as *hyperemesis gravidarum*. Fortunately, it occurs in only 0.3 percent of pregnancies.

A Danish study[27] found that 1 gram of ginger daily (in four divided doses) was extremely effective against hyperemesis gravidarum. In nineteen of twenty-seven women taking ginger, nausea and vomiting became less frequent within the first 4 days of treatment. No side effects appeared.

Ginger should be used only for short periods of time during pregnancy and should not exceed 1 gram of powder daily. Treatment of hyperemesis gravidarum should be undertaken with your doctor's or midwife's supervision.

NAUSEA AND VOMITING FOLLOWING SURGERY

Many people experience nausea and vomiting after surgery—especially when anesthesia is involved (I always thought it was the slop that passes for food in the hospital). Even with the advent of new antinausea drugs, the incidence still hovers around 30 percent. Two studies have found that ginger may be the most consistently effective and safe treatment for this condition. In the first study, the application of 1 gram of ginger before anesthesia cut the rate of postsurgical nausea and vomiting by more than half in women undergoing laparoscopic surgery.[28] Positive results were also seen in sixty women undergoing major gynecological surgery in the other study.[29]

One study found no benefits for ginger in alleviating nausea following anesthesia.[30] This study has been criticized because patients were tracked for only 3 hours following surgery as opposed to the 12 hours in the two positive studies.

If you decide to use ginger before surgery, check with your doctor first. There is concern that ginger may cause excessive bleeding. However, this effect was not reported in either of the postsurgical nausea studies.

OTHER POTENTIAL USES

As mentioned earlier, ginger possesses mild anti-inflammatory and analgesic properties. Published case reports indicate that ginger may help people with rheumatoid arthritis, osteoarthritis, and muscular pain. The daily doses employed in these reports ranged from 3 to 7 grams. The length of treatment varied from 3 months to 2.5 years. Three-quarters of the patients with arthritis enjoyed, to varying degrees, relief from pain and swelling.[31]

Ginger may also offer promise for migraine sufferers. Unfortunately, the only published paper on the topic is mostly theoretical and involves only one case study.[32] More research is needed before ginger can reach the same level of clinical assurance enjoyed by feverfew.

Finally, ginger may be a promising treatment for the nausea following chemotherapy.[33,34] However, larger studies are needed to confirm not only the effectiveness of ginger but also whether it may have any negative interactions with chemotherapeutic drugs. This is definitely one area you need to discuss with your doctor should you decide to take ginger!

How to Use Ginger

The German Commission E monograph recommends 2 to 4 grams of dried rhizome powder daily in two to three divided doses.[35] I like to be a bit more specific. For prevention/treatment of motion sickness, take 500 milligrams half to 1 hour before travel and then 500 milligrams every 2 to 4 hours as needed. Children below the age of 6 years may use half the adult dose. For treatment of nausea of pregnancy, women may use up to 1 gram daily, but they should only use ginger as needed and not on an on-going basis. Use of ginger for nausea associated with anesthesia or chemotherapy should only be done under the supervision of a physician.

Side effects are rare with ginger consumption. Some people may be sensitive to the taste and report some heartburn. The German Commission E monograph suggests that people with gallstones consult a physician before using ginger. Short-term use of ginger to treat the nausea and vomiting of pregnancy appears to pose no safety problems. Long-term use during pregnancy is not recommended.

Use ginger cautiously if you're taking anticoagulant medications (Coumadin®), antiplatelet aggregation drugs (Ticlid®), or aspirin.[36] The combination could increase your risk of spontaneous bleeding.

Related Conditions Discussed in Part 6

- Atherosclerosis
- Migraine headache
- Morning sickness associated with pregnancy
- Motion sickness
- Rheumatoid arthritis

Ginkgo biloba

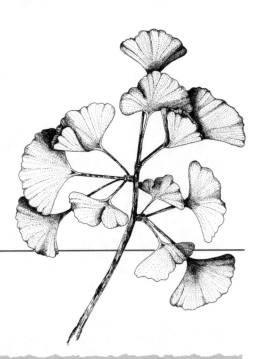

Part Used
The leaves of younger trees

Common/Potential Uses
- Age-related cognitive decline, including memory loss
- Early stages of Alzheimer's disease
- Intermittent claudication (early stage)
- Tinnitus (ringing in the ears) and hearing loss
- Impotence (erectile dysfunction)
- Raynaud's disease
- Altitude sickness

Active Constituents
Ginkgo flavone glycosides (flavonoids) and terpene lactones—ginkgolides and bilobalide

How It Works

Ginkgo extract improves cognitive function in persons with age-related cognitive decline and early-stage Alzheimer's disease. It is associated with improving concentration and focus in healthy persons, particularly those over 50 years of age. Its effect on memory in healthy younger persons is questionable. Ginkgo extract helps improve blood flow to the brain and the extremities. Ginkgo provides antioxidant for the brain, retina of the eye, and the cardiovascular system. It also exerts a protective effect on the cells of the nervous system.

Recommended Use

Standardized extract containing 24 percent ginkgo flavone glycosides and 6 percent terpene lactones—120 to 240 milligrams daily in two or three divided doses. It may take 4 to 8 weeks to notice desired effects.

Side Effects

Side effects are rare with use of the standardized extract. Mild headaches lasting for a day or two and mild gastrointestinal upset have been reported in a very small percentage of people using the standardized extract.

Safety Issues/Drug Interactions

While based on a small number of case studies in the medical literature, there is concern about the use of ginkgo with anticoagulant drugs or aspirin. If you are taking an anticoagulant medication such as Coumadin®, antiplatelet aggregation drugs such as Ticlid®, or aspirin, consult with your health care professional before starting ginkgo. There are no known contraindications to use of ginkgo during pregnancy or lactation.

It is strongly advised that those taking Ginkgo biloba *label the bottle*
"Memory Pills." There is nothing more embarrassing than looking at a bottle
of Ginkgo biloba *and thinking it's a reliquary for a Spanish explorer.*

STEVE MARTIN, *PURE DRIVEL*

FEW herbal medicines better typify the vast potential of plant medicines within the standards of modern medicine as *Ginkgo biloba.* Ginkgo is prescribed daily by thousands of doctors and used by millions of people around the world. It is one of the most commonly prescribed herbal medicines in Germany and France, where is it frequently used for age-related cognitive decline and memory loss as well as circulatory diseases such as intermittent claudication. Over 400 scientific studies have been conducted on standardized ginkgo leaf extracts over the past 30 years.[1] This impressive track record has led to success and mainstream medical interest in the United States as well. In 1998, U.S. ginkgo sales topped $150 million, placing it first on the list of best-sellers.[2] The Office of Complementary and Alternative Medicine at the National Institutes recently announced the funding of a large U.S. clinical trial to see whether ginkgo can prevent dementia in elderly persons.

PLANT FACTS

Ginkgo biloba is a living fossil (my kids will probably be using a similar label for me in a few years!). The last remaining member of the Ginkgoaceae family, its fossil records date back more than 200 million years.[3] The ginkgo tree lives as long as 1,000 years and may grow to a height of 100 to 122 feet. Because of its amazing ability to resist temperature extremes, pollution, and insects, it is commonly grown in urban centers as an ornamental tree. Occasionally referred to as the "maidenhair tree," it produces a fleshy seed that is infamous for a rather characteristic smell (stink is more like it) that may partly explain the reason people, animals, and insects avoid it during certain times of the year. Ginkgo also has characteristic fan-shaped, bilobed leaves. Modern herbal preparations (extracts) of ginkgo employ the leaves of cultivated trees grown on plantations in the United States, France, Japan, and China.

HISTORY

If I tried to cover all the details of ginkgo's history, you'd need some ginkgo just to remember half of it. Ginkgo, which originally grew in North America and Europe, was destroyed in many parts of the world during the Ice Age. It did survive in parts of Asia and was later cultivated in China as a sacred tree.

Ironically, it wasn't the leaves but the fleshy seeds that were first used medicinally. The seeds have been used in China since 2800 B.C. for a variety of ailments, including bronchial complaints. The leaves are reported to be used in present-day Chinese medicine as a dressing for wounds.[4] In 1771, the Swedish botanist Linnaeus christened the tree *Ginkgo biloba*, on the basis of an early description by Dr. Englebert Kaempfer and the bilobed structure of the leaf. Ginkgo made its grand return to America in 1784, when it was planted on the estate of William Hamilton near Philadelphia.[5]

MODERN DEVELOPMENT

The use of ginkgo leaves medicinally is a rather new event that dates back only about 40 years. Spearheaded by the Dr. Willmar Schwabe Company of Germany, pharmacological research into the active constituents and activity of ginkgo leaves began in the late 1950s. Twenty years of research resulted in a standardized, concentrated extract of ginkgo leaves known generically as EGb 761 (European trade names include Tebonin® forte and Rokan®). Using leaves from cultivated trees, the multistep extraction process takes up to 2 weeks to complete and requires approximately 50 pounds of ginkgo leaves to create 1 pound of extract. Most important, the active constituents are measured at various points throughout this process to assure an optimal product (and optimal medical benefits).[6]

Standardized *Ginkgo biloba* extracts (GBE)—especially EGb 761—are among the best-researched herbal medicines in the world, with over 100 clinical studies and several books published to date.

MEDICALLY ACTIVE CONSTITUENTS

The medical benefits of GBE rely on the proper balance of two groups of active components—the ginkgo flavone glycosides and the terpene lactones. The 24 percent ginkgo flavone glycoside designation on GBE labels indicates a carefully measured balance of bioflavonoids, including quercetin, kaempferol, and isorhamnetin. These flavonoids are primarily responsible for GBE's antioxidant activity and ability to mildly inhibit platelet aggregation ("stickiness"). These two actions may contribute to the prevention of circulatory diseases such as atherosclerosis and also GBE's benefits for the brain and central nervous system.[7]

While most plants contain flavonoids, none possess the unique terpene lactone components found in GBE. Conveniently known as *ginkgolides* and *bilobalide,* these components contribute to GBE's ability to increase circulation to the brain and other parts of the body as well as exert a protective effect on nerve cells.

Ginkgolides improve circulation and inhibit the actions of platelet-activating factor (PAF) (see the section "Nerve Protection and Platelet-Activating Factor Inhibition"). These constituents, particularly ginkgolide B, have been widely researched and compose the subject of two textbooks.[8,9]

Bilobalide protects the cells of the nervous system. Animal studies indicate that bilobalide may help regenerate damaged nerve cells.[10,11]

HOW GINKGO WORKS

EFFECTS ON CIRCULATION

Ginkgo biloba extract increases circulation—to both the brain and the extremities. In addition to inhibiting platelet stickiness, GBE regulates the tone and elasticity of blood vessels.[12] In other words, it makes circulation more efficient. This improvement in circulation efficiency extends to both the large vessels (arteries) and smaller vessels (capillaries) of the circulatory system. One study[13] dramatically illustrated increased blood flow through the capillaries: An hour after administration of GBE to healthy adults, there was a 57 percent increase in blood flow measured through the nail-fold capillaries!

This positive effect on circulation extends to the brain. *Ginkgo biloba* extract's ability to increase circulation to the brain and central nervous system (CNS) is documented[14] and has led to its use against depression and memory loss in the elderly.[15] These positive effects on circulation—to both the extremities and the CNS—have made GBE the herbal treatment of choice in both the prevention and management of circulatory disorders in the elderly.

ANTIOXIDANT PROPERTIES

As we will note throughout this book, many herbs have antioxidant capabilities. This means that, like vitamin E, selenium, and vitamin C, some herbal medicines protect parts of the body susceptible to damage by free radicals. This may help combat many age-related diseases of the CNS and cardiovascular system.[16]

Numerous studies demonstrate that GBE exerts antioxidant activity in the brain, retina, and cardiovascular system. Its antioxidant activity in the brain and CNS make it an extremely promising herbal for prevention of age-related declines in brain function.[17] It may also prove useful in the prevention and early treatment of Alzheimer's disease and strokes. *Ginkgo biloba* extract also has therapeutic potential in the prevention of eye disorders such as senile cataracts, macular degeneration, and diabetic retinopathy.[18]

Ginkgo biloba extract's antioxidant activity in the brain is of particular interest. The brain and CNS are particularly susceptible to free radical attack. Free radical damage in the brain is widely believed to be a major factor in many disorders associated with aging, including Alzheimer's disease.[19]

NERVE PROTECTION AND PLATELET-ACTIVATING FACTOR INHIBITION

The terpene lactones in GBE take center stage in nerve protection and platelet-activating factor (PAF) inhibition. At the 1992 Congress for Phytotherapy held in Munich, Germany, GBE's primary benefit to the brain was attributed to its terpene lactone constituents. Protection afforded by ginkgolides arose primarily from their ability to inhibit PAF. Three ginkgolides, A, B, and C, have demonstrated PAF inhibition, with ginkgolide B being the most active.[20]

When platelet-activating factor is released from cells, it causes platelets to aggregate (clump together). High amounts of PAF are associated with damage to nerve cells, poor blood flow to the central nervous system (CNS), inflammatory conditions, and bronchial constriction.[21] Much like the free radicals we discussed earlier, higher PAF levels are associated with increased risk of certain disease associated with aging, including cardiovascular disease and cognitive decline.[22] Thus, in addition to its antioxidant properties, GBE eases another concern of aging.

Ginkgolides A and B, as well as bilobalide, protect nerve cells in the CNS from damage during periods of ischemia (lack of blood flow, and thus oxygen, to body tissues).[23] This quality makes GBE a potentially useful consideration for people who have suffered a stroke. In 1997, I was invited to give scientific lectures on ginkgo in China (kind of like a Beatles cover group playing in Liverpool!). I was amazed at the wide use of GBE for stroke patients among Chinese neurologists. It should also be considered in the treatment of transient ischemic attacks (TIAs), which can be a warning sign of an impending stroke.

The combined actions of GBE on the CNS may also hold promise for persons recovering from brain trauma and injury.[24]

MEMORY IMPROVEMENT AND COGNITIVE ACTIVATION

Having been bombarded with television ads promising better memory for anyone using GBE, I'm sure you'd like to know what to expect when you pop those ginkgo tablets. As we'll note later, the large majority of evidence of GBE's success in improving memory has been with elderly patients with age-related cognitive decline (sometimes called *mild cognitive impairment*) or mild to moderate Alzheimer's disease. Remember that the term *cognition* is used to describe not just memory but also awareness with perception, reasoning, and intuition.

While I have been resistant to these ads because of a lack of studies looking at GBE's effect on the memory of healthy people, a recent study may provide some support for the memory claims. In a study with healthy adults, ages 30 to 59 years, GBE effect on memory and other measures of cognition was measured.[25] Using doses of GBE ranging from 50 to 100 milligrams three times daily to 120 or 240 milligrams all at one time, the study found that GBE was, in fact, useful for improving memory. However, the effect was most notable for persons taking the 120-milligram dose and in those participants over 50 years of age.

Notable in the past few years have been studies showing that GBE does directly affect brain wave activity, resulting in improved cognitive abilities. Two studies with healthy volunteers found that single doses of either 120 or 240 milligrams of EGb 761 increase active brain wave (alpha wave and certain beta waves) activity in the brain while decreasing the amount of slow wave (theta wave) activity.[26,27] This effect was typically noticed within 30 minutes of taking EGb 761, and there was a notable continuation of effect over a 5-day period. Another study, which is unpublished, also noted improved concentration and focus in college students taking EGb 761—particularly as the day wore on and the ol' afternoon slump was expected.[28]

These direct cognitive activating effects for EGb 761 were also shown in a study with persons with mild to moderate Alzheimer's disease.[29] The small study found comparable effects on brain wave activity for both EGb 761 and tacrine hydrochloride (Cognex®). In this study, the higher dose of 240 milligrams of EGb 761 was used. These results are important for Alzheimer's disease and other forms of dementia. One of the hallmark changes in the brains of these patients is a relative increase of slow (theta) wave activity and decrease in the brain waves associated with alertness, focus, and mental sharpness.

Health Care Applications

Age-Related Cognitive Decline

While most of use would probably be less anxious about a little down-swing in our memory if those damn ginkgo ads didn't keep reminding us, some people experience a decrease in their quality of life as their mental sharpness begins to wane. Elderly persons who begin to have consistent impairment of cognitive function and memory that begins to impact their daily lives are often diagnosed as having mild cognitive impairment (I'm calling it *age-related cognitive decline* for ease of description).

GBE has become the herbal treatment of choice for this condition. Studies completed in Europe during the 1980s and early 1990s found that GBE improved memory and overall cognitive function in persons with age-related cognitive decline.[30,31] Most of these studies found success using 120 to 160 milligrams of GBE daily, and most commonly used either the EGb 761 extract described earlier or LI 1370 (Lichtwer Pharma, Berlin).

One study looked at the effects of GBE on patients ages 62 to 85 years with age-related cognitive decline.[32] Participants in the study received either 120 milligrams of EGB 761 daily or placebo for 12 weeks. At the end of 12 weeks, the participants taking EGb 761 showed a significant improvement in cognitive function. Greatly improved reaction times were noted in as early as 4 weeks for the group taking EGb 761.

Two studies using 160 milligrams of EGb 761 daily for 12 to 24 weeks found similar improvements in persons with age-related cognitive decline.[33,34] Side effects were few and those noted mild in both studies. Success was also shown in one study using 150 milligrams of LI 1370 daily for 12 weeks in a similar population.[35] Another study comparing either 120 or 240 milligrams of LI 1370 daily to placebo found that the 120-milligram dose worked best.[36]

Alzheimer's Disease

Momentum has been gathering in the last few years for GBE's potential role in the management of Alzheimer's disease (AD). Studies using the

EGb 761 extract at daily doses ranging from 120 to 240 milligrams for 3 to 12 months have suggested the extract may slow the progression of the disease and improve quality of life in persons with mild to moderate AD.[37]

In 1997, a U.S. study using EGb 761 was published in the prestigious *Journal of the American Medical Association*[38] and catapulted the extract into the awareness of the mainstream medical community in this country. The study enrolled 327 patients 45 years or older with a diagnosis of either AD or another type of dementia known as *multi-infarct dementia.* Patients were assigned to receive either 120 milligrams of EGb 761 or placebo daily for 1 year. While there was a large dropout rate in both groups, analysis of results at the end of 1 year indicated that the use of ginkgo slowed progression of AD and, in many cases, improved quality of life. According to a rating by significant others and caregivers, the patients taking EGb 761 improved slightly as opposed to the expected worsening in those taking placebo. Side effects were few in those taking EGb 761 and consisted mostly of mild gastrointestinal complaints. In an editorial, *JAMA* senior editor Margaret Winkler, M.D., stated that "this agent [EGb 761] is an intriguing addition to the drugs thought to be helpful for patients with AD."[39]

While the U.S. study found success using 120 milligrams of EGb 761 daily, studies out of Europe are suggesting that 240 milligrams of the extract may be the better choice for treating mild to moderate Alzheimer's disease. A 6-month study with 222 patients with either mild to moderate AD or multi-infarct dementia found that 240 milligrams of EGb 761 daily (120 milligrams twice daily) was a safe and effective treatment for AD.[40] In the patients taking EGb 761 who completed the study, significant improvements in cognitive function were noted.

These results have been echoed by two smaller 3-month studies using 240 milligrams of EGb 761 daily.[41,42] GBE's and especially EGb 761's promise for the treatment of AD should stimulate future studies that compare different dosages to arrive at a safe and effective dose. Larger clinical trials are needed to fully understand the potential effectiveness and safety of GBE for the long-term treatment of AD. In the meantime, if you have a loved one with AD, work with your doctor to explore treatment options and be sure that GBE is one that is explored.

RESISTANT DEPRESSION AND SSRI SEXUAL SIDE EFFECTS

Another thing I love about modern medical diagnosis is the labeling of someone as "resistant" when drug therapy fails. Such is the case with many elderly individuals who are being pumped full of antidepressants when, in fact, they aren't getting sufficient blood flow to their brain. Reduction in blood flow to the brain has been found in one study with depressed individuals over the age of 50 years.[43]

Using a daily dose of 240 milligrams of GBE, one study[44] found success in reversing depression among elderly patients who weren't responding to prescription antidepressants. The researchers simply added GBE to the daily regimen of the patients. Significant differences in mood, motivation, and memory were noted after only 4 weeks! The results were even more notable at the end of the 8-week study.

While not responding to antidepressants is a drag, many people taking the new generation of antidepressants known as selective serotonin–reuptake inhibitors (SSRIs) may experience sexual side effects including loss of libido, reduced sensation in the vagina and clitoris, and erectile dysfunction. The SSRIs include commonly prescribed drugs such as Prozac® and Zoloft®. Case reports are beginning to trickle in from doctors who have found success in treating these side effects with GBE.

One report found that doses of GBE up to 240 milligrams daily reduced sexual dysfunction in elderly patients taking SSRIs.[45] The results were noted in both men and women. The second report found success using GBE (180 to 240 milligrams daily) for treating diminished arousal, sexual desire, and altered sensation in the vagina, vulva, and clitoris in a 37-year-old woman taking Prozac.[46]

Reminder: St. John's wort extract (see the chapter in Part 5) may be as effective as SSRIs in treating mild to moderate depression and is not associated with the sexual side effects sometime seen with these drugs.

INTERMITTENT CLAUDICATION

Ginkgo biloba extract is also a leading treatment consideration for intermittent claudication. The condition, which involves severe cramping and pain in the lower legs during walking or exercise, affects primarily the elderly population. It is frequently debilitating and can severely curtail physical activity. Intermittent claudication is more common in persons with atherosclerosis and is also seen frequently in smokers and diabetics (see "Cardiovascular System" in Part 6).

Earlier clinical studies found that 120 to 160 milligrams of GBE daily for 3 to 6 months is successful in the treatment of early-stage intermittent claudication.[47] In these studies, people using GBE typically experienced an increase in pain-free walking distance and an increase in blood flow to the affected leg(s) after about 4 to 8 weeks of treatment, and continued to improve as the study progressed.

A more recent study with 60 patients with intermittent claudication[48] and another with 111 patients[49] both found that the use of 120 milligrams daily of EGb 761 for 6 months resulted in very impressive results. In both studies, pain-free walking distance and maximum walking distance were significantly improved at the 8-week evaluation period. This improvement increased as the study went on, suggesting that ongoing use of GBE is probably best for persons with intermittent claudication.

While the 120-milligram dose may work for many people with intermittent claudication, a new study suggests that 240 milligrams daily may work even better in some cases.[50] In a 6-week study, 74 patients with intermittent claudication were given either 120 or 240 milligrams of EGb 761 daily. At the end of the study, both groups showed improvement when compared to their pain-free and maximum walking distance at the beginning of the study. However, when compared to those taking the lower dose, the group using 240 milligrams of EGb 761 had a far better increase in pain-free and maximum walking distance.

Those of you with intermittent claudication should work closely with your doctor to determine which dose is optimal for you. Remember, it may take a few weeks to notice results, so be patient.

OTHER POTENTIAL USES

According to some studies, GBE may help improve some cases of tinnitus (ringing in the ears) as well as vertigo. The results with tinnitus have been mixed. Studies using 120 milligrams of EGb 761 daily have found some success in treating tinnitus for up to 12 weeks.[51,52] Another study using another ginkgo extract at a much lower dose (29.2 milligrams) did not find success in treating tinnitus.[53]

GBE may prove to be a safe and effective alternative to Viagra® for some men experiencing erectile dysfunction (ED). While more studies are needed before we can get Bob Dole to start doing ginkgo ads for ED, a 9-month study found that 240 milligrams of EGb 761 daily was effective for treating men with ED—particularly those who had been previously responsive to penile injections (ouch!) of drugs such as papaverine and phentolomine.[54] I've had a few patients ask if the GBE helps them get an erection, will it also help them remember how to use it? That's one for the marriage counselor, guys!

Other potential uses for GBE include early-stage macular degeneration, early-stage diabetic retinopathy, Raynaud's disease, and even asthma. For you mountain climbers, one study found that the use of 160 milligrams of EGb 761 essentially eliminated symptoms of altitude sickness in climbers attempting to scale some pretty high peaks in the Himalayas.[55] The EGb 761 also helped reduce cold-related circulatory problems.

How to Use Ginkgo

Choose a GBE standardized to contain 6 percent terpene lactones and 24 percent ginkgo flavone glycosides. My preference is one of the products containing the EGb 761 extract (discussed later). The recommended daily dose is 120 to 240 milligrams in two or three divided doses. I usually recommend an initial 6- to 8-week period to ascertain the effectiveness of GBE.

Ginkgo biloba extract is essentially devoid of any serious side effects. In about 1 to 2 percent of persons studied,[56] use of GBE resulted in mild gastrointestinal upset and a mild transient headache lasting a couple of days. In my experience, the headache will typically resolve within 24 to 48 hours. I have had a couple of patients report dizziness after taking ginkgo. In these cases, it's best to start at a lower dose and build your way up to the higher dose over a period of a few weeks.

The current German Commission E monograph lists no contraindications to the use of GBE by pregnant and lactating women.[57] While I don't know whether many healthy, pregnant women would need ginkgo, those of you in you last trimester that forget why you've got that rather large protuberance in the abdominal area may want to think about a couple of weeks of ginkgo! If you do need the memory boost, be sure to stop ginkgo at least 2 or 3 weeks before the scheduled date of birth.

A great deal of publicity has occurred over the past few years in both the medical and mainstream press about ginkgo's potential to possibly contribute to bleeding. This discussion has been based on two cases of bleeding in persons taking an anticoagulant drug (Coumadin®) or aspirin together with ginkgo[58,59] and two cases in persons taking ginkgo alone.[60,61] While I feel that ginkgo is a healthier insurance policy for the cardiovascular system when compared to aspirin (which many people are using to prevent heart disease and strokes), it's wise to consult with your doctor before choosing to take ginkgo if you're already taking anticoagulant drugs such as Coumadin®, antiplatelet aggregation drugs such as Ticlid®, or aspirin. Also, discuss your use of ginkgo with your doctor if you're scheduled for surgery. It's probably best to stop ginkgo 2 or 3 weeks before surgery.

Hopefully, future studies will help clear the air about ginkgo's effect on bleeding. In the meantime, remember that millions of people to date have used ginkgo safely and that the ginkgo warnings are based on only a handful of case studies that have not definitively proven but only suggested that ginkgo may interact with aspirin or anticoagulant drugs.

It is important to remember that cognitive decline and circulatory conditions in the elderly can involve serious disease. Seek proper medical care and accurate medical diagnosis prior to self-prescribing GBE or other herbal medications

Product update: The EGb 761 extract made by the Dr. Willmar Schwabe company (Karlsruhe, Germany) is used in the following U.S. products: Ginkgold® (Nature's Way) and Ginkoba® (Pharmaton). The LI 1370 extract is sold in the United States as Ginkai® by Lichtwer Pharma.

RELATED CONDITIONS DISCUSSED IN PART 6

- Age-related cognitive decline and early-stage Alzheimer's disease
- Asthma
- Atherosclerosis
- Depression
- Neuropathy (diabetic)
- Diabetic retinopathy
- Impotence
- Intermittent claudication
- Macular degeneration
- Migraine headache
- Raynaud's disease
- Tinnitus
- Uveitis

Asian Ginseng

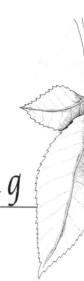

Panax ginseng C.A. Meyer

Part Used
The root

Common/Potential Uses
- Revitalizes those experiencing fatigue and debility with declining concentration and physical endurance
- Supports the hypothalamic-pituitary-adrenal axis of those under stress
- Assists in recovery following surgery or a long convalescence
- May help regulate blood sugar in persons with adult-onset (type II) diabetes
- Supports those undergoing radiation or chemotherapy
- Forms part of the training/recovery program for endurance athletes and body builders
- May help treat male infertility

Active Constituents
Asian ginseng is a complex mixture of many different constituents; the most important, according to research, are the ginsenosides.

How It Works

Ginseng is notable for its ability to support and enhance the normal function of the hypothalamic-pituitary-adrenal axis. This allows for a better overall reaction to stress and possibly more consistent physical and mental energy. Ginseng may sharpen mental acuity and concentration. It maximizes the use of oxygen and glycogen by working muscles, allowing them to function in an aerobic state for longer periods of time and to recover from exercise more efficiently. Ginseng also helps the body regulate blood sugar more effectively.

Recommended Use

The best-researched form of ginseng is extracts supplying 5 to 7 percent ginsenosides. The recommended dosage is 100 milligrams once or twice daily. Crude, nonstandardized extracts require a higher daily dose of 1 to 2 grams. Ginseng is usually used for 2 to 3 weeks continuously, followed by a 1- to 2-week "rest" period before resuming.

Side Effects

Used at the recommended dosage, ginseng is generally safe. In rare instances, it may cause overstimulation and possibly insomnia. Consuming caffeine with ginseng boosts the risk of experiencing overstimulation and gastrointestinal upset. People with uncontrolled high blood pressure should use ginseng with caution.

Safety Issues/Drug Interactions

Long-term use of ginseng may cause menstrual abnormalities and breast tenderness in some women. Ginseng is not recommended for pregnant or lactating women. It may reduce the effectiveness of anticoagulant medications such as warfarin (Coumadin®).

ASIAN ginseng is among the most popular herbal medicines worldwide. Used for centuries in the Orient as a "tonic" herb, it is the perfect embodiment of an herbal adaptogen (see the discussion in Part 4). Hundreds of studies have confirmed its benefit to a variety of body systems. These effects on the body include increased energy, mental alertness, and physical endurance. Along with eleuthero (Siberian ginseng), it offers long-term support of hypothalamic-pituitary-adrenal axis function—a major regulator of our stress response. With antioxidant nutrients and herbal medicines such as ginkgo, it is also a premier "anti-aging" compound.

PLANT FACTS

Asian ginseng is a member of the Araliaceae family, which also includes American ginseng (*Panax quinquefolius*) and Siberian ginseng (*Eleutherococcus senticosus*). It is a perennial herb that reaches heights of 2 feet and produces pale yellowish-green flowers that give way to small, red, berrylike fruit. Because of its long taproots, the harvested root has a look suggestive of a human form.[1]

Asian ginseng commonly grows on mountain slopes in the northeastern provinces of China, adjacent Korea, and also Russia. Ginseng is usually harvested in the fall after the 5th year of growth, when the active ginsenosides are most highly concentrated.[2]

The sheer number of products manufactured from the root of Asian ginseng has led to some confusion; a good example is "white" versus "red" ginseng. There's actually nothing mystical about either. White ginseng is simply the dried, unprocessed root or root powder. Red ginseng is created when the root is steamed for a period of several hours and then dried over a low fire or in the sun. Some sources cite mild differences between the two, the most notable being the slightly greater antioxidant activity attributed to the red version.[3]

In Asia, wild-harvested ginseng is revered—and rare. Take a walk through an Asian herb shop some time and price wild ginseng root. In Hong Kong, the mecca of ginseng trade, a wild-harvested root has been known to sell for as much as $20,000!

HISTORY

Asian ginseng has been a part of Chinese medicine for more than 2,000 years. I defer to my friend Steven Foster when it comes to accurate and heart-felt history. I highly recommend his book (cowritten with Yue Chongxi) *Herbal Emissaries: Bringing Chinese Herbs to the West*. The book, which offers a concise and understandable guide to Chinese herbal medicines, explores ginseng's long and illustrious history in the Orient.

The first reference to Asian ginseng is found in the *Shen Nong Ben Cao Jing*, written around the first century A.D. This work is thought to be the earliest listing of traditional Chinese medicines. S. Y. Hu, in her translation of the text, states that "it is used for repairing the five viscera, quieting the spirit, curbing the emotion, stopping agitation, removing noxious influence, brightening the eyes, enlightening the mind and increasing wisdom. Continuous use leads one to longevity with light weight."[4]

Ginseng acquired the status of "superior" in the Chinese classification of herbs. Reference to ginseng's medical use is listed in the classic Chinese materia medica, *Ben Cao Gang Mu*, written in 1596 by Li Shizhen. Small amounts were noted for improving vitality and again for keeping one slim and trim.[5] Ginseng was commonly used by elderly persons in the Orient to enhance energy and improve memory.

Petrus Jartoux, a Jesuit missionary, is credited with the introduction of Asian ginseng to the West. In 1711, his observations of the plant and its use in China were published.

MODERN DEVELOPMENT

Since the 1940s, ginseng has been one of the most highly researched herbs in the world. Hundreds of scientific studies have attempted to discover what makes this ancient tonic work and what effect it has on the body. Foster and Chongxi have the following to say about the approach to ginseng research in Asia: "Chinese researchers, as is the case with medicinal plants in general, have focused on how ginseng works, whereas Western researchers focus on if it works. This reflects a fundamental difference between the East and West. In Asia, the efficacy of an herb is already established in a cultural context. In the West, we presuppose that traditional or folk uses have no rational scientific basis."[6]

Ginseng's actions make it applicable to treating a vast array of conditions and also optimizing health. Modern research shows that ginseng protects the body from a wide range of harmful influences, including pollution, radiation, and even alcohol. Ginseng protects nerve cells, mildly lowers cholesterol, and is an antioxidant.[7] Its antifatigue and endurance-enhancing actions make it a favorite supplement for athletes.

MEDICALLY ACTIVE CONSTITUENTS

Ginseng's actions in the body are due to a complex interplay of constituents. The primary group consists of ginsenosides. Thirteen ginsenosides have been identified in Asian ginseng. Ginsenosides Rg1 and Rb1 have received the most attention.[8]

The interaction of Rg1 and Rb1 offers a glimpse of the unique synergism that exists among the constituents in ginseng. Rg1 mildly stimulates brain and central nervous system activity. It increases energy, counters fatigue, and enhances intellectual and physical performance.

Rb1, on the other hand, relaxes the activity of the brain and is associated with lowering blood pressure.[9] This balancing effect allows ginseng to adjust various body functions and encourage their return to a healthy, normal function.

Other components beside ginsenosides are also important. A group of constituents known as panaxans help lower blood sugar. Polysaccharides (complex sugar molecules) support immune function.[10]

HOW GINSENG WORKS AND HEALTH CARE APPLICATIONS

Ginseng is the granddaddy of adaptogenic herbs. I. I. Brekhman, the Russian researcher responsible for coining the umbrella term *adaptogen* to describe certain herbs, began with ginseng as his original model (see Part 4 for more information on adaptogens).[11]

Ginseng and other adaptogens work on the premise that the body is in a state of dynamic flux. Wellness depends on the balanced functioning of a number of control centers in the body, including the nervous and endocrine systems. Optimal health depends on keeping these systems in balance.

That's why I've combined the "How It Works" and "Health Care Applications" sections in this chapter, unlike for the other herbs; breaking down ginseng's potential health care applications into nice, convenient categories is difficult because of ginseng's multifaceted actions in the body. *Some* of ginseng's potential uses are as follows:

- Chronic fatigue immunodeficiency syndrome
- Mental and physical fatigue
- Memory loss in the elderly
- Diabetes
- Prevention of atherosclerosis
- Cancer prevention
- Immune system enhancement
- Drug and alcohol withdrawal
- Adjunctive use during radiation or chemotherapy

Another reason that it is hard to categorize ginseng is because of the way its effects overlap: antifatigue, improved mental activity, antioxidant activity, and improved cholesterol metabolism are all important considerations for optimizing health.

ANTIFATIGUE/ANTISTRESS ACTIONS

Most of my patients with chronic fatigue have run-down adrenal glands. The adrenals, which sit atop your kidneys, resemble rechargeable batteries. Highly efficient at helping our bodies react and adapt to stressful situations, the adrenals can become run down if the body is constantly stressed. This stress can come from the daily commute on the Nimitz Freeway, working for Prima Publishing and dealing with authors like me, or chronic illness.

Ginseng supports the adrenals through a unique action. Instead of directly stimulating adrenal action, ginseng influences the control centers that regulate adrenal function—the hypothalamus and pituitary.[12] In traditional Chinese medicine, the hypothalamic–pituitary–adrenal (HPA) axis is not thought of as three separately functioning entities, but rather as one cohesive unit. Ginseng treats the unit as a whole.[13]

This model of indirect support of adrenal function helps us understand ginseng's antifatigue actions. By supporting the function of the HPA axis, ginseng allows the body to adapt more efficiently to stress and thus ease the burden on other systems in the body, including the heart and brain.[14] It also aids in the recovery of physical and mental balance following stress.

One double-blind, placebo-controlled study with 230 people measured the effects of ginseng on general fatigue associated with daily living ("functional fatigue").[15] Compared to the placebo group, persons taking 80 milligrams of the standardized ginseng extract G 115, together with nutrients such as vitamins A, E, C, B_1, B_2, B_6, B_{12}, and manganese, had a significant decrease in reports of fatigue after 42 days of supplementation.

ENHANCED MENTAL PERFORMANCE

Ginseng improves and sharpens mental concentration and performance. One of my favorite nonhuman studies exploring ginseng's effect on memory is a Bulgarian study with rats.[16] According to this study, rats given ginseng showed improved learning and memory. This was in contrast to rats receiving no ginseng. How did they decide the ginseng-taking rats were smarter? My personal image is of the ginseng rats huddled together over afternoon cocktails discussing the works of Sartre while the other rats are drinking Bud Lite and watching arena football!

Human studies show that ginseng improves attention, performance, and memory. One test with sixteen volunteers who took ginseng showed improvement on a wide battery of tests, including arithmetic.[17] Another study found that concentration and performance improved in radio operators and proofreaders taking ginseng.[18]

Ginseng is commonly used in Asia by older individuals showing signs of memory loss. While not as thoroughly researched as ginkgo for this condition, studies have shown that ginseng effectively improves memory and also counters depression in the elderly.[19] Some European phytomedicine supplements have begun to combine ginseng and ginkgo. One study with 64 volunteers ages 42 to 65 years of age found that a combination of

100 milligrams of a standardized ginseng extract (G 115) and 60 milligrams of a standardized ginkgo extract taken twice daily improved memory following the morning dose but not the afternoon dose.[20] After 3 months of use, volunteers reported improved well-being and were able to exercise longer. My guess is that the improvements in memory are most likely due to the ginkgo and the improved physical performance due to the ginseng. This intriguing combination should be the focus of more studies looking at the potential synergy of these herbs for antiaging.

Enhanced Physical Performance

A favorite among endurance athletes and body builders, ginseng may increase physical endurance and speed up recovery time following a workout.[21] Ginseng also builds muscle mass in body builders without the side effects associated with steroids.[22]

Ginseng may improve athletic performance through a number of related actions. First, it may increase the uptake of oxygen by the body.[23] It also lowers the maximum exercise heart rate—an indication that the work load on the heart during exercise is less than before treatment. Last, and perhaps most notable, it enables exercising muscles to maintain glycogen stores more efficiently.[24] Glycogen, a type of sugar, is the primary source of fuel to the exercising muscle. With ginseng use, muscles may stay in an aerobic (nonexhausted) state longer before reaching exhaustion.

Unfortunately, this was not found in a more recent study examining the effects of ginseng on athletic performance. In a study with young males and females not athletically trained, the addition of 200 milligrams per day of ginseng extract led to a small increase in maximal exercising capacity but did not affect endurance overall.[25] This study, as well as those showing a positive effect, has been criticized for poor research design. Clearly, more studies are needed to sort out the value of ginseng for athletic performance.

Effects on Male Fertility

While not exactly a subset of enhanced physical performance, ginseng has been used historically to treat impotence in men and improve sexual drive. There are no modern clinical studies to support this use. However, a study published in 1996 suggests that ginseng may improve sperm count and sperm motility in men with infertility (medically referred to as *oligoasthenospermia*).[26] Supplementation with 4 grams of ginseng daily for 3 months led to an improvement in sperm count, sperm motility, and a rise in serum testosterone levels. It's intriguing to consider the use of ginseng with nutrient shown to improve motility such as L-carnitine and acetyl-L-carnitine as well as antioxidant nutrients (e.g., vitamin E, zinc, vitamin C) shown to enhance sperm health. Used together, men with infertility may join Kramer from *Seinfeld* in declaring, "My boys are swimmers!"

EFFECTS ON BLOOD SUGAR

Ginseng is commonly used in traditional Chinese medicine to treat diabetes. Animal studies show that ginseng enhances the release of insulin from the pancreas and increases the number of insulin receptors.[27] It also has a direct blood sugar–lowering (hypoglycemic) effect.[28, 29]

A double-blind, placebo-controlled clinical study found that 200 milligrams of a ginseng extract daily led to improved blood sugar control and improved energy in adults with a recent diagnosis of diabetes (adult-onset diabetes).[30] The study lasted 8 weeks, and no adverse effects were reported in the persons taking ginseng. Unfortunately, the study is unclear as to what type of ginseng was used.

ANTITOXIN AND ANTIOXIDANT ACTIONS

Ginseng helps remove harmful chemicals and toxins from the body. Ginseng also protects cells from the damaging effects of radiation, including workplace sources and radiation from medical treatment.[31]

An intriguing area of application for ginseng is in drug withdrawal programs. A study with mice indicates that ginseng significantly inhibits morphine dependence.[32] This effect could make ginseng useful for persons trying to withdraw from morphine or similar pain medications.

Ginseng also fights the damaging activity of free radicals in the body.[33] Its antioxidant activities help protect the cardiovascular system, liver, and lungs.[34]

CHOLESTEROL-LOWERING EFFECTS

Ginseng helps the body metabolize and break down cholesterol more efficiently. It mildly reduces total cholesterol and triglycerides while raising the levels of the "good" high-density lipoprotein (HDL) cholesterol. Ginseng also reduces platelet stickiness.[35] High levels of HDL cholesterol and decreased aggregation of platelets are actions that lower the risk of atherosclerosis and cardiovascular disease. While ginseng shouldn't be thought of as a primary treatment for high cholesterol or triglycerides, it may help reduce risk of atherosclerosis.

ANTICANCER AND IMMUNE SYSTEM–SUPPORTING ACTIONS

Imagine feeling more energetic and reducing your risk of cancer, too—where do I sign up? A Korean study[36] indicates that regular intake of ginseng may also reduce the risk of cancer. A survey of more than 1,800 patients at a hospital in Seoul found that people without cancer were more likely to consume ginseng regularly compared to those who had developed cancer. The protective effect applied to men and women equally.

A more detailed and larger follow-up study in Korea found similar results.[37] A total of 4,587 men and women were interviewed about their intake of ginseng intake and then followed for 5 years. Consumption of Asian ginseng was associated with a 60 percent reduction in the risk of dying from any form of cancer! The risk of both gastric and lung cancers were reduced by 67 percent and 70 percent, respectively. The amount consumed made a difference. Persons consuming ginseng more than once a month had a 66 percent overall reduction in cancer risk versus a 54 percent risk reduction in those consuming ginseng less than three times per year.

Animal studies show that ginseng and some of its constituents inhibit the growth of ovarian cancer cells, lung tumors, and liver tumors (treatment of the latter included a chemotherapeutic drug).[38,39] These results have not been tested in humans.

Evidence is mounting that ginseng's anticancer activity stems from immune system support.[40] Ginseng increases the levels of T lymphocytes and natural killer cells, two key components of the immune system's ability to combat viral infections. Particularly noteworthy is ginseng's ability to raise the levels of helper T lymphocytes (also known as *CD4 cells*) and influence the ratio of these cells to suppressor T lymphocytes (also known as *CD8 cells*).[41] Fewer CD4 cells and a decreased CD4/CD8 ratio are features of human immunodeficiency virus (HIV) infection and progression to acquired immunodeficiency syndrome (AIDS). Low natural killer cell activity is common among people with chronic fatigue immunodeficiency syndrome.

This evidence points to using ginseng as a supportive supplement for cancer patients. Much like astragalus and eleuthero (Siberian ginseng), it supports immune function and also helps the bone marrow bounce back and begin producing white blood cells following chemotherapy. This may be helpful for those undergoing treatment for cancer. I lean toward using eleuthero and astragalus for HIV infection, because of the greater research and clinical evidence for these adaptogens.

Finally, ginseng may enhance the effect of flu vaccines. One study with 227 people receiving an influenza vaccine found that the addition of 200 milligrams of a standardized ginseng extract (G 115) for 4 weeks before the vaccination and 8 weeks after significantly reduced the incidence of both colds and flu and improved the activity of the immune system when compared to persons getting just the vaccine.[42]

HOW TO USE GINSENG

Most modern research has been expended on ginseng extracts that supply 5 to 7 percent ginsenosides. The recommended dosage is 100 milligrams once or twice daily. Crude, nonstandardized extracts require a higher daily dose of 1 to 2 grams. I am not a fan of highly extracted ginseng products. Products containing ginsenoside concentrations that exceed 7 percent often lack other important constituents that contribute to immune support and regulation of blood sugar.

Be sure to buy your ginseng supplement from a reputable company. Studies carried out in the United States and Sweden have found dizzying variance in the levels of ginsenosides in both Asian and American ginseng products.[43] Some of this has to do with incorrectly listing the plant as

Panax ginseng when it was actually eleuthero or other unrelated plants. The American Botanical Council is currently wrapping up a detailed study of the quality of various ginseng products in North America, including Asian, American, and Siberian (eleuthero). These results should cast more light on who's giving us the goods!

Use ginseng for 2 to 3 weeks without interruption, followed by a 1- to 2-week "rest" period before resuming. At the recommended dosage, ginseng is generally safe. In rare instances, it may cause overstimulation and possibly insomnia. Consuming caffeine with ginseng, particularly on an empty stomach, increases the possibility of overstimulation and gastrointestinal upset. People with uncontrolled high blood pressure should not use ginseng.

In 1979, the *Journal of the American Medical Association* published a report citing a "ginseng abuse syndrome" caused by long-term consumption of ginseng. Symptoms included high blood pressure, nervousness, insomnia, and morning diarrhea.[44] This report has largely been discredited, because it did not provide information on what type of ginseng was being ingested; furthermore, the amounts of ginseng being consumed (more than 15 grams per day) greatly exceeded what is recommended.[45]

Contrary to the German Commission E monograph on ginseng,[46] I do not recommend its use during pregnancy or lactation. I also urge women of menstruating age to use ginseng with caution, because abnormal periods and cyclical breast pain may occur. Eleuthero (Siberian ginseng) is a good alternative. On the other hand, menopausal women may benefit by adding ginseng to their supplement regimen.

If you are taking warfarin or another anticoagulant medication, it's good to be aware that ginseng may reduce the effectiveness of the drug.[47] Although this has only been reported in one case, it's best to discuss the use of ginseng with your doctor if you're taking an anticoagulant drug. Ginseng was also associated with an increase in vaginal bleeding in two women.[48,49] This may be due to a mild estrogenic effect.

Product update: The G 115 extract produced by Pharmaton is sold in the United States as Ginsana®.

Related Conditions Discussed in Part 6

- Alzheimer's disease
- Atherosclerosis
- Chronic fatigue immunodeficiency syndrome
- Diabetes
- Impotence
- Male Infertility
- Stress and fatigue

Hawthorn

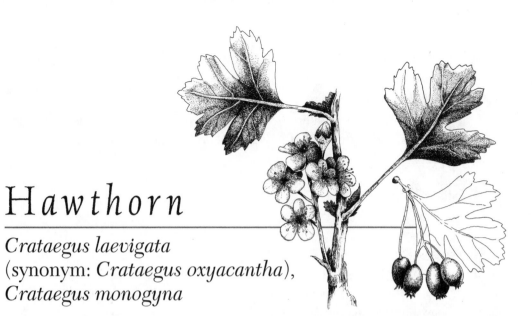

Crataegus laevigata
(synonym: *Crataegus oxyacantha*),
Crataegus monogyna

Parts Used

Modern European extracts use the leaves and flowers. Traditional preparations use the dried fruit.

Common/Potential Uses

- Early stages of congestive heart failure
- Stable angina pectoris
- Long-term recovery from a heart attack

Active Constituents

Oligomeric procyanidins and other flavonoids

How It Works

Hawthorn extract improves the efficiency of the heart by increasing blood supply to the heart muscle. As a result, the heart is able to pump more blood to the body. Hawthorn also lowers the resistance to blood flow in the peripheral vessels.

Hawthorn extracts standardized on total flavonoid (2.2 percent) or oligomeric procyanidin (18.75 percent) content—160 to 900 milligrams daily in two or three divided doses. Traditional berry preparations—4 to 5 grams daily.

Side Effects

None are currently known

Safety Issues/Drug Interactions

There are no documented interactions with other cardiac medications. European monographs list no contraindication to the use of hawthorn during pregnancy or lactation.

WHEN one considers the dizzying array of heart drugs and their potential side effects, the need for gentler and less toxic therapies is obvious. Hawthorn, particularly extracts made from the leaves and flowers, exerts a gentle, measured effect on the heart and circulation, making it useful as an initial therapy for persons with weakened heart function. It is especially useful for early-stage congestive heart failure, particularly before stronger drugs such as digitalis are required.

This represents a rational approach to cardiovascular disease that we need to incorporate into our health care system. Using hawthorn not only gives the heart a fighting chance at some recovery, it may also slow progression of heart disease. As is true with other herbs that slow disease progression, this also equates to incredible savings in medical costs!

PLANT FACTS

Hawthorn is a small, shrublike tree with sharp thorns, often found in woodlands. It is a member of the Rosaceae family. Hawthorn is the popular name given to the plant genus *Crataegus,* which includes more than 100 species. *Crataegus* species are commonly found in Europe, western Asia, and North Africa. The two species most frequently used for medicinal purposes in Europe are *Crataegus laevigata* (often referred to as *Crataegus oxyacantha*) and *Crataegus monogyna*.[1]

Hawthorn has small white or pink flowers that develop a bright, red fruit. Until recently, herbal preparations were made largely from the fruit. In the past decade, standardized extracts from Europe have used primarily the leaves and flowers.[2] These portions of the plant are higher in medically active constituents.

HISTORY

That wild and crazy Greek herbalist, Dioscorides, was using hawthorn medicinally in the first century A.D. Otherwise, the early literature on hawthorn centers on the religious and political symbolism attributed to the plant and details little about its medicinal benefits.

Early medical uses attributed to the plant weren't exactly narrow in scope. Everything from stomach ailments to dropsy were mentioned. Throughout history, however, the heart continued to be the target of use. In *A Modern Herbal*, Grieve mentions the use of the dried fruits (known as "haws") as a tonic for chronic heart ailments.[3]

MODERN DEVELOPMENT

Modern herbal development of hawthorn extracts began with the discovery of certain compounds in the leaves, flowers, and berries that were responsible for the cardiac actions attributed to the plant. Among these was a flavonoid-like complex of oligomeric procyanidins as well as other compounds including the flavonoids vitexin, vitexin 4'-O-rhamnoside, quercetin, rutin, and hyperoside.[4]

The leaves and flowers appear to contain concentrated amounts of these constituents, especially the oligomeric procyanidins.[5] The action of these compounds on the cardiovascular system has led to the development of European hawthorn extracts, which are widely used in general medical and cardiology practices.[6]

How Hawthorn Works

The actions of hawthorn extract[7,8,9,10,11] on the cardiovascular system include the following:

- Improves blood flow through the blood vessels supplying the heart muscle (coronary arteries)
- Improves the contractions of the heart muscle, making it more efficient in pumping blood out to the body
- Increases the tolerance of the heart muscle to oxygen deficiency
- Improves circulation to the extremities by lowering resistance in the arteries. This is partly due to hawthorn's ability to inhibit a substance in the body known as angiotensin-converting enzyme (ACE). ACE is associated with leading to the creation of angiotensin II, a potent constrictor of blood vessels.
- Combats free radicals by way of its potent antioxidant properties. Because of its high bioflavonoid content, hawthorn is very adept at counteracting the damaging effects of free radicals on the cardiovascular system.

In addition, hawthorn extracts are mildly effective in lowering blood pressure. However, medicinal preparations of hawthorn are rarely used as the primary means by which to treat high blood pressure. Some physicians who recommend herbal therapies may incorporate hawthorn into the management of mild high blood pressure and cardiac arrhythmia in elderly patients.

Put simply, hawthorn and its active flavonoid compounds make the heart a more efficient pump. It achieves this partly by increasing blood supply to the heart muscle. It also increases the output of blood from the heart and decreases the resistance of blood vessels to the normal flow of blood. What we're left with is stronger and healthier heart function, as well as better flow of blood throughout the body.

The best news is hawthorn's safety. As opposed to digitalis and other cardiac glycoside drugs that can become very toxic, hawthorn can be used long term without side effects.[12,13]

CONGESTIVE HEART FAILURE

Hawthorn extracts are most commonly used to treat the early stages of congestive heart failure (CHF). Over nine studies have been published on the use of hawthorn for this condition.

People in the early stages of CHF usually do not require stronger heart medications such as digitalis. They are perfect candidates for nontoxic natural medicines such as hawthorn and coenzyme Q_{10}. Because of its ability to strengthen weakened heart muscle and improve blood flow, those with early-stage CHF are able to be more active and enjoy life more. Equally important, hawthorn may slow the progression to more advanced stages of CHF and stave off the need for stronger cardiac medications.

A simple way to see whether a medication is helping people in early-stage CHF is to measure their endurance on a stationary bicycle. Thirty early-stage CHF patients, ranging in age from 50 to 70 years, participated in an 8-week study that required them to exercise on a stationary bicycle.[14] Blood pressure and heart rate were measured, along with exercise tolerance and endurance. Patients were given either the hawthorn extract WS 1442 prepared from leaves and flowers (standardized to contain 18.75 percent oligomeric procyanidins) or placebo. The daily dose of the hawthorn extract was 160 milligrams. After 8 weeks, the patients taking the hawthorn extract were able to perform aerobic exercise longer (relative to the control patients) before reaching exhaustion. They also reported increased endurance and feelings of well-being.

In a similar study, 136 patients with early-stage CHF received either placebo or the hawthorn extract WS 1442 at a daily dose of 160 milligrams for 8 weeks.[15] Results were identical to those found for the study summarized earlier. Another study with early-stage CHF patients used 600 milligrams of the hawthorn extract LI 132 (standardized to 2.2 percent total flavonoids).[16] As before, exercise tolerance improved while shortness of breath and postexercise fatigue lessened. All of the studies mentioned have also shown improved heart function, as measured by electrocardiogram (ECG).

Finally, the LI 132 hawthorn extract (900 milligrams per day) compared favorably with the cardiac drug Captopril (37.5 milligrams per day) in the treatment of early-stage CHF patients.[17] This drug is used to reduce the resistance to blood flow in peripheral arteries. Hawthorn seems to do this as well, with the added benefit of working on the heart.

ANGINA PECTORIS

Hawthorn combats angina, another heart condition that is rampant in Western culture. Often caused by atherosclerosis, angina results from insufficient blood flow reaching the heart muscle. Without enough oxygen, the heart muscle spasms.

Physical exertion or stress often triggers angina attacks. A 1983 study[18] demonstrated the usefulness of hawthorn extract in the treatment of patients with stable angina pectoris. Sixty angina patients were given either 180 milligrams of hawthorn extract or placebo daily for 3 weeks. The patients taking hawthorn exercised for longer periods of time without an angina attack. Their ECG measures improved, and blood flow and oxygen delivery to the heart muscle rose.

HEART ATTACKS AND THE RECOVERY PROCESS

Heart failure patients often have a history of one or more heart attacks. Studies performed on rat hearts indicate that hawthorn extract protects heart muscle during times of oxygen loss.[19] This protection comes primarily in the form of antioxidant activity, which prevents free radical damage to the heart.[20] However, hawthorn's other effects (mentioned earlier) may make it useful in recovery of strength in the heart muscle following a heart attack. This should be a future topic of research on hawthorn.

HOW TO USE HAWTHORN

The extracts used most commonly today are those made from the leaves and flowers. These extracts are standardized on either total flavonoid (2.2 percent) or oligomeric procyanidin (18.75 percent) content, and the daily recommended dose is currently set at 160 to 900 milligrams in two or three divided doses. Persons requiring more intensive treatment should begin at the higher end of this dosage range. If you choose to use one of the traditional hawthorn berry preparations available in the United States, the dosage should be at least 4 to 5 grams daily. Keep in mind, however, that this form of hawthorn is going to be a bit less predictable regarding effectiveness. Hawthorn usually takes 1 to 2 months to provide a maximum effect and should be considered long-term therapy.

As is true of other plant medicines high in flavonoids, hawthorn is extremely safe for long-term use. There are no known interactions with prescription cardiac drugs. You may find mention of hawthorn possibly potentiating the effects of digoxin. However, although reported in one publication,[21] this result is not documented in any of the clinical studies to date and has not been cited as a concern in the German Commission E[22] or American Herbal Pharmcopoeia[23] monographs on hawthorn. Remember, heart disease is something that you should treat in conjunction with your doctor only after proper diagnosis and discussion of treatment options. There are no known contraindications to use of hawthorn during pregnancy and lactation.

Product update: The WS 1442 extract made by the Schwabe company (Karlsruhe, Germany) is sold in the United States under the trade name HeartCare® by Nature's Way. The LI 132 extract from Lichtwer Pharma (Berlin, Germany) is not currently imported into the United States.

Related Conditions Discussed in Part 6

- Atherosclerosis
- Angina
- Congestive heart failure

Horse Chestnut

Aesculus hippocastanum

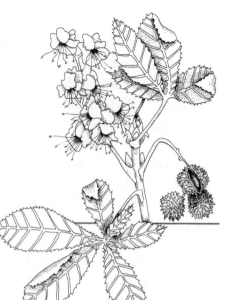

Part Used
The seeds

Common/Potential Uses
- Chronic venous insufficiency
- Varicose veins
- Hemorrhoids

Active Constituents
Aescin (also known as escin)—a complex mixture of saponins

How It Works
Helps promote healthy tone in the walls of the veins and helps strengthen capillaries. The improved tone of the veins promotes more efficient return of blood to the heart, particularly from the veins in the lower extremities. Aescin also has anti-inflammatory actions and reduces swelling when applied topically to injuries such as sprains or strains.

Recommended Use

Internal use: Horse chestnut seed standardized extract containing 16 to 20 percent aescin—300 milligrams (approximately 50 milligrams of aescin) two to three times daily. External use: Gel or cream containing 2 percent aescin—apply topically to affected area three to four times daily.

Side Effects

Side effects with standardized extracts of horse chestnut seed are rare. They can include itching, nausea, upset stomach, and calf spasm. Because of reports of intravenous aescin causing worsening of kidney function in persons with kidney disease, it is probably best for persons with kidney disease to avoid internal use of the extract. Individuals with liver disease should also avoid horse chestnut seed extract.

Safety Issues/Drug Interactions

The literature lists no known contraindications to the internal use of horse chestnut seed extract during pregnancy or lactation. However, you should consult with a doctor before using the extract. While there have been no reports of drug interactions, aescin does have a blood-thinning action and should be probably be avoided if you are taking aspirin or anticoagulant medications such as warfarin (Coumadin®).

THE shiny, nearly round seed of horse chestnut is something many of us have grown up playing with in some children's games. However, recognition of the medicinal benefits of these brown seeds is a relatively recent occurrence in this country. Again, with hats off to our herbally sophisticated friends in Europe, the development of a standardized extract of horse chestnut seeds has led to a safe and effective approach to managing difficult circulatory disorders such as chronic venous insufficiency (CVI). While that's not a condition many of us hear about on a daily basis, consider the following: CVI is one of the most common health care problems afflicting both men and women (please see Part 6 for an explanation of CVI).

Estimates place the prevalence at 10 to 15 percent of men and 20 to 25 percent of women.[1] Early-stage intervention is optimal, but the primary choices used in the United States are compression stockings and diuretic medications. Compression stockings can be inconvenient and uncomfortable, which often leads to low compliance.

The addition of horse chestnut seed extract to the treatment options for CVI as well as varicose veins promises to give many men and women relief from the annoying heaviness and pain that they experience with these conditions. Even as a long-term follow-up to compression stocking therapy (with or without diuretics) for CVI, the extract offers a long-term approach to improving the tone of the veins in the legs and improving blood flow.

PLANT FACTS

The horse chestnut (*Aesculus hippocastinum*) tree is native to parts of Asia and northern Greece but is now widely cultivated throughout Europe and the United States.[2] The tree produces fragrant pink and white flowers in the summer that turn to prickly fruits. These fruits are harvested in September when they become leathery and fall from the trees. The seed inside this fruit is used in modern medicinal extracts. Although the bark and leaves of the tree have been used for centuries by practitioners of traditional herbal medicine, their therapeutic efficacy has not been proven in clinical trials.

HISTORY

Horse chestnut leaves and bark have been used as a cough remedy in the treatment of bronchitis and whooping cough. The bark and leaves have also been used internally in the treatment of intermittent fevers.[3] Horse chestnut has a long history of use for reducing pain and inflammation of arthritis and rheumatism. In fact, superstition suggested that carrying a horse chestnut seed in your pocket would prevent or cure arthritis or rheumatism.[4] The use of horse chestnut seeds for varicose veins, venous congestion, and bruising dates back to sixteenth-century Europe. Extract made from the seeds was being used medicinally in France in the early 1800s, and early clinical reports suggested its use for hemorrhoids.[5]

The development of a horse chestnut seed extract (HCSE) standard-ized to aescin concentration has become a leading treatment in Europe today for chronic venous insufficiency (see "Health Care Applications" later). Additional applications for HCSE consist of internal use for vari-cose veins and capillary fragility. Although hemorrhoids are still listed as an indication for HCSE, this is based on historical use and not modern clinical research. Topical preparations containing aescin are used to treat swelling secondary to trauma such as sprains. Finally, intravenous prepa-rations of aescin are sometimes used in Europe to reduce swelling follow-ing surgery.

MEDICALLY ACTIVE CONSTITUENTS

The dried seeds of the horse chestnut contain a mixture of triterpene saponins collectively called aescin (sometimes shortened to *escin*).[6] Horse chestnut seeds naturally contain about 3 to 6 percent aescin. Stan-dardized extracts of horse chestnut seeds typically contain a much higher concentration of 16 to 20 percent aescin. As we'll note later, aescin is the primary driving force behind HCSE's ability to strengthen and tone veins and capillaries and improve blood flow from the veins in the legs back to the heart.

Other constituents in the seed include coumarins, flavonoids, tannins, allantoin, amino acids, choline, and phytosterols.

HOW HORSE CHESTNUT WORKS

Aescin is a full-service tonic for the veins and capillaries. First and fore-most, it helps improve the strength and tone in the walls of the veins and capillaries.[7] Some researchers call this a "vascular tightening" effect—probably not much different from the effect we get when we put astringent creams on our face. This improves the return of blood to the heart and discourages the pooling of blood and resulting edema (fluid retention) that is often seen in the ankles and lower legs of persons with CVI. This anti-edema effect is also enhanced by aescin's ability to help pooled fluid drain from surrounding tissues back into the capillaries.

The events leading to varicose veins and CVI also include the release of enzymes that attack the walls of the veins and capillaries as well as chemicals that encourage inflammation. Aescin to the rescue again! In addition to leaping tall buildings in a single bound, our herbal hero has also been shown to reduce the activity of the enzymes beta-*N*-acetylglucosaminidase (I think I dated her in high school), beta-glucironidase, and arylsulphatase that break down the compounds needed for healthy vein and capillary walls.[8] Additionally, aescin reduces the actions of other damaging enzymes, elastase (no relation to Elastic Man) and hyaluronidase, which have been found to be high in persons with CVI.[9]

Aescin's anti-edema and anti-inflammatory actions have contributed to its success as a topical treatment for traumatic injuries such as strains and sprains.[10] Since this is an isolation of one constituent from horse chestnut and not an herbal extract, we'll concentrate our focus in the next section on use of HCSE for CVI.

HEALTH CARE APPLICATIONS

In 1998, the *Archives of Dermatology* published an extremely favorable review of the clinical studies on HCSE for CVI.[11] Using predetermined criteria for good-quality studies, the authors narrowed their search to thirteen clinical studies for review. Eight of these studies were placebo controlled, and five were comparisons to other medications (e.g., oxerutins) or standard therapies (e.g., compression stockings and diuretics). The authors conclude that HCSE is a safe and effective treatment for CVI and that future studies should explore the use of HCSE with compression stockings for the long-term management of CVI.

Most of the studies summarized in the *Archives of Dermatology* review used a commercial HCSE known as Venostasin® retard (Klinge Pharma, Germany). The product delivers 50 milligrams of aescin per capsule, typically recommended at a dose of one capsule in the morning and one in the evening with meals.

One of the first studies investigating the action of the product involved 118 patients ages 30 to 70 years with CVI.[12] Patients were given either one capsule of the HCSE or placebo twice daily for 20 days. At the end of the first 20 days, all patients switched treatments—the HCSE folks went over to placebo and vice versa. While taking the HCSE, patients noted significant reductions in edema, pain, and leg cramping. Also noted were reductions in itching, tiredness, and leg heaviness. Persons taking placebo had essentially no improvement. Side effects were rare, with two patients taking HCSE having to stop treatment due to discomfort, and three in the placebo group stopped the therapy due to adverse events.

The success seen in this early study prompted the completion of another placebo-controlled study with thirty-nine CVI patients.[13] Patients were again split into two treatment groups—one receiving two 300 milligram HCSE capsules daily and the other placebo. Treatment lasted for 28 days. Using a device to measure the volume of blood in the lower legs and feet, the researchers found that those taking HCSE had a significantly reduced amount of blood pooling in those areas. In addition, edema was reduced in those taking HCSE, as noted in reduced size of the area around the shinbone and ankle. As was the case previously, symptoms such as pain, itching, and heaviness were also significantly decreased in those using HCSE.

So, you're probably thinking, "All that placebo stuff is nice, Dr. Brown, but how does this stuff really match up to accepted treatment for CVI?" (in other words, "Cut the medical crap and give us the low-down already!"). A 1996 study in the British medical journal *Lancet* compared HSCE with compression stocking/diuretic therapy in 240 patients with CVI.[14] By the way, they snuck a placebo in this one too! Treatment lasted for 12 weeks. Using the same blood volume measure as before (known as *plethysmography*), they found that volume in the lower leg was reduced equally in both the HSCE and compression stocking/diuretic groups. Leg volume increased in the placebo group. This study suggests that HCSE is a logical alternative for those that feel compression stockings are too cumbersome or uncomfortable.

How to Use Horse Chestnut

Remember to use a standardized extract with an adequate concentration of aescin. For treatment of CVI or varicose veins, use 300 milligrams of HCSE (standardized to 50 milligrams of aescin) two to three times daily in the morning and evening (add an afternoon dose if you go up to three times daily—most people do fine at the lower dose) with adequate water or other liquid during meals.[15]

While studies have lasted for at least 12 weeks, persons with CVI or varicose veins should consider HCSE a long-term treatment. For topical use, a gel or cream containing 2 percent aescin can be applied topically three to four times daily until improvement of swelling is noted. Please note that at the writing of this chapter, topical ointments or gels made according to the standards established in Germany and other European countries (e.g. Reparil®, Madaus AG, Germany; and Aesculaforce®/Venaforce®, Bioforce, Switzerland) have not made their way to into the U.S. marketplace.

Please remember that circulation disorders may be the signs of a serious condition. It's important to work with your health care professional to figure out what's going on first, before self-treating with HCSE. Same thing goes for swelling that you may think about using topical HCSE or aescin to treat.

At the recommended dosage, HCSE is generally safe for long-term use. In clinical studies, side effects were reported in 0.9 to 3 percent of the persons taking HCSE and included gastrointestinal upset, itching, nausea, and dizziness.[16] Because of reports of intravenous aescin causing worsening of kidney function in persons with kidney disease, it is probably best for persons with kidney disease to avoid internal use of the extract.[17,18] Persons with liver disease should also avoid horse chestnut seed extract. Topical use of aescin-containing gel has been known to cause skin rashes.[19] Don't use it on broken skin or burns.

It's important to note that safety has only been determined for a standardized extract made from the seeds of horse chestnut. Do not eat the seeds, twigs, or leaves of the tree as they can be poisonous.

The German Commission E monograph for HCSE lists no known contraindications to the use of the extract for pregnant or lactating women.[20] However, I recommend that you consult with your doctor or midwife before deciding to self-treat with HCSE during pregnancy. Because HCSE may have a mild blood-thinning effect (probably due to the coumarin content in the seeds), it's best to avoid using it together with aspirin or blood-thinning medications such as warfarin (Coumadin®) or antiplatelet aggregation medicines such as ticlopidine (Ticlid®).[21] This potential blood-thinning effect means you need to tell your surgeon you're taking HCSE and stop using it a couple of weeks before surgery.

Product update: The Venostasin retard product (Klinge Pharma, Germany) is sold in the U.S. by Pharmaton as Venastat™.

Acknowledgment: I'd like to thank Dr. Ron Reichert for his translation and summary of the German studies on HCSE that he so kindly let me use for this chapter.

RELATED CONDITIONS DISCUSSED IN PART 6

- Chronic venous insufficiency
- Strains and sprains

Kava-Kava

Piper methysticum

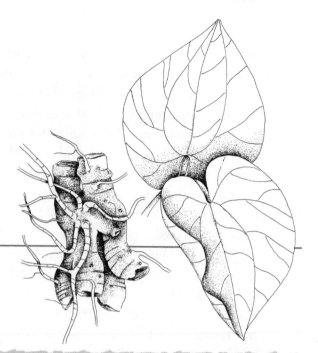

Part Used
The rhizome

Common/Potential Uses
- Anxiety and conditions of tension and restlessness

Active Constituents
Kava lactones (also known as kava pyrones)

How It Works
Kava exerts a relaxing effect on the central nervous system. Kava is noted for promoting relaxation without loss of mental sharpness. This makes it particularly useful for daytime management of anxiety. Kava also promotes normal, restful sleep and exerts a mild, relaxing effect on skeletal muscles.

Recommended Use

Standardized extracts containing 30 to 70 percent kava lactones—the daily dosage should deliver 140 to 240 milligrams of kava lactones in two or three divided doses.

Side Effects

At recommended amounts of the standardized extract, side effects include mild gastrointestinal upset in some people. Kava may turn the skin yellow temporarily and should be stopped if this happens. In rare cases, allergic skin reactions have been reported. Use of crude root and/or rhizome preparations in large amounts may result in impaired reaction time and drowsiness.

The intake of large quantities of nonstandardized kava liquid preparations can lead to a dry, scaly skin rash known as "kava dermopathy." Problems with equilibrium (body balance) have also been reported. Risk of this rash or equilibrium problems occurs only at kava lactone dosages in excess of several grams daily.

Safety Issues/Drug Interactions

Kava is not recommended for use by pregnant or lactating women. The German Commission E monograph on kava also warns against using it with barbiturates, antidepressants, anti-anxiety drugs, or other substances that may act on the central nervous system. Kava has been reported to interact with Xanax®, resulting in grogginess and oversedation in one case.

ALTHOUGH its name could easily be mistaken for a brand of instant coffee, kava-kava is actually a Polynesian and Melanesian herb that has emerged as an effective alternative to drugs commonly prescribed for anxiety. Along with valerian root extracts, kava root extracts in Europe have become an herbal alternative to antianxiety medications such as Xanax and Valium. Kava reduces anxiety and promotes a relaxed, sociable state and heightened mental acuity. Best of all, kava extracts are not associated with the side effects and addictive properties common to prescription antianxiety drugs.

PLANT FACTS

Kava-kava (*Piper methysticum*) is a member of the pepper family and is native to many islands of the Pacific. The plant is a robust perennial shrub that thrives at elevations of 500 to 1,000 feet above sea level. It grows best in stony ground and likes good sun exposure. Although it can reach heights of 20 feet, it is usually harvested at about 7 to 8 feet.[1] Modern herbal preparations of kava primarily use the rhizome or root stock for extraction.

The plant appears to have originated in Papua New Guinea–Indonesia and then spread to other islands through trade and by explorers.[2] For a complete overview of plant origins, traditional use of kava, and its chemical constituents, I highly recommend a book by Vincent Lebot, Mark Merlin, and Lamont Lindstrom entitled *Kava: The Pacific Drug* (Yale University Press, 1992).

HISTORY (CHEWIN', SPITTIN', DRINKIN', AND CHILLIN')

The incredible history of kava and its use in traditional ceremonies of the Pacific islands have been the subject of many lengthy anthropological reports and textbooks.

Introduction of kava to the modern world is attributed to a botanist and artist who accompanied Captain James Cook on his first voyage on the *Endeavor* (1768–1771). Daniel Scholander and Sydney Parkinson are given credit for being the first to describe the plant and its use as an intoxicating drink. The actual botanical name, *Piper methysticum,* was coined by Johann Georg Forster to describe an intoxicating pepper drink.[3]

A nonalcoholic drink made from the root of kava played an important role in a variety of ceremonies in the Pacific islands. The kava ceremonies were a key event to welcome visiting royalty or highly honored guests. It was also a part of smaller meetings among village elders. Less formal kava drinking was a common part of many social gatherings.

The manner of preparation of the kava beverage probably horrified a few of the European explorers. After the root is scraped, designated "chewers" chew cut pieces of the root and spit the macerated root into a bowl. Coconut milk was then added and the mixture strained and decanted into another bowl.[4]

Today, the traditional chewing has largely been replaced by pounding or grating of the root. Special bowls and utensils are used in the ceremony. The kava beverage is placed in a cup by a designated person who, in turn, delivers it to the special guest. The whole cup must be chugged without stopping! The audience claps three times and shouts *maca* ("It is empty"). Others can then be served.

Although the ceremony has been altered and even outlawed on some islands, it continues elsewhere today. Rumor has it that Hillary Clinton took part in a kava ceremony held in her honor by a Samoan community on the Hawaiian island of Oahu.[5] Whether she's continued the ceremony during the rather tumultuous last few years is open to speculation. I have a picture of Pope John Paul sneaking a drink of kava during a traditional ceremony. His look can only be described as heavenly.

So, how do people feel when they drink kava? The drink initially causes the mouth to numb. This is followed by a mellow and tranquil state that encourages socializing (hey, you remember those Grateful Dead concerts, don't you?). As long as the mixture is not too strong, the kava drinker usually attains a state of contentment and often enjoys a greater sense of well-being. Along with relaxation, many people experience sharper mental acuity, improved memory, and heightened sensory awareness.[6]

Excessive consumption can lead to muscle weakness and dizziness. As we'll note later, long-term, excessive use can also lead to a skin rash that will leave one feeling and looking anything but sociable.

MEDICALLY ACTIVE CONSTITUENTS

The search for kava's active constituents spans 130 years. The initial monograph on the chemical components and pharmacological activity of kava was written and published by the pharmacologist Louis Lewin in 1886.

Repeating work that had originally been published in 1860 and 1861, Lewin traced the relaxing properties of kava to a group of constituents in the root and rhizome.[7] These and other compounds discovered later would eventually be called *kava lactones*. The collective action of these constituents is responsible for kava's antianxiety effects.[8]

The kava lactones, sometimes referred to as kava pyrones, have become the focal point of modern kava extracts. These compounds are found in the fat-soluble portion of the root and rhizome. Good-quality kava rhizome contains between 5.5 and 8.3 percent kava lactones.[9] The standard phytopharmaceutical preparation used in clinical research in Europe is known as Laitan®/WS 1490 (Schwabe, Karlsruhe, Germany), with 70 percent kava lactones. Most commercial extracts in the United States are typically standardized to either 30 or 55 percent kava lactones.

HOW KAVA WORKS

In animal studies, kava lactones have shown antianxiety, analgesic (pain-relieving), muscle-relaxing, and anticonvulsant effects.[10] Kava's mode of action on the nervous system appears to differ from that of many sedative and muscle relaxants. Benzodiazepine-based drugs such as Xanax and Valium act by binding to or "turning on" specific receptors in the brain known as *GABA receptors*. By binding these receptors, these drugs promote sedation. Valerian root weakly binds similar receptors, partially explaining its actions as a sedative and antianxiety herbal medicine.

Kava lactones appear to be less selective.[11] Studies suggest that kava may directly influence the limbic system—the ancient part of the brain associated with emotions and other brain activities.[12] This conclusion may partly explain why kava's antianxiety effects seem to extend beyond psychological processes to include muscle relaxation as well. Animal studies also indicate that kava has pain-reducing capabilities.[13]

Kava does not reduce pain by the same pathway as that used by opiate analgesics. Kava is rarely prescribed by modern herbalists to reduce pain, but it has been used extensively for this purpose by native medicine men of the Pacific islands. Kava lactones also have anticonvulsive properties and seem to protect the brain during times of ischemia (reduced blood flow leading to low oxygen supply).[14,15] A focus of some of the recent research on kava lactones has been the treatment of epilepsy. While this certainly has exciting ramifications, it is too early to begin recommending kava extracts for the primary treatment of epilepsy.

HEALTH CARE APPLICATIONS

The primary use for kava is in the treatment of anxiety and nervous tension. In Europe, kava is to anxiety what St. John's wort is to depression. It creates changes in brain activity (as measured by electroencephalogram, or EEG) typical of antianxiety drugs but without their sedative and hypnotic effects.[16,17] Paradoxically, people taking kava show increased attentiveness and concentration while feeling relaxed! This is a remarkable effect for an antianxiety treatment to possess and really places kava in a class all its own.

In one head-to-head study with a benzodiazepine drug, kava fared wonderfully. The study showed that volunteers improved in terms of reaction time and performance on a word recognition test while taking the kava extract WS 1490.[18] Volunteers taking oxazepam (Serax®), the benzodiazepine drug, did not do as well as those taking kava.

How about the treatment of anxiety? One study measured the effect of 100 milligrams of the WS 1490 kava extract (containing 70 percent kava lactones), administered three times daily for 4 weeks, against placebo.[19] Fifty-eight patients suffering from anxiety and tension took part in the study, with half the group getting kava and the other half placebo. Less anxiety was already noted in the kava group after 1 week. By 4 weeks, the difference between the two groups was striking. Patients taking kava had an improved sense of well-being and marked reduction in nervousness and tension. No side effects were noted.

These results were verified in a long-term, double-blind, placebo-controlled study with 101 patients suffering from mild to moderate anxiety.[20] From the 8th week on, there was a significant decrease in anxiety in those persons taking kava. This positive trend was even more significant by the 24th week of the study. Side effects were rare and consisted primarily of mild gastrointestinal complaints. This study is important because it demonstrates both the long-term effectiveness and safety of kava for the treatment of mild to moderate anxiety.

The same extract and dosage were used, in a study with women suffering from anxiety associated with menopause, for 4 weeks.[21] Again, compared to placebo, use of kava led to less anxiety and enhanced well-being. Treatment with kava was well tolerated.

Another important study using the same dose of the WS 1490 extract as in the previously mentioned study compared it head-to-head with two benzodiazepine drugs, oxazepam and bromazepam, for 6 weeks in patients with mild to moderate anxiety.[22] Three treatments led to a similar reduction in anxiety. It's important to note that kava is not associated with the addictive properties or potential withdrawal symptoms associated with benzodiazepines.

Finally, an unpublished study suggests that kava may also be useful for dealing with anxiety and stress associated with the trials and tribulations of everyday life (such as reading long-winded herb books!). In a study completed at the Medical College of Virginia at Virginia Commonwealth University, healthy adults reporting high levels of daily stress and anxiety took place in a 4-week, double-blind, placebo-controlled study to see whether a kava product known as Kavatrol® (Natrol, Chatsworth, CA) could reduce their complaints.[23] Persons in the kava group took one capsule of the product twice daily (equivalent to 240 mg of kava lactones per day). At the end of 4 weeks, all measures of stress and anxiety were significantly reduced in the kava group when compared to those taking placebo. No significant side effects were reported in those taking kava (unless you consider the unexplained surge in West Coast lingo such as "far-out," "cool," and "groovy").

HOW TO USE KAVA

Dosage for use of kava extract for mild to moderate anxiety is typically based on the daily intake of kava lactones. Persons should take a standardized extract that delivers 200 to 250 milligrams of kava lactones per day in two or three divided doses. Work with your health care professional to evaluate the antianxiety effects over 4 to 6 weeks before deciding whether kava works for you. If you're using it for the stress and anxiety of daily living, a similar dose will probably work, but you may want to experiment with a lower dose (e.g., 140 milligrams of kava lactones) first to see whether it works.

At these dosages, the primary side effect reported has been mild gastrointestinal disturbances. Kava may turn the skin yellow temporarily.[24] If this occurs, you should stop taking kava. In rare cases, an allergic skin reaction (rash) may occur.

The intake of large quantities of nonstandardized kava liquid preparations can lead to a dry, scaly skin rash known as "kava dermopathy." Problems with equilibrium (body balance) have also been reported. Risk of this rash or equilibrium problems occurs only at kava lactone dosages in excess of several grams daily. The recommended dosage of a standardized extract listed earlier has been found to have no effect on reaction time while driving.[25]

Kava is not recommended for use by pregnant or lactating women. I also would not recommend it for young children. The German Commission E monograph on kava also warns against using it with other substances that may act on the central nervous system, such as alcohol, barbiturates, and antidepressants.[26] A published case study found that combining kava and the benzodiazepine Xanax® led to oversedation and grogginess in one person.[27] One study did not find any negative effects when kava and alcohol were combined.[28] However, I don't advocate this combination.

Product update: The WS 1490 (Laitan) made by Schwabe (Karlsuhe, Germany) is not currently available in the United States. Kavatrol™ is sold by Natrol.

RELATED CONDITION DISCUSSED IN PART 6

- Anxiety

Milk Thistle

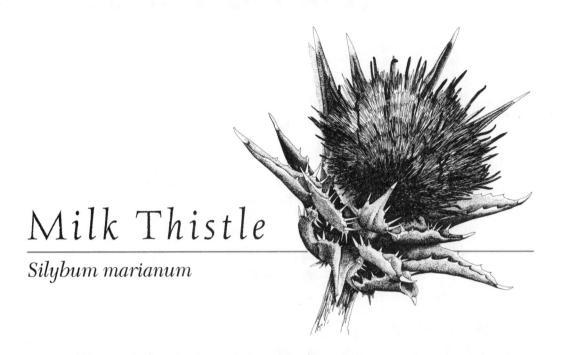

Silybum marianum

Part Used
   The dried fruit (achenes)

Common/Potential Uses
   • Liver disease associated with alcohol abuse
   • Drug-induced liver injury or disease
   • Chronic hepatitis
   • Liver protection for those working with toxic chemicals, pesticides, and other substances that may harm the liver

Active Constituents
   The bioflavonoid silymarin complex and its component known as silibinin

How It Works
   The silymarin complex, particularly the silibinin component, protects the liver through antioxidant activity and stabilization of cell membranes. It prevents certain toxins from entering liver cells and

stimulates regeneration of damaged cells. Silymarin may also prevent fibrotic changes in the liver.

Recommended Use
Concentrated extract standardized to 80 percent silymarin content—420 milligrams of silymarin daily in three divided doses

Side Effects
Milk thistle extract is essentially free of side effects. Because of its stimulating effect on the liver and gallbladder, some people may experience loose stools for the first few days of use.

Safety Issues/Drug Interactions
There are no known interactions with commonly prescribed medications. Current monographs list no reasons to avoid milk thistle extract during pregnancy or lactation.

THE DETOXIFYING capabilities of our bodies face an immense challenge in modern society. Auto exhaust, secondary cigarette smoke, alcohol, drugs, industrial solvents, pesticides, and even some of the water and food we consume burden the cleansing organs of our body. Positive lifestyle choices such as exercise and a healthy diet certainly contribute to strengthening these systems. However, when pushed to the limit or even beyond, these organs of detoxification need support.

The liver, one of the body's major "antipollution" organs, removes toxins that can damage other organ systems, including the heart, blood vessels, eyes, and skin. When its actions are impaired by alcohol or diseases such as hepatitis, the negative effects on long-term health can be staggering.

Milk thistle and its active component, *silymarin,* are nature's offering for optimal liver protection. It is the leader among treatments for chronic liver disease caused primarily by alcohol abuse and may hold promise as a supportive therapy for those with chronic hepatitis. It is also emerging as an important supplement for those desiring to optimize liver function and maximize the detoxifying potential of this important organ.

PLANT FACTS

Also known by its Latin name *Silybum marianum,* milk thistle is commonly found growing wild in a variety of settings, including roadsides.[1] It is a tall plant with prickly leaves and a milk sap. The name *Silybum* is derived from the name given to edible thistles during the first century by Dioscorides. The name *marianum* comes from the legend that the white mottling of the leaves was caused by a drop of the Virgin Mary's milk. Other common names attributed to the plant include Mary thistle, Marian thistle, Lady's thistle, and Holy thistle. Today, extracts are produced from the small hard fruits (often incorrectly referred to as seeds) that have the feathery tuft (known as the *pappus*) removed. These are also referred to as *achenes.*

HISTORY

Medical use of milk thistle can be traced back more than 2,000 years. Pliny the Elder, a first-century Roman naturalist, noted that the juice of the plant mixed with honey was good for "carrying off bile." Culpepper, the well-known eighteenth-century herbalist, cited its use for opening "obstructions" of the liver and spleen and recommended it for the treatment of jaundice.[2] Rademacher, a German physician of the early nineteenth century, gave patients with liver disease a tincture made from the seeds.

Milk thistle was first mentioned in American medical circles in the late nineteenth century. J. U. Lloyd and H. W. Felter, physicians and herbal experts, list the seeds as useful in relieving congestion of the liver, spleen, and kidneys.[3] While liver and onion recipes survived in the United States, milk thistle slowly faded away by the early twentieth century.

Modern Development and Medically Active Constituents

Leave it to Europe to bring back another valuable plant medicine! Over thirty years ago, intensive research on the liver-protecting properties of milk thistle seeds began in Germany. In 1968, a bioflavonoid complex in milk thistle fruit was identified and isolated. Christened *silymarin*, this complex was found to be responsible for the medical benefits of the plant.[4]

The silymarin complex is made up of three parts: silibinin, silidianin, and silicristin. Silibinin, the most active of the three, is largely responsible for the benefits attributed to the silymarin complex.[5,6] Extensive research ultimately led to the approval of a standardized milk thistle extract in Germany for the treatment of alcohol-induced liver disease and other chronic diseases of the liver. The extract, known as Legalon® (Madaus AG, Cologne, Germany), was originally standardized to 70 percent silymarin content. Today, this and other leading milk thistle extracts in Europe are standardized to 80 percent silymarin.

Note: Throughout the remainder of this chapter, the term *silymarin* will be used interchangeably with *milk thistle extract*.

How Milk Thistle Works

Milk thistle extract protects liver cells both directly and indirectly. It also possesses the ability to regenerate liver cells that have been injured and to prevent fibrosis. Let's take a closer look at each of these actions and how they work together to make milk thistle extract a logical choice for persons with liver disease.

Liver Cell Protection

Silymarin, and more specifically silibinin, directly aids liver cells by binding to the outside of the cells and blocking the entrance of certain toxins. This was first noted in experimental studies[7,8] investigating toxins from *Amanita phalloides* (death cap mushroom). Swallowing death cap mushroom causes swift and severe damage to liver cells. Silymarin blocks the receptor sites by which the death cap toxins enter the cells. In addition, toxins that have already penetrated the liver cells are neutralized by silibinin. These actions mean that milk thistle can remain effective even if the initial poisoning occurred several hours earlier. Intravenous preparations of purified silibinin are therefore a mainstay in German hospital emergency rooms for treating death cap mushroom poisoning.

Similar protective effects have been shown in test tube and animal studies against carbon tetrachloride, acetaminophen,[9] and even antipsychotic drugs in one human study.[10]

ANTIOXIDANT ACTIVITY

Silymarin also protects liver cells by boosting their antioxidant activity. As is true with other nutrient and herbal antioxidants, it accomplishes this by helping the cells produce a powerful antioxidant known as *glutathione*.[11,12] Glutathione is the front-line defense against the ravages of free radicals. Silymarin has been shown in animal studies to raise the glutathione level in liver cells by as much as 50 percent![13]

Silymarin also increases the activity of another antioxidant, superoxide dismutase, in red blood cells.[14] This effect, combined with the increase in liver cell glutathione, is a major aid for those with a history of alcohol abuse.

REGENERATION OF DAMAGED LIVER CELLS

Alcohol abuse and viral hepatitis can lead to liver cell injury. Under these conditions, silymarin actually helps the cell synthesize new protein, thus enabling it (and ultimately the liver tissue as a whole) to regenerate.[15,16] This has been demonstrated in studies involving patients with alcoholic liver disease and also chronic hepatitis. Silymarin's protein-regenerating action helps return liver cells to a more optimal, functional state.

Note: Silymarin's regenerative abilities apply only to normal liver cells. It does not appear to stimulate growth of cancerous cells.[17]

ANTIFIBROTIC ACTIONS

In recent years, test tube and animal studies as well as a couple of human clinical trials have indicated that the real protective effects of silymarin for persons with alcohol-induced or viral hepatitis may be its ability to prevent fibrosis. Fibrosis is a process that occurs in the liver cells owing to inflammation. This can be due to alcohol abuse or chronic active hepatitis B or C. Fibrosis is a complex process that requires many steps but basically occurs when collagen invades the normal structure of the liver cell. Helping block this process is a key to keeping the liver of a person with hepatitis from developing cirrhosis.

The ability of silymarin to block fibrosis in the liver was first shown in studies with rats.[18] This important effect was later demonstrated in a study with 998 patients with liver disease due to a variety of factors including alcohol abuse, chronic active hepatitis B or C, drugs, and chemical exposure in the workplace.[19] Use of 140 milligrams of silymarin (equivalent to approximately 60 milligrams of silibinin) three times daily for 3 months led to a significant reduction in a marker of fibrosis known as *amino terminal procollagen III peptide* (PIIINP). In 19 percent of the patients, this measure had dropped to the normal range expected for a healthy person.

HEALTH CARE APPLICATIONS

Milk thistle extracts standardized to 70 to 80 percent silymarin content have been extensively studied and recommended in Europe for supportive or primary treatment of liver diseases.

More than 200 experimental and clinical reports involving more than 5,000 patients have been published to date. Conditions for which silymarin is commonly recommended include alcohol-related liver disease, drug-related liver disease, chronic active hepatitis B or C, and liver damage caused by toxic chemical exposure. Large clinical trials of silymarin, involving a cross-section of "toxic" liver diseases, have shown very good results in reducing damage to the liver and improving the quality of life of patients.[20]

ALCOHOL-RELATED LIVER DISEASE
The leading cause of liver disease in the United States and most Western countries is alcohol abuse. While alcohol recovery programs

have made progress against alcoholism, many alcoholics continue to go untreated. The legal and emotional costs due to this disease are immense.

Silymarin is often prescribed to treat liver disease caused by alcohol abuse.[21] In studies[22,23] exploring silymarin's effect, the daily dose was 420 milligrams. Alcoholic patients generally must take milk thistle extract for 4 to 8 weeks before seeing any signs of reversal of liver damage. Improvement is measured by blood tests comparing before-and-after liver enzyme levels, as well as by liver biopsy. Successful treatment with silymarin results in a significant lowering of elevated liver enzymes (a lowering of these enzyme levels indicates healing of damaged liver cells) over this period of time. Also, patients report a reversal in symptoms such as weakness, loss of appetite, and nausea. In addition to these benefits, one study found that silymarin also reduced the PIIINP marker of fibrosis mention above in patients with alcohol-related liver disease.[24] It should be noted that even with improvement, most alcoholic patients will require several months of treatment with milk thistle extract.

Collectively, these results make silymarin a key to any alcohol recovery program. It would be nice to see alcohol recovery units begin using silymarin as part of their treatment plan for alcoholic patients—particularly those with compromised liver function. For those of you who are consuming alcohol on a regular basis, it's probably wise to start your milk thistle regimen sooner than later.

LIVER CIRRHOSIS

How about patients with advanced liver disease? Some, but not all, clinical studies have suggested a role for silymarin in slowing the advancement of liver cirrhosis (a chronic disease characterized by loss of normal liver cell structure and preceded by fatty infiltration of the liver—particularly in alcoholics). About 20 percent of chronic alcoholics develop cirrhosis, with severe forms often proving fatal. While the liver cell–regenerating capabilities of silymarin do not reverse cirrhosis once it has advanced (cirrhosis appears to be an irreversible process), silymarin may improve quality of life and even extend life expectancy in some patients.

One hundred seventy patients with advanced cirrhosis of the liver participated in a study that compared a daily dose of 420 milligrams of silymarin to placebo.[25] The average length of treatment was 41 months. The silymarin group showed improvements in liver enzyme measures and liver biopsy results. Most impressive, however, was the fact that most of these patients also lived longer due to silymarin therapy!

Positive results were also found in a 12-month study with adult diabetics with alcoholic liver cirrhosis.[26] Using the same dose of silymarin as the prior study, liver enzyme measures improved. However, the real surprise in this study was the finding that ability to control blood sugar was also improved, which led to a reduced need for insulin in those persons taking silymarin. While silymarin is not a treatment for diabetes per se, it may hold some benefit for those persons with diabetes secondary to liver cirrhosis.

A 2-year study in Spain failed to support these two studies.[27] Use of 450 milligrams of silymarin daily failed to influence liver health or survival rate in alcoholic patients with liver cirrhosis. However, patients positive for hepatitis C did seem to fare better when taking silymarin.

CHRONIC HEPATITIS

Silymarin may eventually play a role in the treatment of chronic viral hepatitis B or C. These chronic viral conditions cause ongoing inflammation and impairment of liver function. They are also linked to an increased risk of liver cancer. Current treatment boils down to alpha interferon, alpha interferon with the antiviral drug ribavirin, or watchful waiting. While the combination therapy holds some promise for persons with hepatitis C, the side effects are often debilitating, making long-term therapy difficult. Silymarin does not directly impact the hepatitis virus. Owing to its protective and regenerating capabilities and, most important, its antifibrotic effects, it may be a useful supportive treatment for minimizing the damage to liver cells commonly seen in chronic hepatitis.

In some very small pilot studies in Europe, the same 420 milligrams of silymarin daily, used for an average of 9 months, was shown to reverse liver cell injury effectively (according to biopsy) and led to a decrease in liver enzyme levels in persons with hepatitis B.[28,29] Patients undergoing treatment also noted an increase in appetite and energy. A product combining silymarin and phosphatidylcholine (IdB 1016) found similar results in persons with hepatitis B in two small clinical trials.[30,31]

The big question is whether silymarin is effective for the long-term treatment of hepatitis C. A modern-day epidemic, hepatitis C is being diagnosed at an alarming rate in the United States. While new drug therapies, including combination of alpha-interferon and ribavirin, are being studied, we don't know that much about the long-term prognosis of this disease. While we await the results of long-term studies from Europe looking at the effect of silymarin on patients with hepatitis C, it's my opinion that every person with hepatitis C should consider silymarin as part of their long-term treatment regime.

LIVER SUPPORT DURING DRUG THERAPY

Silymarin may also ward off the damage caused by certain drugs, such as acetaminophen, antidepressants, antipsychotic, cholesterol-lowering, and anticonvulsive drugs. One study showed that adding silymarin to the daily regimen of patients receiving psychotropic drugs reduced the production of potentially damaging free radicals in the liver.[32] According to one report, liver protection by silymarin was also found in patients with acute promyelocytic leukemia taking anthracycline as a maintenance therapy.[33] Silymarin may also block the potential liver-damaging effects of anesthesia and is sometimes used both pre- and postsurgery in Germany.

It's not successful all the time. One study found no liver protection by silymarin in patients taking the drug tacrine (Cognex®).[34]

OTHER POTENTIAL USES

People with multiple chemical sensitivities and workers encountering toxins on the job may benefit by adding milk thistle extract to their daily supplement regimen. I've also noted some improvement in psoriasis patients; this observation is based, however, on isolated case histories. The psoriasis in these patients appeared to be linked to impaired liver function secondary to a history of alcohol abuse, and for them milk thistle extract can be helpful.

While I question the safety of many "cleansing programs" being touted by some health gurus, milk thistle extract may provide support for liver function during a detoxification program. It may assist normal liver clearance of toxins as well as protect liver cells.

How to Use Milk Thistle Extract

For persons with liver disease or those looking to provide extra liver protection from alcohol, drugs or chemicals, the daily dose of milk thistle extract, standardized to 80 percent silymarin content, should deliver 420 milligrams of silymarin in three divided doses. In persons with liver disease, it is recommended that this dose be used until clinical improvement is verified by laboratory tests (don't try to self-diagnose or treat liver disease!). According to research and clinical experience, improvement should be noted in about 8 weeks. However, in persons with chronic liver disease due to hepatitis or cirrhosis, ongoing use of silymarin makes sense.

Milk thistle extract is virtually devoid of any side effects and may be used by a wide range of people, including pregnant and lactating women. Since silymarin does stimulate liver and gallbladder activity, it may have a mild, transient laxative effect in some individuals. This will usually cease within 2 to 3 days.

Product update: The Legalon milk thistle extract (Madaus AG, Cologne, Germany) is sold in the United States as Thisilyn® by Nature's Way.

Related Conditions Discussed in Part 6

- Alcohol-related liver disease
- HIV infection/AIDS
- Psoriasis

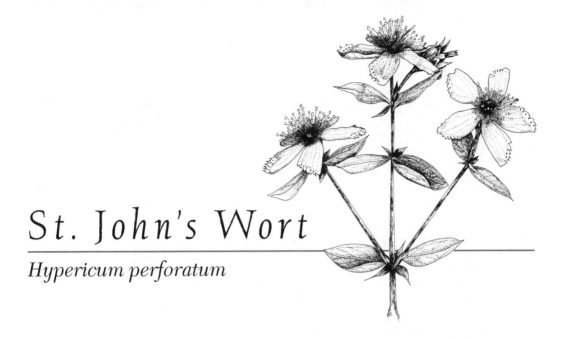

St. John's Wort

Hypericum perforatum

Part Used
   The flowering tops

Common/Potential Uses
   • Mild to moderate depression

Active Constituents
   The exact constituents responsible for the antidepressant action of
   St. John's wort are still unclear, but recent research has focused on
   the constituent hyperforin as well as flavonoids. Although previously thought to be active, the substance hyperforin and related
   dianthrones are unlikely to contribute to the antidepressant actions
   of the herb.

How It Works
   While this topic is still unclear, studies have suggested that St.
   John's wort may inhibit the reuptake of the neurotransmitters
   serotonin, norepinephrine, and dopamine. Other research suggests

that St. John's wort may also work through GABA receptors that modulate the activity of substances with mild antianxiety actions. Contrary to earlier beliefs, the herb does not appear to inhibit the enzyme monoamine oxidase.

Recommended Use

For mild to moderate depression, take 300 milligrams of a standardized St. John's wort extract three times per day. Higher doses may work for more severe depression, but this dosage should only be attempted after consultation with your doctor. Expect results within 2 to 4 weeks.

Side Effects

St. John's wort has a low incidence of side effects compared to prescription antidepressants. Side effects may include mild gastrointestinal upset, dry mouth, nervousness, and skin rash. St. John's wort may make the skin and possibly the eyes more light-sensitive. These reactions are unusual at the doses recommended here. People with fair skin should avoid exposure to strong sunlight and other sources of ultraviolet light (such as tanning lights) when taking St. John's wort.

Safety Issues/Drug Interactions

St. John's wort should not be used at the same time as prescription antidepressants. It may reduce absorption and blood levels of drugs such as digoxin, cyclosporin, indinavir (a protease inhibitor used to treat HIV infection), theophylline, and warfarin. Do not use St. John's wort together with these drugs without first consulting your doctor or pharmacist. In contrast to current European monographs, I believe that St. John's wort should not be used during pregnancy or lactation.

ST. JOHN'S wort has experienced a meteoric rise in popularity during the last decade. It has become the most frequently prescribed medicine for the treatment of mild to moderate depression in Germany, where it far outsells prescription antidepressants. Based on Americans' seeming obsession with depression (note the rise of Prozac® in the early 1990s) and a positive piece on the ABC television news magazine program *20/20*, American consumers sent sales of St. John's wort sky rocketing. While sales have calmed down, medical interest hasn't. The National Institutes of Health in conjunction with Duke University is funding a large clinical trial to assess the effectiveness of St. John's wort for depression.

While we sort through the explosion of information about this herb in the next few sections, remember that to date, the research points to this herb being best reserved for mild to moderate depression as well as mild, situational depression and seasonal affective disorder. Even more important, the explosion of interest in this herb for depression points to the importance of working with your doctor to get a good diagnosis and treatment plan in place before running out to buy St. John's wort.

PLANT FACTS

St. John's wort, also known as *Hypericum perforatum,* is a shrubby perennial plant with numerous bright yellow flowers. Close examination of the flowers reveals small black dots. When rubbed between the fingers, these produce a red stain. This red pigment contains the constituent hypericin. Held up to the light, the leaves of the plant display a number of bright, translucent dots. This perforated look led to the Latin name *perforatum.*[1]

St. John's wort is found in dry, gravelly soil and grows best in sunny areas. It is native to Europe, North Africa, and western Asia and was introduced and naturalized later in parts of the United States (especially northern California and the Pacific Northwest) and Australia. It is currently cultivated for medicinal preparations in Europe, North and South America, Australia, and China.[2] Today, the aboveground parts of the plant are harvested during the flowering season and used in modern, standardized extracts.

HISTORY

St. John's wort has a long and colorful history. Dioscorides, the foremost physician of ancient Greece, as well as Pliny and Hippocrates, recommended the herb for a host of ailments, including sciatica, and for the treatment of poisonous reptile bites. The Latin name *Hypericum* derives from the Greek and means "over an apparition"—a reference to the belief that the herb was so obnoxious to evil spirits that a whiff of it would cause them to depart the premises quickly. Early English lore suggests that the flowers could protect one from the "evil eye" and would banish witches.

The name "St. John's wort" has its origins in Christian folk traditions. One belief held that the red spots appeared on the leaves during the anniversary of St. John's beheading and symbolized his blood. Another legend asserted that if you slept with a piece of the plant under your pillow, the saint himself would appear in a dream, bless you, and prevent some loved one from dying the following year. Whether he gave any odds on the Battle of Hastings is open to speculation.

St. John's wort has a long history of medical use in Europe. It was, and continues to be, very popular for the topical treatment of wounds and burns. It has also been used as a folk remedy for kidney and lung ailments as well as mood disorders.[3]

MODERN DEVELOPMENT

While St. John's wort products have approved since the mid-1980s in Germany for depressed mood and mild anxiety, it wasn't until the early 1990s that things really got hopping.[4] Thanks to the efforts of the German phytopharmaceutical company Lichtwer Pharma (Berlin), a flurry of studies on the pharmacology and clinical effectiveness of St. John's wort began in earnest. While previous St. John's wort products had daily recommended doses in the 400 to 500 milligram range, Lichtwer Pharma focused on a higher dose of 900 milligrams per day. Studies completed on the Lichtwer extract known as LI 160 have established St. John's wort as a viable alternative for the treatment of mild to moderate depression. To date, over thirty clinical trials with thousands of patients suffering from mild to moderate depression have been completed.[5]

MEDICALLY ACTIVE CONSTITUENTS

St. John's wort has a complex and diverse chemical makeup. This has made identification of medically active constituents difficult. While the naphthodianthrones hypericin and pseudohypericin have been the focal point of many earlier studies,[6] there has been increased focus on other constituents in the plant, especially hyperforin.[7]

The early interest in hypericin explains why most standardized extracts of St. John's wort are standardized to this compound. However, because of studies that have suggested that hypericin does not contribute to the antidepressant actions of St. John's wort (see later discussion), many manufacturers are turning their focus to compounds such as hyperforin, xanthone derivatives, and flavonoids in the plant.

HOW ST. JOHN'S WORT WORKS

ANTIDEPRESSIVE ACTIONS

Remember all that stuff I told you in the last edition of the book? Well, forget it! While it was previously thought that St. John's wort inhibits the enzyme monoamine oxidase,[8] new data suggest that St. John's wort acts a little like some of the other antidepressants on the market known as selective serotonin reuptake inhibitors (e.g., Prozac, Zoloft®) and tricyclic antidepressants (e.g., imipramine, amitryptiline). While some of us were tipped off about this in 1996 by Dr. H. D. Reuter during a presentation at an American Chemical Society meeting, Dr. Walter Müller of the Department of Psychiatry at the University of Frankfurt has been responsible for the research that has rewritten the book on how St. John's wort may treat depression. Using test tube studies, Dr. Müller and colleagues found that St. John's wort inhibits the reuptake of not only the neurotransmitter serotonin but also norepinephrine and dopamine.[9] Put simply, "reuptake" means that there's more of these neurotransmitters available to the brain. In the same study, the inhibition of MAO was found to be so weak as to suggest that this action is highly unlikely in the human body. A recent clinical study found that the amount of hypericin in different St. John's wort extracts had no bearing on how effectively they treated depression.[10]

In a follow-up study, Dr. Müller and colleagues found that the compound hyperforin was responsible for the actions cited here.[11] This observation has led to the development of a St. John's wort extract that is standardized to hyperforin content (e.g., WS 5572, Schwabe, Karslruhe, Germany). Hyperforin is very unstable, and thus these extracts employ a technique to stabilize the compound.

ANTIVIRAL ACTIVITY

While they've dwindled on the antidepressant front, hypericin and pseudohypericin are the undisputed champs when it comes to antiviral activity. Experimental studies have found that these constituents exhibit strong antiviral activity against herpes simplex virus types 1 and 2 (the viruses that cause herpes sores on the mouth and genitals) and two different flu viruses (influenza virus types A and B).[12] Hypericin has also shown strong antiviral activity against Epstein–Barr virus.[13] This is the virus that causes mononucleosis. It also has weak antiviral activity against a member of the hepatitis B virus family, duck hepatitis B virus (I think Donald Duck was the test case).[14]

In 1988, hypericin and pseudohypericin drew attention when a report by researchers at New York University Medical Center and the Weizmann Institute of Science (Rehovot, Israel) showed that these constituents could inhibit the activity of animal retroviruses.[15] Since human immunodeficiency virus (HIV) is also a retrovirus, focus quickly shifted to hypericin's effect on the viral cause of acquired immunodeficiency virus (AIDS). The research team demonstrated that hypericin has the ability (in test tubes) to prevent uninfected T lymphocytes (the cells of the immune system targeted by HIV) from being infected by HIV.[16] In addition, the action of hypericin was found to be different from that of drugs used to treat HIV—AZT and ddI.[17]

It is often the case that a plant constituent can look awfully darn good in the test tube and then fail miserably when people use it. This seems to be the story with St. John's wort and hypericin for treatment of HIV infection.

The research at New York University Medical Center led to the widespread use by HIV-infected individuals of St. John's wort extracts with small, measured amounts of hypericin. Early reports in *AIDS Treatment News* indicated some success.[18,19]

However, more extensive studies[20,21] proved disappointing. A major frustration was the inability to pinpoint the suitable dose necessary for an anti-HIV effect. The major effect noted was a decrease in depression! One side effect noted with high doses of St. John's wort was an elevation in liver enzymes (an indication of liver toxicity) in some individuals.

Clinical studies then shifted from a standardized extract to a highly purified hypericin. Studies in Boston, Minneapolis, and New York are using an intravenous preparation of hypericin at very high doses. Unfortunately, human studies with hypericin have hit a dead end due to the fact that the dosages needed to have an antiviral effect have proven to be very toxic to the liver.[22]

WOUND-HEALING PROPERTIES

Oil-based preparations of St. John's wort have been historically recommended for the topical treatment of burns and wounds. Its antibacterial actions are one factor assisting with wound healing.[23,24]

HEALTH CARE APPLICATIONS

The diagnosis and treatment of depression can be a very complex process. If you choose to use a mild antidepressant such as St. John's wort, be sure it is part of a complete program that includes a sound nutritional program, exercise, and counseling.

As mentioned earlier, St. John's wort has been the focus of over thirty clinical trials in depression to date. Analysis of these trials has found that St. John's wort is more effective than placebo and equally effective to low-dose tricyclic antidepressants in the treatment of mild to moderate depression.[25] As we'll note, new studies are also suggesting it might work as well as the selective serotonin reuptake inhibitors (SSRIs) such as Prozac and Zoloft.

In two double-blind, placebo-controlled clinical studies, patients with mild depression showed a positive response to 900 milligrams per day of the St. John's wort extract LI 160. In the first, 105 patients took either the LI 160 or placebo for four weeks.[26] Of the eighty-nine patients completing the study, those taking LI 160 had a significant reduction in all symptoms of depression. Only two patients reported mild side effects.

In the second study, patients with mild to moderate depression taking either the same dose of LI 160 or placebo were followed for 6 weeks.[27] As was the case in the first study, patients taking LI 160 showed a greater drop in depression as assessed by their physicians and also on self-report measures. Side effects were only reported in one patient taking LI 160 (sleep disturbance).

A number of studies have compared St. John's wort head-to-head with prescription antidepressants known as tricyclics. These studies have been criticized a bit because the dose of the prescription antidepressant was well below the amount typically recommended by psychiatrists for depression. It is interesting to note, however, that this criticism may be more about a poor if not total lack of understanding of how to treat mild to moderate depression than it is about the effectiveness of St. John's wort.

The St. John's wort extract LI 160 has compared favorably to the antidepressant imipramine (Tofranil®) in two studies. In the first, patients with mild to moderate depression took either 900 milligrams of LI 160 or 75 milligrams of imipramine per day for 6 weeks.[28] Scores on a standard measure of depression known as the Hamilton Depression Scale (HAMD) dropped slightly more for those taking LI 160. Side effects were not only fewer but also much milder in persons taking LI 160.

Similar results were seen in another study looking at dosages twice as high as those used in the first study.[29] In this study with patients with moderate to severe depression, a dose of 1,800 milligrams per day of LI 160 was compared with 150 milligrams per day of imipramine for 6 weeks.

This dose of imipramine is closer to what would normally be prescribed for depression. A similar drop was noted in HAMD scores, but this time the side effects were more notable in the imipramine group and about the same in the St. John's wort group.

Another St. John's wort extract (STEI, Steiner, Berlin) also compared favorably to imipramine in a recent German study.[30] In this study, patients with moderate depression were given placebo, 1,050 milligrams of St. John's wort, or 100 milligrams of imipramine per day for weeks. As was the case before, the drop in the HAMD score was almost identical for St. John's wort and imipramine. However, side effects in the St. John's group were not only significantly fewer than the imipramine group but also identical to those reported for persons taking placebo.

St. John's wort (900 milligrams per day) has also compared favorably to low-dose (75 milligrams per day) amitriptyline (Elavil®) and maprotiline (a tricyclic antidepressant used in Europe) at the same 75-milligram dose in mildly to moderately depressed people.[31,32]

While comparisons to tryicyclic antidepressants are meaningful, the big question is how does St. John's wort stack up to the SSRIs such as Prozac, Paxil, and Zoloft? While the NIH study should give us some information on how it compares against Zoloft in persons with more severe depression, one study has shown that it matches up pretty well with Prozac in elderly patients with mild to moderate depression.[33] In the study, persons ages 60 to 80 years received either 800 milligrams of St. John's wort extract (Lo-HYP 57, Dr. Loges Co., Winsen, Germany) or 20 milligrams of Prozac daily for 6 weeks. The drop in overall HAMD scores was identical for both groups, while both physician and patient ratings scored both medications equally. Side effects were a bit more similar between the two groups this time. While this outcome points to a need for greater care about side effects in elderly people taking St. John's wort, I have never heard of anyone in this age group complain of the frequent problems with sexual dysfunction (in both men and women) reported with SSRIs such as Prozac.

Finally, as discussed previously in our discussion of active constituents in St. John's wort and how it's thought to work, extracts that provide a standardized amount of hyperforin may be the wave of the future. A study found that a St. John's wort extract standardized to approximately 5 percent hyperforin (WS 5572, Schabe, Karlsruhe, Germany) was more effective in treating mild to moderate depression than another extract with only 0.5 percent hyperforin.[34] It will be interesting to see whether commercial extracts begin an exodus from declaring the percentage of hypericin on extracts and instead move toward hyperforin.

How to Use St. John's Wort

For treatment of mild to moderate depression, you may try 300 to 350 milligrams of a standardized extract three times daily. While results may be noted in as early as 2 weeks, the effectiveness of St. John's wort should be monitored for at least 4 weeks. Higher doses (up to 1,800 mg) have been used for more serious depression, but I encourage people only to consider this option after seeing their doctor.

Although I know people are out there using it for their children, St. John's wort has not been studied in kids, and thus a safe and effective dosage has not been established. If you want to use St. John's wort with your child, consult a doctor trained in herbal medicine first. I'd be very hesitant to use it in any child younger than 6 years old.[35]

While possible side effects with St. John's wort are less than those for prescription antidepressants, they're still a possibility. Clinical studies have reported mild gastrointestinal upset and an occasional skin rash as being the most common.[36] However, there have also been reports of insomnia, dry mouth, and nervousness when using the herb. The good news is that it doesn't cause the sexual side effects such as impotence seen with some prescription antidepressants.

Perhaps the most publicized side effect associated with St. John's wort is photosensitivity. Hypericin makes the skin more sensitive to sunlight and other sources of ultraviolet light, such as sun lamps. In the 1970s, the U.S. Food and Drug Administration (FDA) put an "unsafe" label on St. John's wort. This proved to be overkill. Its warning was based on grazing animals who had consumed huge amounts of St. John's wort and developed a blistering skin disease.[37] The FDA failed to consider the fact that the hypericin content of most St. John's wort extracts is quite low and that most consumers are not "grazing." One study actually took people up to a daily dose of 3,600 milligrams and noticed no increase in photosensitivity.[38] So, if you've got fair skin like me, it's good to be cautious when you spend time in the sun while taking St. John's wort. As hypericin may make your eyes (particularly the lens) more sensitive to sunlight, try to wear some cool shades, too. This is particularly applicable to you retired folks in Florida, Arizona, and California.

The German Commission E monograph for St. John's wort lists no contraindications to its use during pregnancy and lactation.[39] However, I'd like to see a few more safety studies completed on this herb before agreeing. I have had a couple of anecdotal reports of women using St. John's wort for postpartum depression with no adverse effects on the bubelah. Again, best to discuss this with your doctor before self-treating.

It's best to avoid using St. John's wort together with prescription antidepressants. A couple of case studies have suggested that St. John's wort may interact with SSRIs causing side effects (e.g., mental confusion, muscle twitching, sweating, flushing) known collectively as serotonin syndrome.[40,41]

New drug interaction issues have recently emerged for St. John's wort. Case reports and pharmacological studies from Europe and the United States are suggesting that St. John's wort reduces the absorption and blood levels of certain drugs. Among these are digoxin, cyclosporine, theophylline, and warfarin.[42,43,44,45] Recent reports also suggest that St. John's wort may lower blood levels of the AIDS drug indinavir (Crixivan™).[46]

Although far from proven, certain compounds in St. John's wort may interact with enzymes (known as *cytochrome P450 enzymes*) involved in the metabolism of drugs. If you're taking one of these medications, it's best to consult with your doctor or pharmacist before deciding to take St. John's wort. This is particularly important for persons taking antiretroviral drugs for HIV infection as well as persons taking the immunosuppressant drug cyclosporine following an organ transplant.[47]

Product update: The Lichtwer Pharma extract LI 160 is sold in the United States as Kira®. The WS 5572 hyperforin-enhanced product made by Schwabe is sold in the United States as Perika® by Nature's Way and Movana® by Pharmaton.

Related Conditions Discussed in Part 6

- Depression
- Vitiligo

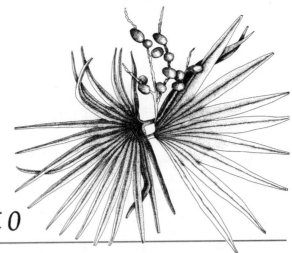

Saw Palmetto

Serenoa repens,
Sabal serrulata

Part Used
The berries of the plant

Common/Potential Use
- Benign prostatic hyperplasia (BPH)

Active Constituents
Free fatty acids and sterols as well as esters and long-chain alcohols in the berry

How It Works
The liposterolic (fat-soluble) extract of saw palmetto berries acts locally in the prostate to reduce the binding of dihydro-testeosterone in the periurethral area (the area of the prostate surrounding the urethra—the tube carrying urine from the bladder) and inhibit the production of growth factors that may contribute to BPH.

Recommended Use

Take 320 milligrams daily of a liposterolic extract rich in the fatty acids from the berry, all at once or in two separate doses.

Side Effects

Side effects are rare with use of the liposterolic extract. Mild gastrointestinal disturbances have been reported on rare occasions.

Safety Issues/Drug Interactions

There are no known contraindications to long-term use of saw palmetto extract. There are no known interactions with commonly prescribed drugs. Use of any medication for BPH should begin only after accurate medical diagnosis and under the supervision of a health care professional. Saw palmetto has not been found to interfere with correct reading of prostate-specific antigen (PSA) levels—an important laboratory marker for prostate cancer. There are no known uses for saw palmetto in women, and it has not been studied for safety during pregnancy and lactation.

BILLIONS of dollars are spent yearly in the United States to manage benign enlargement of the prostate gland, also called *benign prostatic hyperplasia,* or BPH. In Europe, herbs are approved to treat BPH, a condition that largely affects men over 50 years of age. Use of herbal extracts prepared from pygeum bark, nettle root, pumpkin seed oil, African star grass (beta-sitosterol), and saw palmetto berries has resulted in a cost-efficient and effective alternative to drug therapy for mild to moderate BPH. Without a doubt, the most widely recommended and best researched herbal medicine for BPH is a liposterolic (fat-soluble) extract from saw palmetto berries.

Plant Facts

Saw palmetto (sometimes referred to as *Sabal* in Europe) is a native of North America. Primarily found in Florida, Georgia, Louisiana, and South Carolina, it is a member of the fan palm family.[1] Also known by the Latin names *Serenoa repens* and *Sabal serrulata*, the plant grows to 2 to 7 feet tall with leaf clusters that grow to 2 feet or more. The plant produces a brownish-black berry that ripens September through December. These berries are harvested and the extracted oil is used for modern standardized liposterolic herbal supplements.

History

Historical use of saw palmetto berry can be traced to the American Indians, who used it as both a nutritional tonic and a treatment for genitourinary tract disturbances. J. B. Read of Savannah, Georgia, introduced saw palmetto into U.S. medical circles in an 1879 issue of the *American Journal of Pharmacy*.[2] Use of saw palmetto ranged from expectorant to diuretic. Under the title of *Serenoa*, it was an "official" drug in the United States from 1906 to 1950 and was used widely for a variety of genitourinary indications.[3] It was deleted from the *National Formulary* in 1950.

Modern Development

European scientists began studying saw palmetto in the 1960s and discovered that the berry contained approximately 1.5 percent fatty acids. This finding led to the creation of a liposterolic extracts that have become a commonly recommended phytomedicine for benign prostatic BPH in Europe.[4] These purified extracts contain approximately 80 to 95 percent fatty acids and sterols (including beta-sitosterol, campesterol, and stigmasterol).[5] Other constituents include esters, long-chain alcohols, and polysaccharides.

While numerous saw palmetto liposterolic extracts are available in Europe, the leader with regard to research proof is Permixon®, made by

Pierre Fabré of Paris, France. As interest continues to grow in the use of saw palmetto in the United States, we will likely see significantly more research on saw palmetto over the next few years and greater numbers of doctors recommending it for the their patients with BPH.

A BRIEF PRIMER ON BENIGN PROSTATIC HYPERPLASIA

Benign prostatic hyperplasia is a nonmalignant enlargement of the prostate. It can start in men as young as 40 years of age. However, symptoms usually do not develop until after the age of 50. According to U.S. estimates, the incidence of BPH in men 40 to 59 years of age is 50 to 60 percent. Treatment of BPH costs about $1 billion annually.[6]

Enlargement of the prostate leads to a narrowing of the outlet of the bladder, known as the urethra. This results in poor urine flow out of the bladder and a host of other signs and symptoms (known as *lower urinary tract symptoms*, or LUTS). It's interesting to note that some men over 50 actually have LUTS without the enlarged prostate, which has added some dilemma to accurate diagnosis. Please see "Male Health Conditions" in Part 6 for a more detailed discussion of BPH.

It is believed that dihydrotestosterone (DHT), an extremely active form of testosterone, is one of the culprits behind prostate enlargement. High DHT levels have been found in the prostate tissue of men with BPH.[7] High levels are also associated with increased risk of prostate cancer.

A closer look reveals the real cause of high DHT levels. An enzyme known as 5α-reductase (5-AR) converts testosterone to DHT. The activity of 5-AR increases as men age and appears to have a major influence in the development of the disease.[8]

Other hormones may also contribute to the development of BPH. These include estrogen, progesterone, and prolactin. Additionally, growth factors (basic fibroblast growth factor and epidermal growth factor) and inflammatory mediators may also play a role in BPH.

So, with all that going on in that walnut-size gland, guys, no wonder we're getting up at night!

How Saw Palmetto Works

Test tube and animal studies have suggested that saw palmetto helps reduce the contribution of male hormones to BPH.[9] This reaction appears to be due to saw palmetto's ability to reduce the action of the aforementioned enzyme known as 5-AR and its ability to reduce the binding of DHT to prostate tissue.[10,11] According to recent studies, it also helps keep those growth factors mentioned earlier in check.[12,13] This helps shift the balance back toward normal healthy prostate tissue and away from the excessive growth seen in BPH.

I wish I could stop here and tell you that this information says it all. However, there has been debate about saw palmetto's true ability to reduce 5-AR action and reduce DHT binding.[14] To avoid the really boring details and because I may need to go to the bathroom pretty soon, let me summarize by saying that research does weigh in favor of saw palmetto living up to its acclaim.[15,16] The caveat is that saw palmetto, as opposed to the drug Proscar (an aggressive 5-AR inhibitor), appears to act locally in the periurethral portion of the prostate (the area that surrounds the urethra).[17] This may partly explain why prostate size has not been dramtically decreased in clinical studies with saw palmetto but symptom relief has been significant.

According to test tube studies, the extract may also reduce the effects of estrogen and progesterone on the prostate.[18] The antiestrogenic shown directly contradicts recent suggestions that saw palmetto exerts an estrogenic effect in men. It also inhibits the effect of inflammatory substances that may contribute to BPH.[19]

Collectively, these actions make the liposterolic extract of saw palmetto berry one of the most promising interventions for BPH.

Health Care Applications

The goal of any long-term therapy for BPH is first to reduce LUTS and then worry about the size of the prostate. This leads to relief from the common signs and symptoms of BPH, such as increased frequency of urination, increased nighttime urination, dribbling after urination (that's urine, not basketballs!), decreased force and stream of urine flow, and painful urination. Numerous clinical trials have demonstrated that saw palmetto extract is effective in the management of these symptoms, with virtually no side effects. It's also a whole heck of a lot cheaper than the drugs commonly prescribed for BPH!

Optimally, men with BPH should be followed for at least 6 to 9 months to determine whether a medication is truly working on reducing BPH. While many of the early studies with saw palmetto were relatively brief, recently published studies have extended the period of observation to 6 to 12 months. Collectively, they have established saw palmetto as a safe and effective treatment for mild to moderate BPH. In fact, a systematic review of published clinical studies on saw palmetto extracts for BPH was published in the *Journal of the American Medical Association* in 1998.[12] While critical of many studies, the authors concluded that saw palmetto extracts were effective for the treatment of lower urinary tract symptoms associated with mild to moderate BPH.

The short-term studies, however, do indicate that there is a fairly quick response to saw palmetto. One 28-day study[21] with 110 BPH patients found 320 milligrams daily were effective in reducing painful urination (dysuria), nighttime urination (nocturia), and posturination residue in the bladder. There was also a significant improvement in urine flow rate. Forty-seven patients were then followed for 15 to 30 months and found to have continued improvement.

Another study found a 43 percent increase in urine flow rate after only 60 days of treatment with 320 milligrams of saw palmetto extract daily.[22] In a 12-week study, saw palmetto compared favorably with the drug prazosin, another commonly prescribed medication for BPH.[23] Finally, researchers followed 305 BPH patients taking 160 milligrams of saw palmetto extract twice daily.[24] At the end of 90 days, 88 percent of the patients rated the treatment a success. Their physician's evaluation was equally favorable. Urinary flow rate improved significantly, and there was a notable decrease in prostate size.

In the past decade, an increased number of clinical studies have been done over 6 months or longer. Three studies in particular bear mentioning. The first (and probably the best of the bunch) compared the saw palmetto extract Permixon, head-to-head (or is that prostate-to-prostate?) with Proscar®.[25] The study followed 951 men with moderate BPH taking either saw palmetto (320 milligrams per day) or Proscar (5 milligrams/day) for 6 months. At the end of the study, there was a remarkably similar decrease in lower urinary tract symptoms, including urinary frequency, nighttime urination, and painful urination. Urinary flow rates improved equally in both groups. However, side effects, including erectile dysfunction, were reported more frequently by men taking Proscar than those taking saw palmetto.

Another leading product in Europe is a combination of saw palmetto and nettle root (Prostagutt®, forte) manufactured by Schwabe (Karlsruhe, Germany). In a study similar to the one earlier, 543 men with BPH were given either Proscar (same dose as in the prior study) or the saw palmetto/nettle root combination (320 milligrams of saw palmetto and 240 milligrams of nettle root per day) for 1 year.[26] As was the case with the other study, there was a comparable drop in symptoms and similar increase in urinary flow. Again, fewer side effects (particularly erectile dysfunction) were noted in the men taking the herbal product.

A 6-month, placebo-controlled study using the saw palmetto and nettle root combination with forty men also found a significant improvement in urinary flow and a reduction in symptoms that mirrors those found earlier.[27] At the end of 6 months, those patients previously taking the placebo were switched to the herbal combination for another 6 months. Their symptoms improved significantly.

How to Use Saw Palmetto

The liposterolic extract of saw palmetto berries, rich in fatty acids and sterols, is recommended for BPH.[28] The recommended daily dose is 320 milligrams, taken in two divided doses with meals. However, two studies have suggested that a once daily dose of 320 milligrams may work equally well.[29,30] If it's working OK after a couple of weeks, I usually tell patients to use the extract for at least 6 months to determine its effectiveness. If it's working for you at that point, plan on it being a part of your ongoing, daily supplement regimen. Optimally, this decision should be made with the advice of a health care professional.

No significant side effects have been noted in clinical studies with saw palmetto extracts. Mild gastrointestinal disturbances are sometimes reported in clinical studies, although no more so than for men taking placebo. A 3-year study in Germany with 315 men taking saw palmetto (320 milligrams per day) reported only forty-six adverse events in thirty-four patients.[31] Of these, 30 percent were mild gastrointestinal complaints, and the others urological in nature (e.g., urinary tract infections, impotence). As opposed to Proscar, saw palmetto is much less likely to cause problems with erectile dysfunction.

It is important to understand that BPH can be diagnosed only by a physician. You should use saw palmetto extract only after a thorough work-up and diagnosis by your doctor. As far as I can tell, there have been no proof of any benefits of saw palmetto for women, and it certainly hasn't been proven safe during pregnancy and lactation.

The big misconception about saw palmetto bandied about in some medical circles is its potential to mask the correct reading of prostate-specific antigen (PSA)—an important laboratory marker to detect prostate cancer. Well, to put it simply, they're wrong. A test tube study found no effect of saw palmetto on PSA secretion.[32] More importantly, clinical studies have shown no effect on PSA readings after several months of using saw palmetto.[33,34,35]

Product update: The Permixon product is sold in the United States as Elusan® Prostate by Plants and Médicines, Inc. The saw palmetto and nettle root combination made by Schwabe (Karlsruhe, Germany) is sold in the United States by Nature's Way as Prostactive™.

RELATED CONDITION DISCUSSED IN PART 6

- Benign prostatic hyperplasia

Valerian

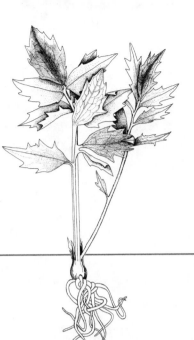

Valeriana officinalis

Part Used
  The root

Common/Potential Uses
  • Insomnia (mild to moderate)
  • Mild anxiety and conditions of restlessness

Active Constituents
  Thought to be the volatile (essential oils) in the root. Some of the volatile oil components portion of the root (e.g., valerenic acid) are occasionally used as markers for quality control during extraction.

How It Works
  Valerian root exerts a mild sedating effect on the central nervous system. It improves the ability of a person to get to sleep and sleep more soundly.

Recommended Use

Concentrated root extract (5:1) containing no less than 0.5 percent volatile oils—300 to 500 milligrams 30 to 60 minutes before bedtime. For anxiety, add a morning dose of 300 milligrams. Alternatively, one may take 2 to 3 grams of unconcentrated powdered root in capsule or 3 to 5 milliliters of a valerian root tincture.

Side Effects

Research has indicated minimal side effects using valerian. A small percentage of persons using the extract may experience mild, transient stomach upset.

Safety Issues/Drug Interactions

Persons currently taking sedative drugs, antianxiety medication, or antidepressants should take valerian only under the supervision of a health care professional. European monographs list no contraindication to use of valerian root during pregnancy or lactation. It should not be used in children under the age of 3 years. Used at the doses listed here, valerian does not lead to dependence or potential addiction. Although some studies suggest no impairment of reaction time following use of valerian, one should use valerian cautiously during the day if driving or operating machinery.

SLEEPING well is an elusive goal for millions of Americans. While a class of drugs known as benzodiazepines (e.g., Valium® and Xanax®) have proven useful in the treatment of severe cases of insomnia and anxiety, they can cause addiction and serious side effects, including withdrawal symptoms. Clearly, there is a need for gentler, nonaddictive medicines for these conditions—particularly in less severe forms of these conditions. There's also a need for alternatives to those over-the-counter sleep aids such as Sominex® and Unisom®. These are simply decongestants and are as safe for long-term use as valerian. For your guys over 50 years old that may have prostate problems, these over-the-counter sleep aids are a definite no-no.

Extracts of valerian root, often in combination with one or two other mild plant sedatives, are often prescribed in Europe as a substitute for benzodiazepines or over-the-counter sleep preparations for the treatment of mild to moderate insomnia and sometimes mild anxiety.

Paired with the historical use of the plant in the United States for insomnia, valerian has become a well-researched herbal sedative that promises to increase in popularity over the next decade.

PLANT FACTS

Valerian is the common name given to the genus *Valeriana*, which encompasses 200 species. In herbal medicine, the species of valerian most commonly used is *Valeriana officinalis*, an upright perennial that grows wild in woodlands, along river banks, and in damp meadows all over Europe. Most of the plants used for medicinal extracts are cultivated. As mentioned earlier, the root of the plant has the sedating properties and is used in herbal preparations.

HISTORY

Our old friend and Greek physician Dioscorides rears his herbal head again! He recommended valerian for a host of medical problems including digestive problems, nausea, liver problems, and even urinary tract disorders. Galen (131–201 A.D.) was the first to note the use of valerian as a treatment for insomnia.

Use of valerian for insomnia and nervous conditions gained momentum in the late sixteenth century. By the eighteenth century, it was an accepted sedative and also used for nervous disorders associated with a restless digestive tract. It was also recommended for a nervous condition in women, referred to as "vapors." This label referred to a hysterical condition involving noises in the head, chills, impatience, and involuntary movements.[1] Use of the label faded away when they figured it was the sexist doctors who were really full of vapors—primarily hot air!

Valerian was listed in medical textbooks in both the United States and England until the 1940s. Currently, it is an approved over-the-counter medicine for insomnia in Germany, Belgium, France, Switzerland, and Italy.[2]

MODERN DEVELOPMENT

Research in Europe led to the discovery that the root of valerian contains volatile oils that may contribute to the sedating properties of the plant. Even though research has pointed to the contribution of constituents known as *valepotriates,* most European medicinal preparations currently focus on the volatile oil content and constituents of these oils such as valerenic acid. This is partially because valepotriates are very unstable chemicals and are unlikely to be present in finished products. According to the standards developed in herbal monographs, the current concentrated extracts contain a minimum volatile (essential) oil content of 0.5 percent.[3]

Combining valerian root with other mildly sedating herbs is common in both Europe and the United States. Chamomile, hops (not the ninety-nine bottles of beer on the wall!), passion flower, and lemon balm are popular choices. Another popular development in Europe has been the creation of odor-controlled valerian root products. For those of you who have had the pleasure of smelling the typical valerian root product, the applause is deafening. For those of you who don't know what I'm talking about, let me just say three words: "old gym socks."

HOW VALERIAN WORKS

Even though studies in the early to mid-1980s found valerian to be an effective treatment for insomnia, no one really knew why it worked. This changed in 1989 when J. Holzl and P. Godau of the Institute of Pharmaceutical Biology (Marburg, Germany) demonstrated that valerian weakly binds the same receptors in the brain as benzodiazepines.[4] In test tube studies, they found that valerian displaced benzodiazepines off these receptor sites.

Follow-up test studies were able to show that constituents of valerian root actually bind $GABA_A$ receptors and influence the uptake and release of GABA in rat brains (OK, we're going to stop the snooze-inducing scientific facts soon!).[5,6] Sedation in the central nervous system and brain is partly regulated by these receptors. Benzodiazepines and barbiturates are known to act on these receptors.

Before you drag this book to the fireplace for recommending something that acts like benzodiazepines and barbiturates, let me finish! The active compounds in valerian *weakly* bind these receptors when compared to drugs like Valium and Xanax. While this activity helps us at least partially understand valerian's action as a sedative, it still lets valerian off the hook as a potential addictive substance. This also makes it an intriguing therapeutic choice for those trying to withdraw from benzodiazepines (discussed later).

HEALTH CARE APPLICATIONS

INSOMNIA

Population surveys have found that approximately one-third of the adult population suffers from initial sleep disorders.[7] While famous insomniacs like Philip Marlowe have turned the condition to their advantage, most people suffer in their personal and professional lives when sleep deprived.

If it works, valerian root makes getting to sleep easier. It increases deep and restful sleep. Best of all, it doesn't cause any morning "hangover"—a side effect common to prescription sleep drugs. As is the case with many treatments for mild to moderate insomnia, the research results have been varied.

In the early to mid-1980s, research completed at the Nestlé Research Laboratories in Switzerland proved the ability of valerian to help a person both get to sleep easier and have a deeper, more restful night's sleep. Concentrated valerian root extract (approximately 3:1) doses of 400 to

450 milligrams helped participants get to sleep quicker and reduced night awakenings. Dream recall was also increased the following day with no morning hangover.[8,9] Unfortunately, chocolate won out, and the jingle "N-E-S-T-L-E-S, Nestlé makes the very best valerian" was never heard.

In another study, taking place at home and later in a sleep laboratory, healthy volunteers were given either 450 or 900 milligrams of a concentrated valerian root extract (approximately 3:1) 30 minutes before bedtime in the home study and only the 900-milligrams dose or placebo in the laboratory study.[10] Paradoxically, the 900-milligram dose seemed to have a somewhat better effect on helping people get to sleep faster and achieve deeper sleep in the study done in the home. At the sleep lab, this dose was not any better than placebo on any of the test parameters.

Based on the negative results found in this study and the use of healthy volunteers instead of persons with insomnia, Dr. Schulz and colleagues in Berlin decided to retest valerian in a group of poor sleepers.[11] For the small study, they chose fourteen elderly women with insomnia. Volunteers received either 450 milligrams of concentrated valerian root extract (approximately 6:1) or placebo three times per day for 7 days. While there was some effect on total sleep time in the first night, analysis at the end of the study showed very little effect for valerian on sleep.

Other studies have found varied success using valerian combined with other herbs. A Swedish study examined the effect of a valerian root combined with lemon balm and hops (in a capsule, not a beer bottle!).[12] Twenty-seven people with sleep disorders were given either one tablet of the combination product (containing 400 milligrams of a valerian root extract) or a weaker preparation containing only 4 milligrams of valerian. Eighty-nine percent of the people taking the full-strength combination reported better sleep; 44 percent reported "perfect" sleep. Nightmares, frequent among many of the patients previously taking prescription sedatives, were nonexistent.

A small German study[13] compared the effect of a combination product (Euvegal® forte) containing a concentrated extract (4.5:1) of valerian root (320 milligrams at bedtime) and extract of lemon balm (*Melissa officinalis*) with the benzodiazepine Halcion. Sleep was monitored for nine nights. The herbal duo matched Halcion in boosting the ability to get to sleep, as well as the quality of sleep in persons with poor sleep. However, the Halcion group reported the old hangover and loss of concentration the next day. People taking the valerian/lemon balm combination reported no negative effect on their daily routine.

The same combination of valerian and lemon balm was compared to placebo in sixty-eight women (ages 22 to 87 years) with insomnia for 14 days.[14] The women were asked to take two tablets (equal to 320 milligrams of valerian root extract and 160 milligrams of lemon balm extract) twice daily, in the morning and before bedtime. The quality of sleep for those women taking the valerian/lemon balm combination was significantly improved at the end of 2 weeks. This effect actually continued for another week after the women stopped the herbal combination! Doctors monitoring the women gave high marks for the herbal combination's ability to reduce the severity of insomnia. Side effects were rare, with eight women taking the valerian/lemon balm combination complaining of nausea, stomach upset, or mild headache.

On the basis of these reports and regular medical use, valerian has become the natural medicine treatment of choice for people suffering from mild insomnia in both Europe and the United States. Valerian's nonaddictive properties make it a logical alternative to the potentially addictive drugs commonly prescribed for sleep in this country and the over-the-counter sleep medications that are simple antihistamines. However, larger, well-designed studies are necessary to give us a better understanding of what dose of valerian works best and how long it's effective.

ANXIETY

It's hard to avoid stress and the anxiety it breeds in our culture. Successfully dealing with anxiety includes stress reduction, proper diet, and support for the adrenal glands. In recent years, kava has emerged as the leading herbal alternative for the treatment of less severe cases of anxiety. Valerian may prove to be a useful back-up for some persons.

One 14-day study with 100 patients suffering from moderate anxiety found that taking a combination of valerian root extract (50 milligrams) and St. John's wort extract (100 milligrams) twice daily compared favorably to low-dose valium for reduction of anxiety.[15] Some patients found that a double dose (100 milligrams of valerian and 200 milligrams of St. John's wort twice daily) was even more effective during the second week. Only 4 percent of people taking the herbal combination complained of dizziness or daytime sedation compared to 14 percent in the Valium group (they also suffered from a strong desire to watch *Valley of the Dolls*).

I've had excellent success using valerian with a number of patients attempting to withdraw from the drug Xanax. Use of valerian at the tail end of the withdrawal process seems to ease the usual withdrawal symptoms and ease the transition off the drug.[16] I will sometimes switch patients over to kava following withdrawal, although some have found ongoing use of valerian to be helpful. I do not advocate the use of kava together with benzodiazepines such as Xanax. Please remember that withdrawal from these medications should only be done under the supervision of a health care professional. Also keep in mind that if you're using valerian or valerian combinations for mild anxiety, the norm is to take it during the morning and before bed at night.

How to Use Valerian

For insomnia, I like to recommend 300 to 500 milligrams of a concentrated (5:1) valerian root extract 1/2 to 1 hour before bedtime. Try to use extracts that contain at least 0.5 percent volatile oils. This will often be designated as a percentage of valerenic acid—one of the key volatile oil constituents. Alternatively, you may choose to use an unconcentrated form of the dried root in capsule form (remember the smell!). The German Commission E monograph recommends 2 to 3 grams if you take valerian this way.[17] As a third alternative, you can also take 3 to 5 milliliters of a tincture. Combination products with lemon balm, hops, and skullcap can also be used. Children ranging in age from 3 to 12 years will usually respond to one-half to three-fourths the adult dose. Valerian is not recommended for children under the age of 3 years.[18]

For mild anxiety, a morning dose of 300 milligrams is recommended in addition to the bedtime dosage listed earlier. I sometimes like to use valerian combined with passion flower for daytime management of mild anxiety.

The current German Commission E monograph on valerian root lists no contraindications on its use during pregnancy or lactation.[19] Avoid taking it with alcohol. Although recent research indicates that valerian does not impair your ability to drive or operate machinery,[20] be cautious if you take valerian during the day as it may cause drowsiness in some persons. Use of valerian root products at the dosages listed here should not lead to addiction or dependence. There are no known drug interactions with valerian.

Product update: The valerian/lemon balm combination (Euvegal® forte) made by Schwabe (Karlsruhe, Germany) is sold in the United States by Nature's Way under the trade name of Valerian Nighttime®.

Related Conditions Discussed in Part 6

- Anxiety
- Insomnia

Vitex
agnus-castus

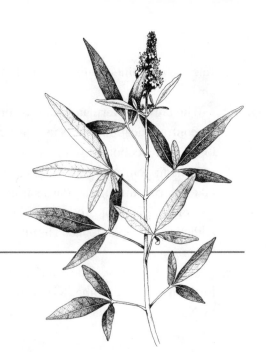

Chaste tree, Chasteberry,
Monk's pepper

Part Used
The ripe, dried fruit

Common/Potential Uses
- Premenstrual syndrome (PMS)
- Breast tenderness/pain associated with the menstrual cycle
- Amenorrhea (lack of menses)
- Infertility

How It Works
Vitex stimulates the pituitary gland to produce more luteinizing hormone, which leads to greater production of progesterone during the second half (luteal phase) of a woman's cycle. Vitex also reduces high levels of prolactin in the second half of the menstrual cycle.

Recommended Use

Dried or liquid preparations delivering 30 to 40 milligrams of the crushed fruit daily. Use vitex over a period of several months continuously. Once improvement occurs, continue treatment for an additional 4 to 6 weeks.

Side Effects

Side effects are rare using vitex. Minor gastrointestinal upset and a mild skin rash with itching have been reported in less than 2 percent of the women monitored while taking vitex.

Safety Issues/Drug Interactions

Vitex is not recommended for use during pregnancy. It should not be taken together with hormone therapy.

NATURAL therapies have made a dramatic contribution to women's health care. Growing numbers of women are opting for safe and effective natural medicines to manage gynecological conditions for which drugs offer short-term relief but threaten long-term health. This is particularly true for women with menstrual abnormalities stemming from hormonal imbalances. Nutritional and herbal interventions such as vitamin B_6, magnesium, vitamin E, black cohosh, dong quai, and evening primrose oil offer relief for women with menstrual cycle abnormalities such as premenstrual syndrome.

The unique ability of vitex to correct female hormonal imbalances in a gentle manner makes it effective against premenstrual syndrome, amenorrhea (lack of a period), and even infertility.

PLANT FACTS

Vitex agnus-castus, also known as chaste tree, is a shrub with finger-shaped leaves and slender violet flowers. The plant grows in creek beds and on river banks in valleys and lower foothills in the Mediterranean and central Asia. The plant blooms in high summer. After pollination, it develops dark brown to black fruit the size of a peppercorn. The fruit possesses a pepperlike aroma and flavor. The ripe, dried fruit of *Vitex agnus-castus* is the part of the plant used in medicinal preparations today.

HISTORY

Vitex belongs to the official plants of antiquity (although I'm not sure whether it was ever featured on *American Bandstand*). Hippocrates, Dioscorides, and Theophrast mention the use of the plant in their writings. In the fourth century B.C., Hippocrates wrote that vitex was effective for a wide variety of conditions, including hemorrhaging following childbirth, and also assisted with the "passing of afterbirth." Decoctions of the fruit and plant were also used in sitz baths for diseases of the uterus.

Vitex was also believed to inspire chastity. This is the source of one of its common names—"chaste tree." This name partially developed from the ancient Greeks, who used it in festivals honoring the goddess Demeter. During the festival, young women were expected to refrain from sexual activity and were adorned with blossoms of vitex to demonstrate their chastity.

The Christian church in Europe later developed a variation on this theme by placing the blossoms along the path leading to the monastery at the initiation of novice monks. The vitex blossoms supposedly suppressed libido and served as a deterrent to the temptation to run off to town and lose one's monkhood! Monks were also responsible for another common name for vitex—"monk's pepper." This name is derived from the fact that the fruits, which taste and smell like pepper, were commonly used as seasoning by the chef in residence at the monastery.[1]

Modern Development

Modern medical work with vitex began with the introduction of a concentrated extract of the dried vitex fruit in the 1950s. Produced by Madaus of Cologne, Germany, the extract (Agnolyt®) was concentrated so that 100 milliliters of the solution contained 9 grams of the fruit. This is the form that has been employed in modern clinical research. Another European vitex-based product (Mastodynon®) has also been the focus of many studies—particularly in the area of prolactin inhibition and the treatment of breast pain associated with a woman's menstrual cycle.

The German Commission E monograph (see Part 2 for an explanation of the German monograph system) lists the whole extract as "medicinally active."[2] This term implies a cooperative effort among the different components of the fruit. Contrast this with an herbal extract such as milk thistle, which has very specific active compounds.

A Brief Primer on Luteal Phase Defect

If you are a woman with menstrual cycle irregularities or imbalances, there's a good chance you're not producing enough progesterone during the second phase of your cycle (also known as the *luteal phase*). This means that estrogen, the dominant female hormone during the first phase of the cycle (*follicular phase*), continues to dominate the second half. The result leads to a shortening (by as much as 50 percent) of the luteal phase, or "luteal phase defect."

The net effect of luteal phase defect and low progesterone production is a host of menstrual cycle abnormalities. These include heavy periods (hypermenorrhea), abnormally frequent periods (polymenorrhea), and also lack of menstruation (amenorrhea). Luteal phase defect may also contribute to premenstrual syndrome.[3]

Another problem frequently found with luteal phase defect is overproduction of the pituitary hormone prolactin. Prolactin, which assists with lactation in nursing mothers, has been shown to be abnormally elevated in 70 percent of women with luteal phase defect.[4] High levels of prolactin in the latter part of a woman's cycle can lead to breast tenderness and pain. More important, high levels are associated with infertility in some instances.

HOW VITEX WORKS

Vitex does not contain hormones. Its benefits stem from its actions on the pituitary gland.[5] Vitex increases the pituitary's production of the regulating hormone luteinizing hormone (LH).[6] LH boosts the secretion of progesterone during the luteal phase. The resulting increase in progesterone production leads to a normal balance between estrogen and progesterone and a normal two-phase cycle.

Vitex also keeps prolactin secretion in check.[7] This effect appears to be modulated by the ability of vitex to bind to dopamine receptors and thus inhibit prolactin release.[8] This action is an important focal point of the success of vitex in the treatment of breast pain and swelling associated with the menstrual cycle, and often a component of PMS.

HEALTH CARE APPLICATIONS

PREMENSTRUAL SYNDROME AND CYCLICAL BREAST PAIN

Following more than 1,500 women for an average of 166 days, a survey of gynecology practices in Germany[9] found vitex to be a valuable treatment for premenstrual syndrome (PMS). Women were placed on a daily dose of 40 drops of a vitex liquid extract (Agnolyt), taken once in the morning with some water. The success of treatment with vitex was determined through questionnaires given to both gynecologists and their patients.

Physicians rated the treatment as very good or good 92 percent of the time. Fifty-seven percent of the patients reported improvement, while another 33 percent had complete symptom relief. Mild side effects (mild upset stomach and short-term skin rash with itching) were reported in only 2 percent of the women. These results have been verified in another study with PMS sufferers.[10]

Another study with women suffering from PMS found that vitex matched up very well with the ol' standby vitamin B_6 in the reduction of symptoms.[11] One hundred seventy-five women were given either vitex (approximately 30 to 40 milligrams per day in capsule form) or 200 milligrams of vitamin B_6 for three consecutive menstrual cycles. At the end of the study, women in both groups and their doctors reported success. However, the vitex group reported a greater decrease in overall symptoms and specifically breast tenderness, bloating, and depression. Thirty-six percent of the women taking vitex reported being symptom-free at the end of three cycles, compared to 21 percent of women taking vitamin B_6.

Another benefit for women taking vitex for PMS has been reduced cyclical breast pain, a result of elevated prolactin and possibly progesterone levels.[12] A liquid product known as Mastodynon® (Bionorica, Neumarkt, Germany) combines 32.4 milligrams of vitex with assorted homeopathic ingredients. The product (not yet available in the United States) has been widely researched for cyclical breast pain[13] and is approved in Germany and other countries specifically for that indication. Expect the same three or four cycles for vitex to work for this condition as well. It may be interesting for women with cyclical breast pain to use vitex and evening primrose oil together.

SECONDARY AMENORRHEA AND INFERTILITY

Research and clinical experience have also pointed to vitex as useful in a host of other menstrual cycle imbalances and irregularities. These include amenorrhea (no menstrual cycle at all) and some cases of infertility. In one study, ten of fifteen women with secondary amenorrhea began having a normal period after 6 months of treatment with vitex.[14] Hormone measures indicated a rise in progesterone and LH levels.

Vitex has also shown some promise in the treatment of infertility—particularly those cases with established luteal phase defect and high prolactin levels. Forty-eight women diagnosed with infertility, 23 to 39 years of age, were given vitex once daily for 3 months.[15] Forty-five women completed the study.

Seven women became pregnant during the study. In twenty-five women, progesterone levels were restored to normal—a factor that bodes well for potential pregnancy. Seven women had a rise in serum progesterone that did not reach normal levels during the 3 months of treatment.

However, the upward trend in their progesterone levels probably means they'd achieve normal levels in another two to three cycles.

A double-blind, placebo-controlled study with eighty-nine women with infertility, luteal phase defect, or secondary amenorrhea looked at the effect off Mastodynon® on progesterone, LH, prolactin, and conception rates over a 3-month span.[16] Of the sixty-six women evaluated at the end of the study, thirty-one had normal hormone values. More important, fifteen women (seven with amenorrhea, four with infertility, and seven with luteal phase defect) conceived during the 3-month study.

High Prolactin Levels

As mentioned previously, vitex exerts a modulating effect on prolactin levels in the body. One study found that vitex was able to lower levels after 3 months of use.[17] It is interesting that the fifty-two women in this study also had luteal phase defect. A lengthening of the luteal phase and increased progesterone were also noted. No side effects were noted, and two women actually became pregnant during the study. Please remember that vitex is not a substitute for drugs such as bromocriptine that are used in severe cases of hyperprolactinemia, which are often secondary to a pituitary tumor.

How to Use Vitex

With its emphasis on long-term balancing of a woman's hormonal system, vitex is not a fast-acting medication. If you have PMS or frequent or heavy periods, use vitex continuously for 4 to 6 months. Women with amenorrhea and infertility should remain on vitex for at least 12 to 18 months unless pregnancy occurs during treatment. Vitex should not be used once a woman becomes pregnant. Use of vitex with hormone therapy is not recommended. Because of its actions on dopamine receptors, vitex is probably best avoided during lactation.

The best news for women taking vitex is the one-a-day dosage. The recommended daily dose is an encapsulated or liquid product delivering 30 to 40 milligrams of the dried fruit daily.[18] Take this dose first thing in the morning with some liquid. Some women may experience increased menstrual flow for the first couple of periods while using vitex. This effect will usually stop by the third or fourth cycle.

While there are no known drug interactions with vitex, it is probably best to avoid using it with drugs that block dopamine receptors, including haloperidol.

Product update: Agnolyt (Madaus AG, Cologne, Germany) is available from Nature's Way under the trade name Femaprin™.

RELATED CONDITIONS DISCUSSED IN PART 6

- Acne
- Fibrocystic breast disease/cyclical breast pain
- Infertility
- Premenstrual syndrome

part 6

HERBAL PRESCRIPTIONS FOR COMMON HEALTH CONDITIONS

REMEMBER all that stuff I told you at the beginning of Part 5? Well, it's applicable here, too. Many of the conditions that we're about to discuss require accurate medical diagnosis and careful monitoring by your doctor. Many of them may also require a combination of standard medical treatment along with your complete natural health care plan.

This section is organized by body system. So, if you're having problems with angina, look under "Cardiovascular System." If you have diabetes, refer to the appropriate section under "Endocrine System."

Each section (with the exception of a few miscellaneous conditions) begins with a brief description of the condition and then offers herbal prescriptions to consider. The "Herbal Prescriptions" section is reserved for those herbs that I highly recommend. My recommendations are based on research and history of effective use for that particular ailment. Herbs under "Other Herbal Considerations" either support the primary herbal prescriptions or warrant some mention because of traditional use.

I've also added sections on nutritional supplements, diet, and lifestyle. The "Nutritional Supplement Considerations" section includes key vitamins, minerals, or other dietary supplements you should consider adding to your comprehensive natural health care program. I've tried to supply you with one or two key references for each recommendation. Please note that this presentation is not intended to be a complete overview of the nutritional research literature.

In both the nutrition and herbal suggestions, I've added research references for all entries except those herbs that have already been mentioned in Part 5.

The recommendations offered here are not an exhaustive overview of all complementary or alternative therapies. They represent my attempt to offer what I think are some good options. For a thorough look at natural medicine approaches to various conditions, please see *The Natural Pharmacy,* second edition (Prima Health and Healthnotes, 1999). Alternatively, you can get the same information on CD-ROM by purchasing *The Natural Pharmacy: Complete Home Reference to Natural Medicine* (Healthnotes, 1999).

A good diet and positive lifestyle changes (e.g., stress reduction and exercise) are the cornerstone of any wellness program. Although herbal treatments can play a critical part in your attempt to get well, how you eat and live your life should form the foundation of your wellness program.

Cardiovascular System

ATHEROSCLEROSIS (PREVENTION)

Atherosclerosis, the primary villain in most major cardiovascular disease, contributes to angina, congestive heart failure, and intermittent claudication. It also may contribute to strokes as well as some of the mental decline we associate with aging. So, even though it's not first alphabetically, we need to talk about it first.

Let's start with arteriosclerosis. *Arteriosclerosis* is a hardening of the arteries. The hardening results when the arteries lose their elasticity and begin to thicken. This condition leads to narrowed arteries and less blood flow to many parts of the body.

When fatty plaques build up on the walls of these narrowed arteries, we call it *atherosclerosis*. If blood vessels that supply the heart (coronary arteries) become atherosclerotic, the condition is known as *coronary artery disease* (CAD). Coronary artery disease contributes to angina, congestive heart failure, and even heart attacks.

You've all been beaten over the head with some of the requirements for reducing your risk of atherosclerosis. Diet, exercise, and stress reduction all are important tools for reducing risk. Herbs, particularly those that are a common part of our normal diets, also play a key role in reducing your risk.

By altering your eating habits and lifestyle and using prudent supplementation as described further on in this chapter, you'll:

- reduce the levels of cholesterol and triglycerides in the bloodstream,
- reduce the "stickiness" of platelets in the blood,
- improve the strength of blood vessel walls,
- reduce homocysteine levels,
- improve the flow of blood through the body, and
- provide antioxidant protection to the cardiovascular system.

The payoff: a reduced risk of atherosclerosis.

HERBS AND HERBAL CONSTITUENTS THAT MAY REDUCE YOUR RISK OF ATHEROSCLEROSIS
Bilberry
Bioflavonoids (including quercetin and oligomeric procyanidins)
Evening primrose
Fenugreek
Garlic (along with bioflavonoids, this may be your best herbal/dietary deterrent to atherosclerosis)
Ginger
Ginkgo biloba
Ginseng
Green tea
Guggul
Hawthorn
Psyllium
Red yeast rice
Resveratrol
Rosemary
Turmeric

NUTRITIONAL SUPPLEMENTS THAT REDUCE YOUR RISK OF ATHEROSCLEROSIS

Vitamin C
Vitamin E
Vitamin B_6
Vitamin B_{12}
Folic acid

Note: Folic acid and vitamins B_6, and B_{12} reduce the level of homocysteine; a high homocysteine level is associated with increased risk of cardiovascular disease.

Niacin
Selenium
Carotenoids such as lycopene
Carnitine
Essential fatty acids (e.g., evening primrose oil and fish oil)

Note: For more specific recommendations, please see the "Hyperlipidemia" section.

DIETARY RECOMMENDATIONS THAT REDUCE YOUR RISK OF ATHEROSCLEROSIS

- Increase your intake of complex carbohydrates from vegetables, grains, and fruit sources. This diet will provide you with more dietary fiber and valuable antioxidants such as flavonoids and carotenoids.
- Reduce your dietary fat from animal sources. This includes red meat and milk. Some kinds of fats are healthier than others. Avoid heating polyunsaturated fats that may be transformed to saturated fats. A good bet is to cook with olive oil, which doesn't change when heated. The fat from fish and nuts is also preferable.
- Reduce food that contains trans fatty acids (margarine, some vegetable oils, and many processed foods containing vegetable oils).

- Increase your dietary sources of the herbs listed earlier. These include garlic and ginger. Also, don't forget turmeric, onions, and green tea.

LIFESTYLE CONSIDERATIONS THAT WILL REDUCE YOUR RISK OF ATHEROSCLEROSIS

Stress Reduction

Seek an outlet for your frustrations and anger so your cardiovascular system doesn't have to bear the brunt. Above all, try to avoid writing any lengthy herb books!

Regular Exercise

Regular exercise helps work off stress and also keeps weight down. Best of all, it strengthens and builds up the efficiency of your cardiovascular system.

ANGINA

Atherosclerosis can disrupt blood flow to many parts of the body. When it harms the arteries that supply the heart muscle (the coronary arteries), a lack of oxygen to the heart results. This leads to *angina*—a squeezing or pressurelike pain in the chest.

Angina attacks are most common during exercise, when the heart is forced to work harder. Stress can also bring on an attack. In addition to pressure in the chest, pain may radiate to the left shoulder and arm. Angina can sometimes be a warning sign of a heart attack.

Angina caused by atherosclerosis occurs most commonly; this type is called *secondary angina*. Another, less common form of angina results from spasms of the coronary arteries. Known as *primary* or *Prinzmetal's variant angina*, this form commonly occurs when a person is at rest.

When angina becomes more severe, drug therapy is usually needed. with medications such as nitroglycerin, beta-blockers, and calcium channel blockers. These relieve symptoms but do not address the key problem, which is insufficient blood flow to the heart muscle.

Herbal and nutrient interventions work best in the early stages of angina. By increasing blood flow to the heart muscle and improving the work efficiency of the heart, they may actually slow the progression of angina.

HERBAL PRESCRIPTION

- Hawthorn extract (standardized to 18.75 percent oligomeric procyanidins or 2.2 percent flavonoids)—160 to 900 milligrams daily in two to three divided doses. Individuals initially requiring more intensive treatment should use the higher end of the dosage range.
  Action: Increases blood flow and oxygen to the heart muscle

OTHER HERBAL CONSIDERATIONS

See the recommendations listed under "Atherosclerosis (Prevention)."

NUTRITIONAL SUPPLEMENT CONSIDERATIONS

- Coenzyme Q_{10}—100 to 150 milligrams daily in two to three divided doses[1]
- L-Carnitine—1 gram two to three times daily[2,3]
- Vitamin E—300 to 400 IU daily[4]
- Magnesium—300 milligrams twice daily[5] (*Note:* This dosage is only an educated guess, as the studies on magnesium for angina have used an intravenous form.)

DIETARY RECOMMENDATIONS

See the recommendations under "Atherosclerosis (Prevention)."

LIFESTYLE CONSIDERATIONS AND OTHER ALTERNATIVE THERAPIES

Stress reduction is critical. Try yoga, meditation, or biofeedback. Settle on a method of relaxing that works for you and stick with it. I like listening to *Kind of Blue* by Miles Davis.

Regular exercise is important, but ease into it. Too much, too soon can worsen the problem. Try reducing caffeine consumption and stopping smoking.

Acupuncture has been shown in some studies to help persons with angina reduce their symptoms as well as their medication.[6] One study found the combination of acupuncture, Shiatsu massage, and lifestyle changes a very promising therapy.[7]

BRUISING

If you're a perfectly healthy person who suddenly begins to develop bruises on the thighs, buttocks, or upper arms, it may be that your small blood vessels (primarily the capillaries) are fragile. It's not uncommon for people experiencing such bruising to seek the help of their doctor, only to be told that there's nothing wrong—just avoid bumping into things and take aspirin. Easy bruising does not mean you've got a terrible bleeding disorder.

Easy bruising is often more noticeable with aging. The capillaries become more fragile, and pressure on the skin is more likely to create a bruise. In older individuals, these bruises may linger longer than in younger people. Again, this is not a serious medical condition.

HERBAL PRESCRIPTIONS
- Bilberry extract—80 to 160 milligrams three times daily
  Actions: Strengthens and stabilizes the walls of the blood vessels such as capillaries
- Grape seed extract (high in oligomeric procyanidins [OPCs]—50 milligrams two times daily[1]
  Actions: Similar to those shown for bilberry

OTHER HERBAL CONSIDERATIONS
You can choose from a host of flavonoid products, including rutin, quercetin, hesperidin, and pycnogenol; these are all excellent options. Like bilberry, these compounds will assist in strengthening blood vessels. Remember, it's best to use flavonoids together with vitamin C. A recent example from the medical literature found success combining 1,000 milligrams of vitamin C and 1,000 mg of rutoside (a type of rutin) daily in three women with progressive pigmented purpurea—a form of progres-

sive bruising that is difficult to treat and tough on the person cosmeti-
cally.[2] This approach led to improvement in 2 weeks and complete resolu-
tion of bruising within 4 weeks in all three women!

NUTRITIONAL SUPPLEMENT CONSIDERATION
- Vitamin C (preferably with bioflavonoids)—500 to 1,000 milligrams
  twice daily

DIETARY RECOMMENDATIONS
Increase your intake foods high in flavonoids, such as green tea,
onions, blueberries, cherries, and apples.

CHRONIC VENOUS INSUFFICIENCY

Many people will complain of a feeling of heaviness and swelling around
their calves, ankles, and feet after standing all day. This sometimes can be
an early warning of chronic venous insufficiency (CVI). This condition
can result from the valves in the veins of the legs failing to hold blood
back against gravity, which leads to sluggish flow of blood through the
veins in the lower leg. The swelling and dull ache are the common symptoms of the early stages of CVI. As it progresses, the skin can often darken
in the lower legs and skin ulcers can occur. CVI sometimes follows varicose veins. The following recommendations may also reduce your risk or
help manage varicose veins.

HERBAL PRESCRIPTIONS
- Horse chestnut seed extract (standardized to 16 to 21 percent
  aescin)—One capsule of the extract containing 50 milligrams of aescin
  twice daily
  Actions: Aescin helps improve the tone of the veins for more efficient
  blood flow. It also strengthens capillaries so swelling is reduced.
- Grape seed extract (high in oligomeric procyanidins [OPCs])—150 to
  300 milligrams daily in two to three divided doses[1]

Actions: As is the case with other flavonoids, OPCs help strengthen the walls of blood vessels, including capillaries, improving blood flow and reducing swelling.

OTHER HERBAL CONSIDERATIONS

- Butcher's broom—Standardized extract delivering 15 to 30 milligrams of ruscogenins (the active constituents in butcher's broom) three times daily[2]
- Flavonoids—In Europe there have been studies on synthesized rutin known as "oxerutins."[3] While naturally occurring flavonoids such as rutin or quercetin have not been studied, they are known to strengthen capillaries and improve blood vessel tone—important features for managing CVI.

LIFESTYLE CONSIDERATIONS

Try to avoid sitting or standing in one place for prolonged periods of time. Put some Sly and the Family Stone on and dance or get involved in regular aerobic exercise such as walking or jogging. Regular massage on the legs may also help.

CONGESTIVE HEART FAILURE

When a weakened heart fails to provide adequate blood flow to the extremities of the body, the condition is called *congestive heart failure* (CHF). A number of factors can lead to CHF, including a history of heart attack(s). As the condition progresses, fluid can accumulate in the lungs and around the ankles. Once the condition reaches this stage, the prognosis is poor.

The New York Heart Association has defined four stages of CHF. Medical treatment is sometimes reserved for Stages III and IV. Digitalis is a common treatment in these later stages. Table 6.1 lists the four stages and their characteristics.

How about Stages I and II? Typically, treatment is not recommended during these stages, owing to the potential side effects of digitalis. This is where herbal and nutritional interventions play an important role. By

Table 6.1
STAGES OF CONGESTIVE HEART FAILURE AS DEFINED
BY THE NEW YORK HEART ASSOCIATION

Stage	Symptoms
Stage I	Patient is symptom free when at rest and on treatment.
Stage II	Patient experiences impaired heart function with moderate physical effort. Shortness of breath with exertion is common. There are no symptoms at rest.
Stage III	Even minor physical exertion results in shortness of breath and fatigue. There are no symptoms at rest.
Stage IV	Symptoms such as shortness of breath and fluid around the ankles (edema) are present when the patient is at rest.

improving the heart's efficiency in supplying blood to the body and by enhancing circulation to the extremities, natural medicines offer an opportunity to slow the progression of CHF and improve a person's quality of life.

HERBAL PRESCRIPTION

- Hawthorn extract (standardized to 18.75 percent oligomeric procyanidins or 2.2 percent flavonoids)—160 to 900 milligrams daily in two to three divided doses. Individuals requiring more intensive treatment initially should use the higher end of the dosage range.
  Actions: Hawthorn improves the efficiency of the heart muscle, which means greater blood flow throughout the body. It also reduces the resistance to blood flow in the blood vessels of the extremities of the body.

NUTRITIONAL SUPPLEMENT CONSIDERATIONS

- Coenzyme Q_{10}— 90 to 150 milligrams daily in two to three divided doses[1,2]
- Propionyl-L-Carnitine—500 milligrams three times daily[3,4]

- Taurine—2 grams three times daily[5]

  Note: This one's expensive. I usually start my CHF patients on Hawthorn and coenzyme Q_{10} with carnitine as a third option.
- Magnesium—300 to 400 milligrams daily in two divided doses[6]

  Note: Only use magnesium under the supervision of your doctor. While it can be extremely useful in persons with CHF taking potassium- and magnesium-depleting diuretics and digitalis, those of you taking potassium-sparing diuretics want to use magnesium cautiously or not at all.

DIETARY RECOMMENDATIONS

See the recommendations listed under "Atherosclerosis (Prevention)."

HYPERCHOLESTEROLEMIA (HIGH CHOLESTEROL)

While not the only major risk factor for atherosclerosis and coronary artery disease, high cholesterol in the blood is clearly associated with a higher risk of cardiovascular disease. Sometimes, when we talk about a high cholesterol level, we're also talking about high levels of another set of fats in the blood known as *triglycerides*.

In Western culture, the primary culprit causing high cholesterol is diet. The atherosclerosis prevention program outlined earlier is intended to prevent high cholesterol. Incorporate those recommendations into your cholesterol-lowering program.

Most doctors suggest that we keep our serum cholesterol below 200 milligrams/deciliter. It's also important to note the distinction between different types of cholesterol. LDL cholesterol is thought to increase risk of heart disease and is referred to as "bad" cholesterol. HDL cholesterol is the good guy and is associated with decreasing risk of heart disease. Therefore, the ratio between these two types of cholesterol is often more important than the actual total amount of cholesterol measured in your blood.

A small percentage of people are genetically predetermined to have high cholesterol and/or triglycerides. Because their levels of blood fats can rise to dangerous heights, an aggressive cholesterol-lowering drug (e.g., Mevacor®, Lipitor®) is sometimes best at first. Following a drop in cholesterol, long-term treatment should focus on gentler medications, such as red yeast rice, guggul, or garlic, and the atherosclerosis prevention program outlined earlier. Remember that these drugs don't impact triglycerides significantly. So if your triglycerides are also high, look at adding some pantethine or fish oil to your supplement regimen.

HERBAL PRESCRIPTIONS

- Red yeast (*Monascus pupureas*) rice—1.2 grams twice daily[1]
  Action: A relative newcomer on the block, red yeast rice may lower cholesterol like HMG-CoA reductase inhibitors such as Lipitor and Mevacor as it contains small amounts of these inhibitors including lovastatin. While certainly not as aggressive as these drugs, it may be an ideal choice for those of you in the 200 to 280 milligrams/deciliter cholesterol arena and for long-term management of mild to moderately elevated cholesterol levels. The brand of red yeast rice proven to lower cholesterol is Cholestin® sold by Pharmanex.
- Gugulipid (*Commiphora mukul*)—Extract standardized to provide 25 milligrams of guggulsterones three times daily
  Actions: Standardized extract of an ancient Ayurvedic herbal remedy (the name is easily pronounced by 2-year-olds). It lowers cholesterol and triglycerides in amounts comparable to clofibrate. It also raises the HDL cholesterol level and reduces platelet stickiness[2]

OTHER HERBAL CONSIDERATIONS

- Garlic (standardized garlic powder product containing 1.3 percent aliin and providing 5,000 to 6,000 micrograms of allicin potential daily)—600 to 900 milligrams daily in two to three divided doses
  Note: I don't consider garlic to be a primary consideration for lowering cholesterol. However, its ability to prevent atherosclerosis as well as improve blood vessel health and circulation makes it a great choice of any program aimed at lowering risk of cardiovascular disease.
- Psyllium—5 to 10 grams daily (typically added to the diet in cereal)[3]
- Fenugreek seed—4 to 5 grams three times daily[4]

Nutritional Supplement Considerations

- Niacin—1 to 3 grams daily in two to three divided doses[5]
  Note: Research indicates that the immediate-release form of niacin is the safest. Time-release forms are more likely to cause harm to the liver.[6] However, immediate-release niacin can cause severe flushing in some individuals that can be quite uncomfortable.

Even with use of immediate-release niacin, you should have your liver enzymes checked by your doctor every few months. I will often recommend milk thistle extract with niacin therapy to add some liver protection

One form of niacin, known as *inositol hexaniacinate,* is supposed to be safer without the flushing associated with regular niacin.[7] However, the evidence that it lowers cholesterol is very slim at this time. Remember that if you decide to try inositol hexaniacinate, it's still important to have your liver enzymes checked by your doctor.

- Folic acid—400 to 800 micrograms daily
- Vitamin B_6—12.5 to 25 milligrams daily
- Vitamin B_{12}—500 micrograms daily

Note: These three nutrients are our protection against high levels of homocysteine—a substance linked to cardiovascular disease.[8,9]

- Chromium—200 micrograms daily[10]
- Vitamin E—400 IU daily[11]
- Vitamin C—500 to 1,000 milligrams daily

For lowering triglycerides, try:

- Pantethine—300 milligrams two to four time daily[12]
- Fish oil (high in EPA and DHA)—Daily dose providing 3,000 milligrams of total EPA and DHA[13]

Dietary Recommendations

See the recommendations listed under "Atherosclerosis (Prevention)."

INTERMITTENT CLAUDICATION

Atherosclerosis can also harm blood flow to the extremities, causing poor oxygen supply to the muscles. This often results in a condition known as *intermittent claudication,* characterized by pain or aching in the calf muscles on exertion. It is relieved by rest but returns as soon as exercise begins again. As the condition becomes more severe, the pain limits a person's walking distance.

Treatment of intermittent claudication in its early stages can prevent the condition from worsening. It will also allow greater freedom to exercise and help you maintain an active lifestyle.

HERBAL PRESCRIPTION

- *Ginkgo biloba* extract—120 to 240 milligrams daily in two to three divided doses
  Action: Improves blood flow to the extremities

OTHER HERBAL CONSIDERATIONS

- Garlic (standardized garlic powder product containing 1.3 percent aliin and providing 5,000 to 6,000 micrograms of allicin-potential daily)—600 to 900 milligrams daily in two to three divided doses
  Action: Makes platelets less sticky, which results in more efficient blood flow
- Padma 28—560 milligrams twice daily[1] (Padma 28 is a combination of twenty-eight herbs and is based on an ancient Tibetan formula)

NUTRITIONAL SUPPLEMENT CONSIDERATIONS

- Vitamin E—400 to 600 IU daily[2]
- Inositol hexaniacinate—2 grams twice daily[3]
  Note: This form of niacin will not cause flushing. However, your doctor should monitor your liver enzymes while you are taking the high dose recommended here.

- Propionyl-L-Carnitine or L-Carnitine—2 to 4 grams twice daily[4,5]

DIETARY RECOMMENDATIONS
See the recommendations listed under "Atherosclerosis (Prevention)."

LIFESTYLE CONSIDERATIONS
Don't stop exercising! You should try to walk at least an hour daily. When the pain starts, stop walking, allow it to disappear, and then resume walking. The distance you are able to walk pain-free tells you how successfully your treatment program is progressing.

RAYNAUD'S DISEASE

Raynaud's disease is characterized by a spasm of the midsized blood vessels, known as *arterioles*, in the hands. This interrupts blood flow to the fingers and causes a loss of color in the hands. Raynaud's disease is not usually painful but leads to a lack of sensation in the hands. It's triggered by exposure to cold or by emotional upsets. Color and sensation will return to the hands after they are warmed up. It usually affects both hands and is most common in younger women.

A related condition, Raynaud's phenomenon, is often due to connective tissue diseases such as scleroderma, lupus, and rheumatoid arthritis. Other conditions associated with the nervous and cardiovascular system can also contribute to Raynaud's phenomenon. This condition frequently involves only one hand. The herbal approach to treatment is similar with both forms.

HERBAL PRESCRIPTIONS
- *Ginkgo biloba* extract—120 to 240 milligrams daily in two to three divided doses
  Actions: Improves circulation to the small blood vessels in the extremities and has a mild dilating effect on the blood vessels

- Evening primrose oil—4 to 6 grams daily with meals in two divided doses[1]

  Action: Reduces prostaglandins, which may contribute to vasospasm and inflammation

NUTRITIONAL SUPPLEMENT CONSIDERATIONS

- Inositol hexaniacinate—3 to 4 grams daily[2]
- Fish oil (high in EPA and DHA)—8 to 12 grams daily[3]

Digestive System

RELATED CHAPTERS IN PART 5

- Chamomile
- Eleuthero (Siberian Ginseng)
- Ginger
- Milk Thistle

ALCOHOL-RELATED LIVER DISEASE

Alcohol abuse can lead to gastritis (inflammation of the stomach), pancreatitis (inflammation of the pancreas), malabsorption of important nutrients, nerve disorders, heart disease, and liver disease.

The area of the body most directly affected by alcohol abuse is the liver. The major detoxifying organ of the body, the liver is responsible for clearing alcohol and some other drugs from the body. Overconsumption of alcohol wears down the liver, lessening its ability to clear toxins and eventually leading to destruction of liver cells.

Alcohol disrupts the membrane surrounding liver cells. Inflammation of the liver cells (i.e., *hepatitis*) follows, and this condition leads to infiltration of fat into the liver cells. The final stage in liver destruction is known as *cirrhosis*. Once this stage is reached, alcohol-related liver disease becomes irreversible. Cirrhosis is topped only by cardiovascular disease and cancer as a cause of death in the 45 to 65 age group in the United States. Remember, the goal here is to stop progression of the inflammation (hepatitis) to cirrhosis.

Treatment of alcohol-related liver disease needs to begin with abstinence from alcohol. Get into a good alcohol rehabilitation center, and stick with the initial withdrawal program and follow-up. Remember, alcoholism involves addiction: Long-term treatment is necessary.

Treatment should then aim to reestablish normal liver function. The chapter on milk thistle in Part 5 covers the functions of the liver and offers a glimpse at the importance of reestablishing optimal liver function.

HERBAL PRESCRIPTION

- Milk thistle extract (standardized 80 percent silymarin)—420 milligrams of silymarin in three divided doses

  Note: It's easy to figure out silymarin content. If it's a milk thistle extract that contains 80 percent silymarin, take 175 milligrams of the extract three times daily.

  Actions: Milk thistle regenerates injured liver cells and helps them reestablish normal function. Silymarin has also been shown to prevent fibrosis in the liver cells. It also strengthens the liver cells' antioxidant defense system, which is impaired by alcohol abuse. While the goal is to start treatment before cirrhosis occurs, there is some evidence that milk thistle can improve the quality of life and life span of persons with alcohol-related cirrhosis.

OTHER HERBAL CONSIDERATIONS

- Eleuthero (Siberian ginseng)—Standardized dry extract of the root and rhizomes—300 to 400 milligrams daily; dried, powdered root and rhizomes, 2 to 3 grams daily in two or three divided doses[1]

  Note: Eleuthero is recommended for use during an alcohol-withdrawal program. It is noted for decreasing the recurrence of alcoholism.

- Schizandra—2 grams three times daily[2]

NUTRITIONAL SUPPLEMENT CONSIDERATIONS

Alcoholism can lead to a number of nutritional deficiencies. It is important that you work closely with a health care professional trained in nutrition to establish and treat any nutritional deficiencies. Then use supplements to help maintain normal liver function. Some considerations are the following:

- Multiple vitamin/mineral supplement
- Vitamin E—400 to 800 IU daily
- Selenium—100 to 200 micrograms daily
- Chromium—200 micrograms daily

Other nutrients that may help persons with cirrhosis include S-adenosylmethionine (SAMe), phosphatidylcholine, zinc, and branched-chain amino acids.

Note: Self-treatment of cirrhosis is not advised. Choose your treatment program with the assistance of your doctor.

DIETARY RECOMMENDATIONS

Liver disease hinders the digestion of fats. It's wise, therefore, to reduce fats in your diet and increase sources of complex carbohydrates (leafy green vegetables, legumes, and fruit). Get your protein from low-fat and easy-to-digest sources such as soy. Use the "hypoglycemic" diet outlined in the discussion on stress and fatigue under "Endocrine System" to help with proper blood sugar balance.

ADDITIONAL NOTES ON LIVER DISEASE

One of the biggest challenges facing health care professionals today is reliable treatments for hepatitis C. As drug therapies such as interferon and ribavarin continue to show inconsistent results in treating the disease, it is imperative that research monies be made available to explore the adjunctive use of herbal and nutritional therapies. I am extremely positive about the benefits offered by milk thistle extracts to persons with hepatitis C (see the chapter on milk thistle in Part 5). Other candidates that should be looked at more closely include vitamin E, thymus extracts, glycyrrhizin from licorice, and Chinese herbs such as buplerum and schisandra.

COLIC

A distressing experience for new parents is their first encounter with a colicky baby. Infant colic is characterized by bouts of crying, abdominal pain, and irritability. Infants will often draw their legs up and have excessive gas and a tight abdomen. A gentle stomach massage will often relieve some of the abdominal distress.

Even though a colicky infant can turn your otherwise tranquil world upside down, the condition usually doesn't cause long-term difficulty for a child. Most colicky infants eat and gain weight normally.

Herbal Prescription

- Chamomile—2 to 3 milliliters of a liquid extract in warm water three to four times daily

  Actions: Eases intestinal cramping and exerts a mild sedating effect, aiding sleep

  Note: Peppermint tea is often listed as a potential treatment for infant colic. However, I don't recommend it because infants and young children may have breathing difficulties due to the menthol content in peppermint. Stick with chamomile or other soothing, carminative herbs such as lemon balm, fennel, or licorice.

Dietary Recommendations

A few general considerations:

- If your colicky baby has a strong sucking urge when eating and then fusses after stopping, he or she may need to feed longer.
- If they're bottle feeding, make sure that the hole in the nipple is not too big. Also, some infants swallow air with bottle feeding if allowed to suck on an empty bottle after feeding.
- If your infant has started on formula and becomes colicky, the problem may be an intolerance to lactose in the cow's milk formula or an allergy to the milk proteins. Try substituting a soy formula for the cow's milk formula. However, about 40 percent of infants with cow's milk allergies also react to soy. If this occurs, then try a nonallergenic formula such as Nutramigen.

CONSTIPATION

The urge to be "regular" has resulted in a multimillion-dollar industry. Laxatives have become one of the biggest-selling over-the-counter medications in our society.

Constipation implies a difficulty in having bowel movements or a decreased frequency of bowel movements. Right off the bat, you should notice that this is very subjective. What's normal for one person may be totally unacceptable to another (case in point, the father in the novel *Portnoy's Complaint*).

Here are some of the possible causes of constipation:

Diet high in refined foods and low in fiber
Inadequate fluid intake
Physical inactivity
Pregnancy
Drugs such as anesthetics, antacids, antidepressants, and muscle relaxants
Iron supplements
Low thyroid function
Irritable bowel syndrome
Nerve disorders of the bowel
Overuse of enemas and laxatives

It's interesting that the first few items listed concern diet and physical activity. We'd probably cure a lot of constipation by focusing on more fiber in the diet and a regular exercise program!

Chronic constipation is a major concern among the elderly, particularly those in rest homes and among people who are bedridden. Loss of intestinal tone results from inactivity and also from impaired nerve control of the bowels. Bowel health ranks high in an overall wellness program. Sluggish movement of food through the digestive tract can lead to irritation and cause a harmful buildup of bacteria in the intestines.

HERBAL PRESCRIPTIONS
Stimulant Laxatives

For people with severe constipation, stimulant laxatives are a good short-term consideration. Long-term use of stimulant laxatives can lead to sluggish bowel function and dependence on the laxatives for a normal bowel movement (see discussion of laxatives in Part 4).

- Senna or *Cascara sagrada*—These are the most commonly used stimulant laxatives, with cascara being somewhat more gentle. These herbs are approved over-the-counter medicines, so the dosage is fairly consistent. Carefully follow the instructions on the product you decide to buy.

Action: These herbal laxatives produce anthraquinone glycosides that increase bowel motility.

Bulk-Forming Laxatives

Bulk-forming laxatives, when consumed with sufficient liquid, expand in volume and stimulate the bowels to move. They are considered safer for long-term use than the stimulant laxatives.

- Psyllium seeds—7.5 grams of the seeds (2 teaspoonfuls) or 1 teaspoon of the husks one to two times daily. Mix it up with some water or juice and down the hatch! Be sure your intake of fluids remains regular throughout the day.

Combination Products

Over the past few years, research has indicated that a combination of senna and psyllium is the best choice for treatment of chronic constipation in the elderly. Please see the discussion at the end of "Laxatives" in Part 4.

NUTRITIONAL SUPPLEMENT CONSIDERATION
- Magnesium—300 milligrams twice daily[1]

DIETARY RECOMMENDATIONS

Increase your consumption of vegetables, grains, and fruit. These are all sources of dietary fiber. Decrease red meat, cow's milk, and fried foods. Work with a health care professional trained in nutrition to rule out food allergies. Be sure to drink plenty of liquids during the day—especially with increased fiber intake. Reduce coffee intake.

DIARRHEA

Diarrhea is the result of irritation or inflammation of the intestinal tract. This condition is often due to an infection in the intestinal tract owing to bacteria or viruses. One of the most common forms of diarrhea is traveler's diarrhea. In these cases, the diarrhea can be frequent and explosive. During serious bouts, make sure you have close medical monitoring.

Proper amounts of fluid and electrolytes must be administered, or life-threatening dehydration can occur.

Diarrhea can also be a symptom of inflammatory bowel conditions such as ulcerative colitis or Crohn's disease. It is a frequent complaint of irritable bowel patients as well. It can also result from the foods that we eat—particularly if we are allergic to them. A classic example is mild diarrhea and loose stools in infants who are allergic to cow's milk. Finally, remember that some medications can cause diarrhea (e.g., antibiotics in children and protease inhibitors taken by persons with HIV infection/AIDS).

Note: The following recommendations should be used for more serious cases only after proper medical monitoring takes place.

HERBAL PRESCRIPTIONS

- *Croton lechleri* latex (standardized to 70 percent proanthocyanidin [SP-303])—350 to 700 milligrams two to four times daily
  Note: A newcomer to the herbal supplement market in the United States, this product is from the latex of a tree grown in the Amazon and is standardized to high amounts of proanthocyanidins shown to have antidiarrheal properties. The isolated proanthocyanidins (SP-303) have been studied for traveler's diarrhea[1] and diarrhea in AIDS patients.[2] A standardized extract of the latex that contains 70 percent SP-303 (SB-300 Normal Stool Formula, Shaman Botanicals.com) is currently sold and has shown results in treating twenty HIV-positive men with chronic diarrhea.[3]

Note: The following substances are all rich in tannins, which have an astringent action in the intestines. Please see the discussion on astringents in Part 4.

- Carob powder—1 to 2 tablespoons mixed with applesauce three to four times daily (particularly useful for diarrhea in young children and infants)[4]
- Other common astringents used for diarrhea—Blackberry leaves, blackberry root bark, blueberry leaves, and raspberry leaves[5]

OTHER HERBAL CONSIDERATIONS

- Psyllium—See directions in the section on constipation.

Note: Treating diarrhea with something recommended for constipation? You're probably thinking I've got mental diarrhea! Actually, psyllium has been shown to help make stool better formed and more solid in persons with chronic, noninfectious diarrhea (e.g., irritable bowel syndrome).[6]

- Chamomile—Reduces cramping and helps ease irritation of intestinal tissue (see the instructions for use provided in "Irritable Bowel Syndrome")
- Marshmallow root—1,000 milligrams two to three times daily
  Action: Soothing effect on irritated intestinal tissue
- Goldenseal—3 to 4 grams of the dried root daily in two or three divided doses or 3 to 5 milliliters of tincture three times daily
  Action: Due to its antimicrobial alkaloids such as berberine, it may be beneficial for persons with infectious diarrhea such as traveler's diarrhea.[7]

NUTRITIONAL SUPPLEMENT CONSIDERATIONS

Acute and chronic diarrhea can lead to a host of nutritional deficiencies, especially zinc and the fat-soluble vitamins, vitamins A and D. This is of particular concern in children and infants. Work closely with a health care professional trained in nutrition to avoid loss of nutrients. This precaution is particularly important for infants recovering from diarrhea.

- Acidophilus/bifidus supplements—Excellent for use during diarrhea and also for long-term use afterward. An excellent preventive of traveler's diarrhea and diarrhea in children after taking antibiotics.[8,9,10]
  Note: While there are many probiotic products on the market, the one with the most impressive body of clinical studies is a strain known as *Lactobacillus GG*. It's currently sold under the trade name Culturelle™. Another organism that is widely used in Europe for antibiotic-related diarrhea, traveler's diarrhea, and even diarrhea associated with Crohn's disease is *Saccharomyces boulardii*. Products containing this organism are becoming available in the United States through dietary supplement companies selling directly to health care professionals.

In some cases, foods with sugars that absorb slowly, such as fructose in fruit juice and sorbitol, can cause diarrhea. If you're drinking a lot of fruit juice or diet soda with sorbitol, reduce or eliminate these from your daily regime. Lactose intolerance can cause loose stools and diarrhea. If you react to milk products (with the exception of yogurt), have your doctor check to see whether you should supplement with lactase to help with this problem. Remember, as mentioned earlier, food allergies or intolerance to food additives can also be a cause of loose stools and diarrhea. Again, work with your health care professional trained in nutrition to rule this out.

Remember, too, that some vitamins and minerals can cause diarrhea as can many herbs. High amounts of vitamin C and magnesium are classic examples. Finally, if you're drinking lots of coffee and experiencing loose stools or diarrhea, cut back!

HEARTBURN

Heartburn involves a backflow of stomach contents and acid into the esophagus. It often results in a burning pain in the chest that may radiate to the neck, throat, and face. It frequently occurs following meals or when a person is lying down.

Heartburn is a symptom and not an actual disease. It is most commonly a sign of gastroesophageal reflux, a condition caused by an inability of the lower esophageal sphincter (a valve between the lower esophagus and the stomach) to properly block the reflux of stomach contents into the esophagus. Repeated reflux of stomach contents into the esophagus leads to inflammation and often ulceration. If you're experiencing repeated heartburn, seek the attention of a physician for proper diagnosis and treatment.

HERBAL PRESCRIPTIONS
- Deglycyrrhizinated licorice (chewable tablets)—One to two tablets 5 to 10 minutes before major meals during the day and before bed at night

Action: Soothes irritation of the tissue on the inside of the esophagus. Please see the note on deglycyrrhizinated licorice in the section "Peptic Ulcer Disease."
- Chamomile—Follow the instructions for preparing a tea as outlined in the chapter on chamomile in Part 5.
Action: Anti-inflammatory and soothes irritation of tissue inside the esophagus

Nutritional Supplement Considerations
- Vitamin B complex—50 milligrams daily[1]
Note: A deficiency of vitamin B_3 (niacin) should be ruled out by your health care practitioner
- Calcium carbonate (either liquid or chewable tablet)—600 milligrams every 2 to 3 hours during an acute attack of heartburn

Dietary Recommendations
Eliminate caffeine, alcohol, and chocolate. Reduce saturated fats in your diet from meat and dairy products. A diet high in fiber and complex carbohydrates from vegetables, fruits, and grains will stimulate normal emptying of stomach contents, reducing reflux into the esophagus. Be sure your doctor checks for lactose intolerance.

Irritable Bowel Syndrome

Irritable bowel syndrome (IBS) affects one in seven people and accounts for half of all referrals to outpatient gastroenterology clinics. It is characterized by pain in the abdomen, accompanied by a change in bowel habits. This change can be either diarrhea or constipation. Increased flatulence is also common.

Since IBS affects more women than men, our sexist medical community has presumed that the condition is 90 percent psychological. However, research in Great Britain has indicated that IBS patients have no higher levels of anxiety than persons suffering from intestinal conditions with similar symptoms.

HERBAL PRESCRIPTIONS

- Peppermint oil (enteric-coated)—One to two capsules (0.2 milliliters of oil per capsule) three times daily between meals[1,2]

  Action: Carminative action eases intestinal cramping and soothes irritation.

  Note: Be sure to use the enteric-coated form for the most direct symptom relief. It is released in the intestines and not the stomach, where it would cause irritation. More recent studies in Germany have also found that combining peppermint oil with caraway oil in an enteric-coated capsule is also very effective in treating the symptoms of IBS.[3,4] Some people may experience a burning sensation in their rectum with regular use of the enteric-coated form (affectionately known as "irritable buns syndrome"). They may be better off opting for psyllium or chamomile.

- Psyllium (or another high-fiber, bulk-forming laxative)—See the previous instructions for use of psyllium seeds under "Bulk-Forming Laxatives."

  Action: Helps regulate normal bowel activity and reduce the alternating constipation/diarrhea noted with IBS patients.[5]

OTHER HERBAL CONSIDERATIONS

- Standardized Chinese Herbal Combination (twenty different herbs combined, Mei Yu Imports, Sydney, Australia)—Five capsules three times daily.[6]

  Note: This study got a lot of press because it was published in the *Journal of the American Medical Association*. It combines herbs such as wormwood, ginger, buplerum, schizandra, and dang shen. I advise consulting with a well-trained Chinese herbalist if you can't find the product.

- Chamomile—Chamomile is typically taken in a tea form. Pour boiling water over a heaping tablespoon of dried flowers, cover it, and after 5 to 10 minutes pass it through a tea strainer. Drink a cup of freshly brewed tea three to four times daily between meals. An alternative is to take a dried, encapsulated product or alcohol-based tincture and mix it with hot water. The dosage should be 2 to 3 grams of the encapsulated product or ½ to 1 teaspoon of the tincture three times daily between meals.

DIETARY RECOMMENDATIONS

Please refer to the dietary recommendations under "Constipation." Rule out food allergies and lactose intolerance by consulting a health care professional trained in nutrition.

LIFESTYLE AND MEDICAL CONSIDERATIONS

Hypnotherapy and relaxation techniques have proven successful in the treatment of IBS.[7,8] Stress reduction should also be a part of your long-term approach to IBS.[9] Be sure to ask your doctor to check your thyroid function to see whether it is low.

NAUSEA ASSOCIATED WITH MOTION SICKNESS

Please refer to the chapter on ginger in Part 5 for a discussion of nausea associated with motion sickness.

HERBAL PRESCRIPTION

- Ginger—500 mg ½ to 1 hour before travel and then 500 mg every 2 to 4 hours as needed. Children below the age of 6 years may use half the adult dose.

PEPTIC ULCER DISEASE

Peptic ulcer disease describes ulceration of either the stomach or duodenum (the first part of the small intestine). Duodenal ulcers are the most common, occurring about five times more frequently than gastric ulcers. Duodenal ulcers are about four times more common in men than in women. Gastric ulcers can occur with overconsumption of alcohol, aspirin, and nonsteroidal anti-inflammatory drugs (NSAIDs).

People with duodenal ulcers have a fairly consistent pain pattern. The pain is usually absent first thing in the morning. By midmorning, it begins to rear its ugly head and can sometimes be relieved by food. This is only temporary, as pain returns 2 to 3 hours later. Pain will often wake a person afflicted with a duodenal ulcer at 1 or 2 A.M. Pain may occur daily for one to several weeks and then resolve without treatment. Recurrence, however, is normal.

Gastric ulcers do not follow the same pattern. Eating will often make symptoms worse, producing heartburn, bloating, or nausea. Gastric ulcers are often preceded or accompanied by a condition known as *gastritis,* or inflammation of the stomach lining. The treatment for gastritis is virtually the same as that for ulcers.

Recently, high levels of a bacterial species known as *Helicobacter pylori* have been linked to gastritis and ulcers. This has led to the use of bismuth and antibiotics in the treatment of these conditions.

Note: Peptic ulcer disease can be a dangerous condition, especially if it's causing bleeding. The following herbal and nutritional recommendations should be used only following proper medical diagnosis. These recommendations may also be helpful for those with gastritis.

HERBAL PRESCRIPTIONS

- Deglycyrrhizinated licorice (DGL) (chewable tablets)—250 to 500 milligrams 15 minutes before meals and 1 to 2 hours before bedtime[1,2]
  Actions: Heals the tissue lining of the duodenum and stomach and promotes protection against stomach acid and other irritants. The flavonoids in the herb may also inhibit growth of *H. pylori.*
  Note: Deglycyrrhizinated licorice is an extract of licorice root that has had the constituent glycyrrhizin removed. This is the portion of licorice that has been blamed for increasing blood pressure in some individuals who consumed large amounts of licorice root supplements or licorice tea. By removing the glycyrrhizin, the healing portion of the licorice root remains and the risk of side effects is erased. Deglycyrrhizinated licorice is an approved treatment for ulcers in Great Britain and is widely used in this country by alternative practitioners as a substitute for cimetidine (Tagamet®).
- Catechin—1,000 milligrams five times daily[3]
  Action: As is true with other bioflavonoids, catechin reduces the formation of histamine, a pro-inflammatory substance in the body.

OTHER HERBAL CONSIDERATIONS
- Chamomile—See the instructions for use under "Irritable Bowel Syndrome."
- Marshmallow root—1,000 milligrams two to three times daily
- Mastic (gummy extract of *Pitachia lentiscus*)—1 gram daily[4]

NUTRITIONAL SUPPLEMENT CONSIDERATIONS
- Zinc (monomethionine or citrate)—25 to 30 milligrams daily[5,6]
- Vitamin A—5,000 IU daily[7]

  Note: The amount of vitamin A used in one clinical trial was 150,000 IU daily. This dose is potentially toxic and is especially dangerous to women of childbearing age, as it can potentially cause birth defects.
- Vitamin C—1,000 milligrams daily[8]
- Manuka honey[9]

  Note: Research suggests that this New Zealand honey inhibits the growth of *H. pylori*, the bacterial species associated with ulcers and gastritis. The effect is likely due to the high flavonoid content in the honey. You may get the same results from DGL and chamomile.

DIETARY RECOMMENDATIONS
Increase your consumption of foods high in fiber and complex carbohydrates (leafy green vegetables, fruits, and legumes). These foods will also be higher in antioxidant nutrients such as beta-carotene, vitamin A, and vitamin C. Reduce your intake of sugar, saturated fats (primarily from meat, milk, and cheese), coffee (including decaffeinated) and black tea (green tea is fine), and alcohol. Increase your consumption of garlic, thyme, and cinnamon. All three of them have been associated with inhibiting growth of *H. pylori* in test tubes. With the help of a health care professional, identify and eliminate potential food allergens. Don't use milk to treat your ulcer!

LIFESTYLE CONSIDERATIONS
Reduce risk factors including smoking, aspirin, and NSAIDs such as ibuprofen. Stress reduction through meditation, relaxation training, and so on, is essential.

ULCERATIVE COLITIS

Ulcerative colitis is a serious condition due to inflammation of the lining of the intestine. It often results in bloody diarrhea and, as it progresses, can lead to severe weight loss. Conventional drug therapies are usually aimed at symptom relief (e.g., sulfasalazine) and keeping the inflammation in check (e.g., corticosteroids). Side effects often hamper the long-term effectiveness of these drugs. These limitations in conventional approaches lead many persons with ulcerative colitis to look to herbal and nutritional approaches. However, this approach should be done only under the careful guidance of a health care professional trained in herbs and nutrition and close monitoring by a qualified gastroenterologist.

HERBAL PRESCRIPTIONS

- *Boswellia serrata* extract (standardized to 37.5 to 65 percent boswellic acids)—150 milligrams of boswellic acids (which means 400 milligrams of an extract standardized to 37.5 percent boswellic acids) three times daily

  Actions: Boswellia extracts are made from the resin of an Indian tree and have been proven to have anti-inflammatory properties. One small pilot study found the extract to be as effective as the drug sulfasalazine in improving symptoms of ulcerative colitis.[1] Remember, these are only preliminary findings

- Psyllium seeds—10 grams twice daily[2]

  Action: Helps support the production of short-chain fatty acids (e.g., butyrate) by intestinal bacteria in the intestine

NUTRITIONAL SUPPLEMENT CONSIDERATIONS

- Fish oil (MaxEPA)—Five capsules three times daily (equivalent to 3.2 grams of EPA and 2.2 grams of DHA)[3]

- Folic acid—800 to 1,000 micrograms daily[4]

  Note: Folic acid has been shown to reduce the risk of colon cancer in persons with ulcerative colitis. Be sure to take some vitamin B_{12} at the same time (about 500 micrograms daily is fine).

OTHER CONSIDERATIONS

- Butyrate enemas—Administer twice daily and retain for 30 minutes.[5]
  Note: Butyrate is a short-chain fatty acid manufactured by intestinal bacteria that serves as a fuel for the cells that line the intestines. These enemas are not available over the counter. If you decide to try them after consulting with your doctor, you can obtain them from a compounding pharmacist with a prescription from your doctor.

DIETARY RECOMMENDATIONS

Reduce the amount of sugar in your diet as well as animal fats and margarine. While food allergies are often hard to link to ulcerative colitis, it is worthwhile to work with your nutritionally trained health care professional to rule out any foods that may be contributing.

Ears, Nose, Throat, and Respiratory Tract

Related Chapters in Part 5

- Echinacea
- *Ginkgo biloba*

Asthma

> **Vegetarian Diet and Natural Medicines**
> **Combine to Improve Asthma**
>
> A 1985 Swedish study looked at the effect of a vegetarian diet and lifestyle changes on thirty-five adult asthmatics.[1] The treatment regimen included
>
> - Vegetarian diet: mainly raw foods and soups with no meat, fish, eggs, or dairy products
> - Fresh spring water
> - No chocolate, coffee, caffeinated tea, sugar, or salt
> - Initial 7-day juice fast
> - Herbal teas from licorice and marshmallow
> - Vitamin C, garlic, nettles were added as supplements
> - Fresh, unpolluted air
> - Regular physical activity
>
> Twenty-four patients completed the study. The results indicated a 71 percent improvement after 4 months and a 92 percent improvement after 12 months.

Asthma is a tightening or spasming of the bronchial tubes that leads to wheezing and difficulty in breathing. While the precise cause of asthma is unclear at this point, we do know that many stimuli or stresses can induce an asthma attack. These include viral infections, exposure to allergens such as pollen or food, inhalation of cold air, airborne irritants (pollution, cigarette smoke), emotional distress, and exercise. Antibiotic use during the first 2 years of life may also contribute.[2] As is the case with ear infections, nursing for the first few months of life is also associated with a lower risk of asthma in children.

Standard drug treatment of asthma focuses on combating acute asthma attacks and reducing bronchial tightness between attacks. Unfortunately, these medications often must be taken for many years. While they're potentially lifesaving in some situations, recent research has found that regular use of bronchodilating medications such as Alupent and albuterol may harm cardiovascular health.[3,4]

Research in the United States, England, and Australia has shown that medicine is failing miserably in the long-term treatment of asthma. The rate of death among asthmatics actually *rose* during the 1980s![5] One finger potentially points at the choice of medications for long-term treatment of asthma, although the rise in environmental pollution and increased use of food additives are also potential contributing factors.

While natural medicine has little to offer for the treatment of a serious asthma attack, it does possess tools that may improve the long-term outlook and serve as supportive therapies for standard medical approaches. Remember, asthma can be life threatening, and it's important to work closely with your doctor as you make choices on how to best manage your asthma or that of your children.

HERBAL PRESCRIPTIONS

- *Ginkgo biloba* extract—120 to 240 milligrams daily in two to three divided doses. For children 6 to 12 years old, reduce the dosage to 80 to 120 milligrams daily. For children under 6 years, use 40 to 80 milligrams daily.[6]

  Note: These doses are based on personal clinical experience using a standardized extract of ginkgo. While tylohora and ivy leaf may act more quickly, ginkgo seems to be a good choice for long-term treatment. In children with asthma, I've observed a noted decrease in need for bronchodilators over time when using ginkgo. One Chinese study with adult asthmatics used a highly concentrated ginkgo tincture with some success.[7] However, the product is not available in the United States and probably does not have the quality control standards of extracts from Europe such as EGb 761.

Actions: In test tube studies, ginkgolides (see the ginkgo chapter in Part 5 for an explanation of these compounds) inhibit the substance platelet-activating factor. Platelet-activating factor increases the tightness (hyperresponsiveness) of bronchioles. Ginkgo is also a scavenger of free radicals (i.e., an antioxidant).

- Ivy (Hedera helix) leaf extract—25 drops twice daily.[8]

Action: While much more widely used for coughs and bronchitis in Europe, ivy leaf extract contains saponins that act as expectorants and seem to possess antispasmodic actions that may contribute to its potential benefit in asthmatics.[9]

OTHER HERBAL CONSIDERATIONS

- Ma Huang (*Ephedra sinica*)—1 to 2 grams of the dried herb in two to three divided doses (this represents about 15 to 30 milligrams of ephedrine)[10]

Note: This Chinese herb provides two constituents commonly used in over-the-counter medications for hay fever and asthma. The first, pseudoephedrine, is used as a nasal decongestant. The second, ephedrine, is included in products assisting with bronchodilation and providing relief from asthma attacks. The dosage of ephedrine should not exceed 150 milligrams in a 24-hour period for adults and children over 12 years old. While it provides excellent results, ephedrine can also strain the heart and adrenal glands. I do not favor prescribing it for children less than 12 years old. I will occasionally use Ma Huang in cough formulations to add a mild bronchodilating and decongestant effect. However, I am a strong opponent of its long-term use and do not think it is a suitable substitute for the treatment of acute asthma attacks.

- *Tylophora indica*—200 to 400 milligrams of the dried, powdered leaf

Action: It appears to have some short-acting bronchodilating effects and immune system effects that may or may not contribute to its actions for asthmatics.[11,12,13]

Note: While this herb has become popular over the past few years, most of the clinical work is older and lacking in clear dosage or consistent effect. More clinical studies are needed to give me a greater comfort with tylophora as a treatment alternative for asthma.

- Quercetin—500 milligrams two to three times daily

  Action: Like other bioflavonoids, quercetin is a natural antihistamine. It may be helpful if your asthma is linked to an airborne or food allergy.[14]

- Marshmallow root—2 grams three to four times daily

  Note: Mucilage-containing herbs are sometimes helpful for irritated airways. Other herbs that may have a soothing effect are mullein, hyssop, and licorice.

NUTRITIONAL SUPPLEMENT CONSIDERATIONS

Note: The recommended dosages listed here are for adults. Appropriate reductions should be made for children, under the supervision of a health care practitioner. All supplements should be free of additives and potential allergens.

- Vitamin B_6—50 to 100 milligrams twice daily[15]
- Vitamin C—500 to 1,000 milligrams twice daily[16]

  Note: If your asthma gets worse when you exercise, try taking 1,000 milligrams of vitamin C about 15 minutes before you start exercising.

- Magnesium—200 to 400 milligrams daily in two three divided doses
- Selenium—200 micrograms daily[17]

DIETARY RECOMMENDATIONS

Identify and eliminate food allergens under the supervision of a health care practitioner. Omitting cow's milk from the diets of children with asthma makes sense, but be sure to make up for the loss of calcium and vitamin D. Avoiding food additives, particularly sulfites, and food colorings is essential. The following list includes commonly used food additives and colorings:

Benzoic acid	EDTA derivatives
Formic acid	Sulfites
Sodium benzoate	Tartrazine
Food Red 14	Sunset Yellow
Propionic acid	4-Hydroxybenzoic acid
Malic acid	Acetic acid
Nitrate compounds	Benzaldehyde
Carminic acid	Cyclamate

And here are some foods high in sulfites:

Commercially baked products	Beer
Canned seafood	Canned soups
Corn sweeteners	Dried fruits
Food starches	Gelatin
Maraschino cherries	Mushrooms
Salads (in restaurants)	Sausage meats
Shrimp (uncooked;	Wine
outside the United States)	Vinegar

Keeping down saturated fats, primarily from animal products, will also assist in lowering the amount of pro-inflammatory mediators being produced. I hate to sound like a broken record, but we're talking a whole-foods, low-processed-food diet here, folks!

Eat lots of onions and garlic unless you're allergic to them. Onions have been shown to be an excellent antiasthma food![18]

Last but not least, asthma is another of those childhood diseases that goes down dramatically when breast-feeding is a part of a child's first 9 to 12 months of life.[19]

LIFESTYLE CONSIDERATIONS
A lot of stigma is attached to childhood asthma. Work with your child on relaxation and breathing exercises. I like to use visualization that encourages the asthmatic child to "open up," both physically and mentally. Breathing exercises are fabulous and can be a lot of fun. Try huffing and puffing and blowing your house down.

For adults, research has shown that yoga breathing exercises and relaxation are great for reducing asthma attacks.[20] Acupuncture may also help some persons with asthma.

Children exposed to secondhand cigarette smoke have a greatly increased chance of asthma. Stop smoking around your kids![21]

Also, remember that some asthma medications can deplete adrenal reserves. Use eleuthero (Siberian ginseng) or Asian ginseng to support adrenal function if you're taking inhaled corticosteroids for the long term.

COUGHS

Instead of trying to give you the medical details on different kinds of coughs, let me just say to be careful with coughs. A tight cough that makes breathing difficult should always be monitored by your doctor—particularly if it's a child who is having problems. If a large amount of phlegm and mucus are being produced, it may be a sign of bronchitis or pneumonia. While some of the recommendations here (e.g., ivy leaf extract) are great for treating coughs and bronchial congestion, bronchitis and pneumonia often need to be properly diagnosed and treated with antibiotics. Chronic coughs that aren't resolving should also be brought to your doctor's attention.

The categories of coughs listed here have a lot of overlap. So don't be afraid to mix and match from different categories. These remedies are my personal favorites.

MILD, IRRITATING COUGH

- Loquat syrup—1 to 2 tablespoons every 2 to 3 hours for short-term relief of cough. This is excellent for young children.
- Marshmallow root, mullein flowers, and slippery elm—Equal parts of each, either from liquid extracts or prepared in a tea from the dried product. In the liquid extract, take 2 tablespoons every 2 to 3 hours. As a tea, combine 2 to 3 teaspoonfuls of each herb and brew for 10 to 15 minutes. Strain the preparation, and drink 8 to 10 ounces every couple of hours.[1]

DRY, SPASMODIC COUGH

- Drosera (sundew) and thyme—Equal parts of both herbs either as liquid extracts or as the dried herbs prepared in a tea, or 1 tablespoon of the liquid extract preparation every 3 to 4 hours. With the tea, brew 1 to 2 grams of each herb and then strain. Drink 8 to 10 ounces three to four times daily.[2,3]

  Note: Drosera and thyme are grossly underused in this country. Call your favorite herb company and tell them you want cough syrups with these ingredients!

COUGH WITH CONGESTION

- Ma Huang, thyme, licorice root—This combination includes a bronchodilating herb (Ma Huang), an antispasmodic and expectorant herb (thyme), and a soothing and expectorant herb (licorice root). It also tastes bad, so combine it with some honey or glycerin to sweeten it. Follow the instructions given for the preceding drosera and thyme combination. Remember that Ma Huang should be administered only to older children and is intended for short-term use.

  Note: I'll usually recommend a steam with either tea tree oil or eucalyptus oil as another means to loosen mucus and help clear the airways. Place ¼ teaspoon of either oil in a pot of boiling water and steam for 10 to 15 minutes. For younger children, use a hot-air vaporizer at night.

BRONCHITIS

- Ivy leaf extract—A great expectorant and cough suppressant for chronic inflammatory bronchial conditions. Just now starting to be recognized in the United States, it's been a mainstay in Europe for years. For children, use the dosage listed under "Asthma." For adults, 5 milliliters of the liquid three times daily.[4]

- Sinupret herbal combination—For adults, take one tablet three times daily. For children ages 6 to 12, take one tablet twice daily.

  Note: For more details on this fascinating herbal combination from Germany (sold in the United States as Quanterra™ Sinus Defense; see the section on sinus infections). While it's more widely noted for treating persons with acute or chronic sinusitis, it also seems to be useful for helping to clear mucous in the airways of persons with bronchitis.[5]

General note: Don't forget your echinacea and vitamin C! While the herbs listed here may help with cough relief and expectoration of mucous, supporting your immune system is important during any infection, whether it be viral or bacterial.

Ear Infections (Recurrent)

Chronic ear infection, also known as *otitis media with effusion* (OME), is a chronic inflammation of the middle ear. Loss of hearing can result from the prolonged buildup of fluid behind the tympanic membrane (the membrane separating the middle ear and external ear). Otitis media with effusion is a major cause of hearing loss in young children, especially those 3 years of age and under.

Fluid buildup results from obstruction in the eustachian tube, the canal draining the middle ear. The eustachian tube of young children sits in a somewhat horizontal position, which hinders drainage of fluid. Obstruction occurs as a result of inflammation caused by repeated acute ear infections, frequent colds, and allergic reactions starting in the nose. When the eustachian tube does not drain and fluid builds up, the eardrum does not move properly in response to sounds. It is then that hearing is damaged.

The following are important questions if your child has OME:

- Does your child have allergies? Environmental allergies to animal dander, dust, and pollen can cause inflammation in the nose and impair proper draining. Also, food allergies are very important. Early weaning and introduction of cow's milk are linked to an increased risk of OME.
- Does your child get frequent colds or upper respiratory tract infections? A sluggish immune system can make children more susceptible to these infections, particularly if they attend day care. Also, chronic use of antibiotics can contribute to a sluggish immune response.[1]

- Does either parent smoke? Secondhand smoke increases the risk of OME.[2]
- Finally, does your child drink out a bottle lying flat on their back or use a pacifier? Interestingly, there appears to be a link between pacifier use and incidence of ear infections.[3]

HERBAL PRESCRIPTION

- *Echinacea purpurea* (expressed juice of the herb—preferably alcohol free)—20 to 40 drops of the juice three times daily for 10 to 14 days
  Actions: Strengthens the immune response and decreases the risk of colds and upper respiratory tract infections. This serves to lower the risk of ear infections recurring.

NUTRITIONAL SUPPLEMENT CONSIDERATIONS

- Vitamin C

  In children less than 1 year of age—100 to 200 milligrams daily
  In children 1 to 3 years of age—250 milligrams daily
  In children 3 years of age and older—250 milligrams twice daily

- Zinc (citrate or monomethionine)—The typical adult dose of 25 mg daily should be adjusted based on the child's weight. For instance, a 30-pound child could be given 5 milligrams of zinc.
- N-Acetyl-L-cysteine (NAC)—400 to 600 milligrams daily[4]
  Note: N-Acetyl-L-cysteine is a mucolytic. This means it thins the mucus and helps with drainage from the middle ear. (It's also useful for chronic sinus congestion.) N-Acetyl-L-cysteine tastes horrible! Try to hide it in sweet potatoes or applesauce. It also can cause loose stools or diarrhea in some children.

DIETARY RECOMMENDATIONS

Breast-feeding is the best preventive medicine. Children breast-fed for at least 9 to 12 months have a greatly reduced risk of OME.[5,6] Children with OME should be evaluated for food allergies as part of an entire treatment program involving environmental allergens.[7] Once specific food allergens are identified, a systematic elimination should be carried out under the supervision of a health care practitioner. Major allergens to consider include cow's milk, eggs, wheat, soy, citrus, and peanut butter. Make an attempt to decrease sugar and simple carbohydrates in your child's diet. These can contribute to a sluggish immune system.

SINUS INFECTIONS (RECURRENT)

Sinusitis is an inflammation of the sinus passages that can occur due to bacterial infections or as a result of viral upper respiratory infections such as the common cold. The inflammation leads to mucous buildup and congestion in sinuses, which in turn can result in pain and tenderness over the sinus areas on the face. While acute sinusitis can cause more severe discomfort, chronic sinusitis is usually milder and can include postnasal drip, bad breath, and cough. Sinusitis can also be triggered by hay fever, food allergens, and dental infections. The goal of managing the condition is eliminating any bacterial infections, reducing inflammation, and keeping the sinus passages clear and draining.

HERBAL PRESCRIPTION
- Sinupret herbal combination (gentian root, elder flowers, European vervain herb, primrose flower, sorrel herb)—For adults, take one tablet three times daily. For children ages 6 to 12 years, take one tablet twice daily.[1]

  Actions: This fascinating herbal combination has become the number one selling herbal product in Germany over the past decade (it's sold in the United States as Quanterra™ Sinus Defense).[2] It's used there primarily as a supportive therapy for persons with acute sinusitis taking antibiotics. It's also widely used for stubborn cases of chronic sinusitis. The combination naturally supports mucous drainage and helps reduce inflammation in the sinus passages. It isn't a decongestant, and it doesn't have the side effects associated with those drugs. I've been recommending it for a wide variety of sinus-related problems associated with congestion, including hay fever and the common cold. For acute sinus conditions, 1 to 2 weeks of use is fine. For chronic conditions, you can take it continuously for several months.

OTHER CONSIDERATIONS

The following recommendations are listed under "Ear Infections (Recurrent)." For adults, the doses should be adjusted as follows:

- *Echinacea pupurea* (expressed juice of the herb)—40 drops of the juice three times daily or one capsule of the dried juice three or four times daily for 10 to 14 days
- N-acetyl-L-cysteine (NAC)—500 milligrams three times daily[3]
  Note: I think the Sinupret works better and should be your first choice for getting that stubborn mucous to drain.
- Bromelain—Potency is usually listed as "milk clotting units" (MCUs). Try to take a supplement delivering 3,000 MCU three times daily between meals.[4]
- Vitamin C—2 to 3 grams daily

And now, something completely different:

- Tea tree oil or eucalyptus oil—Place $\frac{1}{4}$ to $\frac{1}{2}$ teaspoon in boiling water and breathe in the steam for 15 minutes.

TINNITUS AND HEARING LOSS

Tinnitus is simply a ringing or buzzing noise in the ear. However, the complexity of managing the condition can be overwhelming. Part of the frustration is the fact that an underlying disease is identified only about 5 percent of the time (my father-in-law says it's a natural defense against the nagging of my mother-in-law).

One person out of ten has some form of hearing impairment or ear problem; 85 percent of these sufferers have tinnitus. Tinnitus affects more than 37 million Americans. It's most common in elderly persons but can occur at any age. The most common causes are noise-induced damage to the inner ear and age-related hearing loss. Contributing factors to tinnitus include smoking, caffeine, aspirin, some prescription drugs (examples include indomethacin, Elavil, and Gantrisin), and stress.

Tinnitus may be a sign of conditions such as Meniere's disease and sensorineural hearing loss (hearing loss originating in the inner ear). In addition, tinnitus may indicate circulation problems to the inner ear, high blood pressure, hyperthyroidism, or high cholesterol.[1]

You should consider the following suggestions for possible treatment of tinnitus, sensorineural hearing loss, and Meniere's disease.

HERBAL PRESCRIPTION

- *Ginkgo biloba* extract—120 to 240 milligrams daily in two or three divided doses[2]

  Action: Improves blood flow to the inner ear. Ginkgo seems to be effective in a subset of persons with tinnitus (most likely those with tinnitus caused by noise damage or atherosclerosis).

NUTRITIONAL SUPPLEMENT CONSIDERATIONS

- Vitamin B_{12}—1,000 micrograms daily (sublingual lozenges are best if used orally). Be sure to take with at least 400 micrograms of folic acid. If you have a health care professional willing to help out, the better option is to have an intramuscular injection of 1,000 micrograms (1 milliliter) of B_{12} weekly for 4 to 5 months.[3]
- Zinc (monomethionine or citrate)—50 milligrams three times daily between meals. Use for 12 to 24 weeks. Additional supplementation of copper should take place during this time (2 to 3 milligrams daily).[4]

DIETARY RECOMMENDATIONS

Reduce your dietary sources of saturated fats, such as beef and dairy products. Also lower your dietary intake of sodium (salt is usually the culprit) as well as sugar and other simple carbohydrates. Eating more frequent, smaller meals that are higher in protein and complex carbohydrates helps regulate sugar metabolism.[5]

LIFESTYLE CONSIDERATIONS

There appears to be some correlation between stress and tinnitus. Stress reduction through meditation, biofeedback, or yoga should be part of your long-term strategy to combat tinnitus.[6]

Other Ear, Nose, and Throat Conditions

Hay Fever
- Nettle herb—450 milligrams two to three times daily[1]
- Quercetin—500 milligrams two to three times daily[2]
- Vitamin C—2 to 3 grams daily[3]

Sore Throat

Note: The following recommendations are for symptom relief. A sore throat can indicate a more serious infection (e.g., strep throat). Please seek medical attention if you have a sore throat accompanied by swollen lymph glands in the neck or if you've been exposed to someone with strep throat.

- Slippery elm—One or two lozenges every couple of hours for symptomatic relief
- Goldenseal root (liquid extract or tincture)—2 milliliters every 2 to 3 hours for 7 to 10 days. Gargle with the preparation before swallowing.

Other Herbal Considerations
- Cayenne
- Garlic
- Echinacea

Nutrient Considerations
- Zinc lozenges
- Vitamin C

Endocrine System

DIABETES

Diabetes mellitus is a chronic disease caused by insufficient production of insulin by the pancreas. This causes blood sugar to rise. Chronically high blood sugar leads to a host of complications in other parts of the body. Examples include retinopathy (see the following chapter on eye conditions), neuropathy (see the chapter on nervous system conditions), cardiovascular disease, and kidney disease. Diabetes is one of the leading causes of blindness and kidney disease in our country.

More than 11 million people have diabetes in the United States. Each year, 500,000 new cases are reported. Treatment of diabetes and its eye, nerve, cardiovascular, and kidney complications leads to a yearly medical cost of approximately $20.4 billion!

Diabetes mellitus comes in two forms. Type I, also known as *juvenile-onset diabetes*, begins in childhood or adolescence. It is the most serious form and requires a lifetime of daily injections of insulin to maintain normal blood sugar levels. In type I diabetes, the immune system attacks the cells in the pancreas that produce insulin—hence the need for an external source of insulin. Another term for this type of diabetes is *insulin-dependent diabetes mellitus*. Type I diabetics represent less than 10 percent of the cases of diabetes in the United States.

Type II diabetes is called *adult-onset* and affects older people. The most common characteristic of the adult-onset diabetic is obesity. Type II diabetics have a lower rate of complications, and their condition can sometimes be controlled with diet and noninsulin medications that lower blood sugar (also known as *hypoglycemic drugs*). In medical circles, this form of diabetes is referred to as non-insulin-dependent. It represents more than 90 percent of diabetes cases nationwide.

So, where does herbal medicine fit into the picture? Type I diabetics require insulin. It should not be assumed that they'll ever be able to do without it. However, diet, nutritional supplements, and occasionally herbal medicines play an important supporting role. Research is showing that these may prevent complications and even lower the requirement for insulin.

Dietary and herbal prescriptions also directly benefit type II diabetics. In many cases, healthy changes in a diet and sticking to a good exercise plan can work wonders in lowering blood sugar. Nutritional and herbal supplements can sometimes serve as primary therapies with type II diabetes. *Gymnema sylvestre* leaves and fenugreek seed can reduce the need for antidiabetic (hypoglycemic) medicines, which have well-known side effects.

As we'll see in the discussion of HIV (human immunodeficiency virus) infection under "Immune System," diabetics need to become the captain of their health care ship. Create a team of health care providers that addresses the condition from different and yet complementary perspectives. The complex and chronic nature of diabetes requires an eclectic approach.

Remember that chronically high blood sugar is dangerous! Every optimal health care plan for diabetes needs to start with regular monitoring of blood sugar and include other important laboratory measures. Regular visits to your doctor not only will keep an eye on these measures but will also give you direct feedback about the effectiveness of your dietary and supplement program. Finally, if you are using an herbal supplement that lowers blood sugar while taking insulin or oral hypoglycemic drugs, be very careful that your blood sugar doesn't get too low.

HERBAL PRESCRIPTIONS

The list of herbs that may lower blood sugar is never ending. Cultures around the world have depended on plant medicines to treat diabetes. So, the list here is just a sprinkling of what's used in herbal medicine around the world.

HERBAL MEDICINES THAT MAY HELP LOWER BLOOD SUGAR

- Fenugreek seeds (defatted)—10 to 15 grams (1 to 3 ounces) with each meal[1,2]

  Action: Effectively lowers blood sugar following meals

  Note: Defatted fenugreek seeds are available in capsules. At the recommended doses, you may simply want to add it in with your food. Remember that other sources of fiber such as psyllium, guar gum (found in beans), and oat bran have also shown benefit in helping improve glucose tolerance in diabetics.

- *Gymnema sylvestre* leaf extract (GS4)—400 milligrams daily[3,4]

  Actions: Enhances the ability of the pancreas to produce insulin in type II diabetics. It also helps insulin work more effectively in lowering blood sugar in both type I and type II diabetes, which may provide a substitute for oral blood sugar–lowering drugs in some type II diabetics.

  Aloe vera juice—1 tablespoon twice daily[5,6]

  Note: Small clinical studies have noted benefit for type II diabetics and similar blood sugar–lowering effects as the drug glibenclamid.

- Asian ginseng—Extract supplying approximately 5 to 7 percent ginsenosides—100 milligrams twice daily

  Actions: This adaptogenic herb has been used historically in the long-term management of diabetes. According to a study with type II diabetics, it promote normal blood sugar balance (see chapter on Asian ginseng in Part 5).

HERBAL MEDICINES THAT LOWER THE RISK FOR OR CAN BE USED TO TREAT DIABETIC COMPLICATIONS
Diabetic Cataracts

- Quercetin—500 milligrams two to three times daily[7]

  Note: Since bilberry is also high in bioflavonoids and useful for prevention of retinopathy, I usually recommend bilberry so that prevention of both conditions is covered.

Diabetic Retinopathy

See the section on herbal prescriptions in the treatment of diabetic retinopathy in the following chapter ("Eyes").

- Bilberry extract
- *Ginkgo biloba* extract

Diabetic Neuropathy

Please turn to the chapter on nervous system conditions and review the herbal recommendations for the treatment of diabetic neuropathy (they're near the end of the chapter).

- Evening primrose oil
- *Ginkgo biloba* extract
- Capsaicin (from cayenne pepper) ointment (topical use only)

NUTRITIONAL SUPPLEMENT CONSIDERATIONS

Start with a good multiple-vitamin and mineral supplement. The following recommendations are total daily doses, so don't forget to include the amount in your multiple-vitamin/mineral supplement. Work with a nutritionist or nutritionally trained doctor to fine tune your daily supplement regime. Taking every nutrient that may be potentially helpful can get to be quite a burden on the bank account.

- Vitamin C—1 to 3 grams daily[8,9]
  Note: People with type I diabetes often have low vitamin C levels. Vitamin C may improve glucose control in type II diabetics and possibly reduce the risk of cataracts and neuropathy in both types of diabetes.
- Chromium (polynicotinate or picolinate)—200 micrograms once or twice daily[10,11]
  Note: Chromium may help improve glucose tolerance and increase the ability of insulin to its job more effectively. It may also lower the risk of cardiovascular disease.
- Magnesium—300 to 400 milligrams daily[12,13]

Todd Bell—A Friend and Hero

Storytellers are always indebted to the characters who shape their stories. Many of my stories are richer because of people who've woven their experiences with mine. Todd Bell, my friend and brother-in-law, enriched my life greatly during the short time I knew him.

Todd was diagnosed with diabetes at the age of 11. After battling with retinopathy and other complications, Todd had kidney failure in December 1985. After a successful kidney transplant in June 1986, we all breathed a sigh of relief and assumed Todd would get back to his life in the restaurant business.

One of the most determined and stubborn people I've ever met, Todd decided only one year after his transplant to ride a bicycle across the country to increase public awareness of organ donation. He set about raising money through connections in Florida, as well as New York.

His route took him from Los Angeles to Miami. Todd completed the trip with flying colors. Newscasts along the way carried the story of his trip and his message, "Don't take your organs to heaven; heaven knows we need them here."

He became the president of the Southwest Florida Branch of the National Kidney Foundation in 1990 and continued to increase awareness about organ donation. He also participated in the National Transplant Olympics in the same year. He won a bronze medal for swimming.

After the transplanted kidney failed in early 1993 and chronic hepatitis dealt another blow to his health, Todd began his final journey with the courage and stubborn determination that were his trademarks. He died December 27, 1993.

The National Kidney Foundation created a research grant in Todd's name in June 1994.

OK, Todd, I'll join the battle cry, "BE AN ORGAN DONOR!!"

Note: Diabetics may have low magnesium. Supplementing magnesium may help improve the ability of insulin work more effectively and thus lower the amount needed. It may also reduce the risk of retinopathy.

- Zinc (monomethionine or citrate)—25 milligrams daily[14] (be sure copper is also supplemented)
  Note: Diabetics tend to be low in zinc, a critical nutrient for healthy immune system function.
- Vitamin E—800 to 900 international units (IU) daily[15,16]
  Note: May help improve cardiovascular health and nerve function
- Biotin—9 to 16 milligrams daily[17]
  Note: Biotin is an essential nutrient for processing glucose in the body.
- Alpha-lipoic acid—800 milligrams daily[18]
  Note: Research suggests that, like EPO, alpha-lipoic acid may treat early-stage diabetic neuropathy.

OTHER NUTRIENT CONSIDERATIONS

- Vitamin B_1
- Vitamin B_3
- Vitamin B_6
- Vitamin B_{12}
- Coenzyme Q_{10}
- Carnitine

DIETARY RECOMMENDATIONS

Research suggests an ideal diet is a cross between a whole-foods, high-complex carbohydrate diet and a Mediterranean diet high in monounsaturated fats such as olive oil. To tell you the truth, I'd rather have my complex carbohydrates with some olive oil and garlic than without!

It's critical to increase your dietary fiber. High-complex carbohydrate foods (vegetables and fruits) are high in dietary fiber. Fiber from beans, peas, and oats have all been shown to reduce blood sugar and prevent diabetic complications such as retinopathy and neuropathy.

Avoid processed grains and white bread. Drink fruit juice in moderation, and definitely avoid soda pop, candy, and other sugary junk foods.

Reducing protein intake may reduce risk of kidney damage caused by diabetes and also improve glucose tolerance. Get your protein from cold-water fish (e.g., salmon), soy, and other healthy sources. Avoid red meat and other animal sources of protein and fat. Eliminate fried foods and other sources of saturated fats.

LIFESTYLE CONSIDERATIONS

If you have type II diabetes, get on an exercise program immediately! Exercise increases the body's response to insulin and also reduces your risk for heart disease. Type I diabetics also benefit from exercise, but they should be careful about overdoing it and disrupting blood sugar control.

Stress can affect your ability to monitor blood sugar. Try yoga, meditation, or any other favorite method—listening to *Impressions* by John Coltrane is a favorite of mine—to keep stress in check.

STRESS AND FATIGUE (ADRENAL EXHAUSTION)

Stress is usually defined in terms of impaired balance. It can be triggered by both mental and physical stimuli. When stress occurs, it shifts your body's equilibrium or balance. How efficient you are at rebalancing often determines how little or how much effect stress will have on your body.

In the 1930s, Hans Selye developed a model for the way we react and adapt to stress. His model, referred to as the general adaptation syndrome (affectionately abbreviated "GAS"), is divided into three stages.[1]

The first stage is called the *state of alarm*. During this phase, a person is ready to react ("fight or flight"). The hypothalamic–pituitary–adrenal (HPA) gland axis in the endocrine system kicks into high gear. The adrenal glands begin producing hormones, including epinephrine and cortisone-like substances. This explains the keyed-up feeling a person gets when reacting to stress. Fat stores are also mobilized to offer extra energy. All of these factors contribute to a nonspecific resistance to stress.

The second stage is the *state of resistance*. After trying either to make the stress go away or to avoid it during stage 1, our body begins to adapt to the stress, and the adrenals and other glands start to return to a normal, balanced state. The resistance thus becomes specific to the stress and not a generalized reaction.

The third stage, termed *exhaustion*, represents the body finally breaking down under the pressure of stress. Selye observed in animal studies that damage to organs in the body occurred during this phase.

The organs most directly affected by constant stress are the adrenal glands. When your body is regularly bombarded with stress, your adrenal glands can become run down. This is often secondary to the endocrine stress center of the body getting out of whack. That center is known as the HPA axis. What happens then?

In the late 1940s, John Tintera, a medical doctor living in New York, picked up where Selye left off. Tintera began to look at patients in his practice who complained of chronic fatigue and unexplained aches and pains. He observed that many of these people had been experiencing recurring stress and had poorly functioning adrenal glands. The term *hypoadrenocorticism* was created to describe their condition.[2]

Tintera then assembled a list of specific symptoms common to people with sluggish adrenal function:

Excessive fatigue
Nervousness and irritability
Depression
Anxiety
Excessive weakness
Inability to recover from exercise
Insomnia
Headaches
Inability to concentrate
Increased allergies
Enlarged lymph nodes on the neck

What's fascinating is the remarkable similarity of these signs and symptoms to those associated with what is now called *chronic fatigue immunodeficiency syndrome* (CFIDS) (please see "Immune System" for a discussion of CFIDS). Anxiety and depression are also components of this condition. Tintera also noticed that people with low adrenal function were likely to have problems with hypoglycemia (low blood sugar).

Tintera's solution for reestablishing normal adrenal function was to give his patients regular injections of an extract made from animal adrenal glands. He found that this treatment gave the adrenal glands some rest and recuperation time, which allowed them to build up some reserves. He also placed these patients on a diet similar to the one I outline here and used nutritional supplements such as vitamin C and pantothenic acid, which help support normal adrenal function.

Unfortunately, Tintera didn't know about adaptogenic herbs such as eleuthero (Siberian ginseng) and Asian ginseng (see "Adaptogens" in Part 4). These herbs are the perfect fit for both treating and preventing adrenal exhaustion. It's interesting to note that the term *adaptogen* implies an ability to help the body adapt to stress in its various forms. So, when you've got Selye's GAS, try a little herbal tonic!

HERBAL PRESCRIPTIONS

Choose one of the following adaptogens:

- Eleuthero (Siberian ginseng)—Standardized, concentrated extract of the root and rhizomes, 300 to 400 milligrams daily; dry, powdered root and rhizomes, 2 to 3 grams daily in two or three divided dosages; alcohol-based extract, 8 to 10 milliliters in two to three divided doses. Use continuously for 4 to 6 weeks with a 1- to 2-week break before resuming.
  Action: Promotes and supports healthy communication in the HPA axis and normal adrenal function. Eleuthero is my personal favorite for long-term support of adrenal function.
- Asian ginseng—100 milligrams twice daily of an extract standardized to contain 5 to 7 percent ginsenosides. Use for 4 weeks continuously with a 1- to 2-week break before resuming.
  Action: Promotes and supports healthy communication in the HPA axis and normal adrenal function

OTHER HERBAL RECOMMENDATIONS

See the chapter "Nervous System" for recommendations for management of anxiety and mild depression.

NUTRITIONAL SUPPLEMENT CONSIDERATIONS

- Vitamin B complex—50 to 100 milligrams daily
- Pantothenic acid—250 milligrams daily
- Vitamin C—2 to 3 grams daily
- Chromium (polynicotinate or picolinate)—200 micrograms once or twice daily

DIETARY RECOMMENDATIONS

Low adrenal function often leads to low blood sugar (hypoglycemia). A good way to counter low blood sugar is to eat smaller, more frequent meals. In addition to your three major meals, try a midmorning and midafternoon snack. Snacks don't mean a candy bar or diet soda! Try fruit, a salad, or a bag of mixed nuts. Breakfast is an important meal. Don't skip it! Move your dietary focus away from simple carbohydrates (primarily sweets) toward complex carbohydrates and dietary fiber found in vegetables and fruits. Keep your protein intake at a normal level by consuming soy, fish, and nuts.

Eyes

RELATED CHAPTERS IN PART 5

- Bilberry
- Chamomile
- Evening Primrose
- *Ginkgo biloba*

CATARACTS

Cataracts result when the normal transparency of the eye degenerates. As the eye (usually the lens or capsule) becomes less transparent, it turns cloudy or opaque. The cardinal symptom of cataracts is a progressive and painless loss of vision. Cataracts may occur because of injury or surgery, diseases such as diabetes, overexposure to X-ray and ultraviolet light, and even some medications.

Cataracts afflict 50 million people worldwide. In the United States, it is a leading cause of blindness. Conservative estimates indicate that 18 percent of people from 65 to 75 years of age have cataracts. This figure jumps to 46 percent for people more than 75 years old.[1] In the United States, more than 541,000 surgeries for cataracts are performed annually at a cost of over $3.8 billion. It has been estimated that if cataract formation could be delayed by only 10 years, the need for lens surgery could be cut in half.[2]

As will be noted in the following discussion of macular degeneration, free radical damage to the lens of the eye is a major factor. Thus, prevention centers on using antioxidant supplements to block free radical buildup.

Note: These recommendations are made with the understanding that herbal and nutritional interventions are preventive in nature. Those of you with documented cataract formation should be under the close care of an ophthalmologist.

Herbal Prescription
- Bilberry extract (25 percent anthocyanosides)—120 to 240 milligrams daily in two or three divided doses (prevention)[3]
  Action: Potent antioxidant for the eyes

Nutritional Supplement Considerations
- Vitamin C—1 gram daily[4]
- Vitamin E—400 international units (IU) daily with meals[5]
- Riboflavin (vitamin B_2) and Niacin (vitamin B_3)—In a Chinese study, 3 milligrams of riboflavin and 40 milligrams of niacin daily were found to protect against cataracts.[6] You may be able to find these levels of these nutrients in a good multiple-vitamin and mineral formulation.

Dietary Recommendations
To keep free radicals from forming, avoid fried foods and animal products such as red meat and milk. Add leafy, green vegetables and also yellow and orange veggies that are high in carotenoids such as beta-carotene and lycopene to your diet. Increase your consumption of fruits—particularly berries and others high in bioflavonoids.

Lifestyle Considerations
I'm probably going to cause rioting in Scottsdale and Boca Raton, but I've got to say it anyway: Reduce sun exposure to avoid ultraviolet radiation. This is one of the major sources of eye-related free radical damage. Get some good sunglasses or start thinking of places like Seattle and London as new retirement havens.

Diabetic Retinopathy

The leading cause of blindness among diabetics is retinopathy. This condition causes the capillaries in the eye to become fragile and begin leaking, which in turn leads to swelling in the retina and eventual loss of normal vision. Advanced complications include scarring and retinal detachment.

The onset of diabetic retinopathy appears to be linked to how long a person has had diabetes. It most commonly appears around the 10th year following diagnosis of diabetes. Two factors that are important in delaying onset are control of blood sugar level and keeping blood pressure down. Yearly retinal exams should begin 5 years after diabetes has been first diagnosed.

Note: With the exception of bilberry, the recommendations given here are for prevention. Please review the general nutritional and dietary recommendations given in the section on diabetes in "Endocrine System," as well as the nutritional supplement recommendations cited later for macular degeneration. Particular emphasis should be on vitamin E supplementation.

HERBAL PRESCRIPTIONS

- Bilberry extract (25 percent anthocyanosides)—120 to 240 milligrams daily in two or three divided doses (prevention); 480 to 600 milligrams daily in two or three divided doses (treatment of early-stage diabetic retinopathy)
  Actions: Strengthens capillaries and reduces hemorrhaging in the retina
- *Ginkgo biloba* extract—120 to 240 milligrams daily in two to three divided doses
  Action: Protects the retina of the eye, primarily by antioxidant properties[1]

MACULAR DEGENERATION

Also known as *age-related macular degeneration* (AMD), this condition is the leading cause of irreversible blindness in adults over 50 years of age. The incidence of AMD in persons over 65 years of age is 10 percent and increases to more than 28 percent in those over 75 years old. Cases in the United States are predicted to rise from 2.7 million in 1970 to more than 7.5 million by the year 2030. Approximately 20 percent of new cases of blindness in the United States are due to AMD.

AMD refers to a degeneration of the macular disk—the portion of the retina of the eye responsible for precise vision. Technically speaking, AMD is a type of retinopathy. It destroys central vision and affects the ability to read or do close work, drive, and differentiate colors and faces. A classic early symptom of AMD is a person complaining that door frames appear bent or wavy. The condition can often be aggravated by high blood pressure, diabetes, and high cholesterol.[1]

A major focus of research on AMD over the last few years has been the role of free radical damage in the macula caused by high sun exposure and ultraviolet B light. As with cataracts, AMD occurs more frequently in areas of year-round sunlight.

HERBAL PRESCRIPTIONS

Prevention and Treatment of Early-Stage Macular Degeneration

- *Ginkgo biloba* extract—120 to 240 milligrams daily in two to three divided doses[2]

  Actions: Protects the retina of the eye and slows the progression of macular degeneration in the early stages. Please note that studies to date have been very small and must be considered preliminary.

- Bilberry extract—120 to 240 milligrams daily in two or three divided doses (prevention); 480 to 600 milligrams daily in two or three divided doses (treatment of early-stage AMD)

  Note: A new kid on the block is grape seed extracts high in oligomeric proanthocyanidins (OPCs). Like bilberry, these flavonoid-rich supplements may also help in the treatment of mild forms of retinopathy.[3] The recommended dose is 100 milligrams of OPCs three times daily.

NUTRITIONAL SUPPLEMENT CONSIDERATIONS

In addition to the recommendations listed previously for the prevention/treatment of cataracts (with the exception of riboflavin and niacin), consider the following:

- Lutein and zeaxanthin (members of the carotenoid family)—Oral supplement providing approximately 6 or 7 milligrams per day (this is usually listed as just lutein even though the zeaxanthin is in there, too)[4]

- Zinc (monomethionine or citrate)—30 milligrams daily[5]

  Note: The research study cited used 80 milligrams of zinc daily. I think this amount is too high for long-term use.

DIETARY RECOMMENDATIONS

Please review the dietary recommendations in the "Cataracts" section. For prevention of macular degeneration, it's best to get plenty of vegetables high in carotenes—especially lutein and zeaxanthin. Examples include kale, spinach, and collard greens.[6] Also, it's important to note that high intake of saturated fat may increase your risk of AMD.[7]

EYE GEAR RECOMMENDATION

If you have AMD or are at risk for AMD, you should consult an ophthalmologist to obtain protective eye wear for use in bright sunlight.

OTHER EYE CONDITIONS

BLOCKED TEAR DUCT

Note: A common condition in young infants is a temporary blockage of the tear duct in one or both eyes. This can lead to an infection and often requires antibiotic treatment and dilation of the tear duct. The recommendations made here are early measures, meant for use before infection sets in.

- Chamomile—Place a warm chamomile tea bag over the eye for 5 to 10 minutes. Repeat every 2 to 3 hours. Be sure the tea bags are not too hot!
- Breast milk—Many mothers and midwives tell me that the best cure for a blocked tear duct is simply to squirt breast milk into the child's eye. I hear this is a good cure for the ol' Oedipus complex in boys!

POOR NIGHT VISION
- Bilberry extract—See dosage instructions under "Cataracts."
- Vitamin A—5,000 IU daily
- Zinc—30 milligrams daily

Dry Eyes Associated with Sjögren's Syndrome

- Evening primrose oil—3 grams daily with meals[1]
- Vitamin C—1 gram three times daily
- Vitamin B6—50 milligrams twice daily

Uveitis (Chronic and Acute)

- *Ginkgo biloba* extract—Follow the instructions under "Macular Degeneration."
  Action: Ginkgo counters a pro-inflammatory substance known as platelet-activating factor. This factor is elevated in the eyes of people with chronic uveitis.[1]
- Curcumin (from turmeric)—375 mg three times daily[2]
- Vitamin C—500 milligrams twice daily
- Vitamin E—200 to 400 IU daily

Note: In one study, combining vitamin C (1,000 milligrams) and vitamin E (200 IU) daily for 8 weeks with standard therapy (cortisone eye drops) led to improved visual acuity in people with acute anterior uveitis.[3] Please remember that acute uveitis should be treated only under the supervision of a qualified ophthalmologist.

Female Health Conditions

RELATED CHAPTERS IN PART 5

- Black Cohosh
- Echinacea
- Evening Primrose
- Garlic
- Ginger
- *Vitex agnus-castus*

FIBROCYSTIC BREAST DISEASE/CYCLICAL BREAST PAIN

Fibrocystic breast disease (FBD) is a benign (noncancerous) condition that affects approximately 40 percent of premenopausal women. This makes FBD the most common breast disease.

It is characterized by the formation of cysts within the breasts and usually involves both breasts. There are often multiple cysts, and, if located near the surface of the breast, they can be freely moved and are usually tender to touch. Pain often accompanies cyst formation and can range from mild to severe. Some women with FBD have no pain and discover cyst formation only by breast self-examination.

Women with FBD who have a family history of breast cancer should be under the close supervision of a physician and have regularly scheduled breast examinations and mammography.

Note: For a more comprehensive look at prevention and treatment of breast cancer, I highly recommend *Breast Cancer: What You Should Know (But May Not Be Told) about Prevention, Diagnosis, and Treatment* by Steve Austin and Cathy Hitchcock (Prima, 1994).

HERBAL PRESCRIPTIONS

See the recommendations for vitex and evening primrose oil in the section on premenstrual syndrome (PMS) later in this chapter. While these treatments have been proven most effective for pain and tenderness associated with a woman's period, they may provide some benefit for women with FBD.

NUTRITIONAL SUPPLEMENT CONSIDERATIONS

Please see recommendations for vitamin E and vitamin B_6 in the section on PMS.

DIETARY AND LIFESTYLE RECOMMENDATIONS

For FBD, the first step is to eliminate methylxanthines (caffeine), common in coffee, tea, colas, and chocolate.[1,2] Reduce dietary fats, especially red meat and dairy products, and follow the rest of the dietary instructions for PMS. Exercise may also reduce breast tenderness associated with a woman's cycle and reduce risk of FBD.[3]

HOT FLASHES (ASSOCIATED WITH MENOPAUSE)

Menopause technically means the cessation of the monthly female menstrual cycle. Women who have not had their period for a year or more are considered postmenopausal. Menopause typically begins in the late 40s or early 50s and is sometimes heralded by hot flashes, vaginal dryness, and loss of libido.

While many hormonal (or as my preadolescent daughter calls them, "harmonial") changes occur, the primary focus is on the decrease in estrogen. Many women are pressured to consider hormone replacement therapy (HRT) to reduce their risk of cardiovascular disease and osteoporosis. However, HRT is not without its downsides (e.g., increased risk of certain forms of cancer), and you should definitely discuss the pros and cons with your doctor.

There's been a huge amount of attention in the past few years on the potential role of foods and specifically phytoestrogens as potential replacements for HRT. While foods such as soy that are high in phytoestrogens have noted health benefits—particularly for the cardiovascular system—we have a ways to go (e.g., clinical studies) before we can definitively call them replacements for HRT.

My focus in this section is primarily on reducing acute symptoms associated with menopause such as hot flashes. For more details, I highly recommend reading *Perimenopause: Preparing for the Change* by Nancy Lee Teaff and Kim Wright Wiley (Prima, 1995). It provides a thorough overview of the symptoms associated with perimenopause and also evaluates issues such as hormone replacement therapy. Another excellent book for women is *Women's Encyclopedia of Natural Medicine* (Keats, 1999) by my good friend Dr. Tori Hudson. She provides an excellent overview of the pros and cons of HRT and describes where nutrition and herbal options fit into your personalized approach to menopause.

HERBAL PRESCRIPTION

- Black cohosh root extract—20 milligrams twice daily
  Actions: Contrary to popular belief, it does not have estrogen-like actions. Think of black cohosh as herbal relief for hot flashes.

NUTRITIONAL SUPPLEMENT CONSIDERATIONS

Note: While vitamins C and E may help hot flashes, these nutrients and the ipriflavone are primarily focused on promotion of cardiovascular and bone health.

- Calcium (citrate malate)—1,200 milligrams daily
- Magnesium—600 milligrams daily
- Vitamin C—1 to 2 grams daily[1]
- Vitamin E—400 800 IU daily with meals[2]
- Ipriflavone—600 milligrams daily[3]

DIETARY RECOMMENDATIONS

Increase your consumption of foods high in isoflavones (phytoestrogens) (see the following discussion on phytoestrogens). The all-purpose one here is soy. One cup of soy beans daily delivers close to the equivalent amount of conjugated estrogens as one tablet of Premarin.[4] However, the isoflavones from soy are only about 1 percent as potent as estradiol. Other constituents in soy also appear to be health promoting, including the soy protein, which has benefits for the cardiovascular system. In studies with menopausal women, daily consumption of approximately 60 grams of soy protein was associated with a decrease in hot flashes.[5] (Please note that this was dietary soy and not pills.) Remember, soy is not the only food with phytoestrogens. Chickpeas and other legumes also contain these constituents.

Reduce your intake of saturated fats from animal sources and eat plenty of complex carbohydrates and fiber from vegetables, fruits, and legumes. Add green tea to your daily beverage intake.

A NOTE ON PHYTOESTROGENS

The term *phytoestrogen* implies a plant or food that has estrogen-like constituents and actions. These are flavonoid compounds known as *isoflavones*. The most popular example is soy, which contains a substance known as *genistein*. Currently, the most we can say about phytoestrogens is that eating foods high in these compounds offers promise against breast cancer, osteoporosis, and many of the maladies that women suffer from in the United States.

Herbs that qualify as phytoestrogens include red clover, licorice root, and Asian ginseng. Dong quai is often mistakenly listed as a phytoestrogen.[6] As noted earlier, so is black cohosh. One of the more interesting isoflavone supplements developed is from red clover. Sold in the United States as Promensil® (Novogen, Stamford, CT), the extract delivers 40 milligrams of isoflavones per tablet. While the research thus far suggest some benefit for cardiovascular health in menopausal women,[7] effects on treatment of hot flashes has been somewhat disappointing.[8]

As previously mentioned, we don't know whether these plant estrogen sources can replace Premarin for the prevention of osteoporosis and heart disease in menopausal women. In the meantime, increase soy, other legumes, and flaxseed in the diet. It's my guess that the real benefit of these foods is preparing women for a healthier life following menopause.

That means placing focus on these foods long before menopause while reducing those foods that will increase risk of cardiovascular disease and osteoporosis, such as saturated fats from animal sources.

INFERTILITY

Please see the related discussion in the chapter on vitex in Part 5. I'm limiting the focus here to infertility caused by high production of prolactin by the pituitary and an abnormal estrogen-to-progesterone balance during the second phase of the menstrual cycle. Also, please review the section on infertility in the "Male Health Conditions" section. Remember, in couples with problems conceiving, it's as likely to be a problem with the male partner as it is with the female.

HERBAL PRESCRIPTION
- *Vitex agnus-castus*—Dried or liquid preparations delivering 30 to 40 milligrams of the crushed fruit once daily in the morning with some water. Use vitex over a period of several months continuously. *Actions:* Restores normal balance of progesterone and estrogen; also reduces excess prolactin production in the latter part of the luteal phase.

NUTRITIONAL SUPPLEMENT CONSIDERATIONS
- Zinc (monomethionine or citrate)—50 to 75 milligrams daily[1]
- Vitamin B_6—100 milligrams twice daily[2]
  Note: The two nutrients listed here may help reduce prolactin levels. There is no specific research using them in women with infertility.

DIETARY AND LIFESTYLE RECOMMENDATIONS
Reduce your daily consumption of caffeine. Smoking and excessive alcohol intake have been associated with delayed conception. Finally, auricular (ear) acupuncture has been found to help some women who are having difficulty conceiving.[3]

MORNING SICKNESS DURING PREGNANCY

Please refer to the discussion in the chapter on ginger in Part 5.

HERBAL PRESCRIPTION

- Ginger root powder—1 gram daily as needed for nausea
  Actions: Decreases nausea and improves digestion. Ginger has also been used in the treatment of hyperemesis gravidarum, a more serious condition characterized by severe vomiting and nausea. This should be considered only after proper medical consultation.

NUTRITIONAL SUPPLEMENT CONSIDERATIONS

- Vitamin B_6—30 to 75 milligrams daily[1]
- Vitamin K (5 milligrams) and vitamin C (25 milligrams)—This combination (daily dosage for each is listed) was found to successfully treat morning sickness within three days in one older clinical study.[2]

DIETARY RECOMMENDATIONS

Smaller, more frequent meals will sometimes help. My midwife friends also recommend some dry toast upon rising in the morning (yummy!).

PREMENSTRUAL SYNDROME

If you're a woman 30 to 40 years of age, there's a better than even chance you've suffered premenstrual syndrome (PMS). Premenstrual syndrome is a condition marked by nervousness, irritability, mood swings, depression, and often headaches, water retention, and breast tenderness. Other symptoms that appear include nausea, constipation, backache, and abdominal bloating. Symptoms usually start 7 to 10 days before the onset of your period and will often resolve with the onset of menstrual flow. Symptoms can vary in severity from month to month.

The exact cause of PMS is unknown and probably involves a number of different factors. These factors also vary from woman to woman. One area of focus has been the production of high estrogen and low progesterone as well as high prolactin during the luteal or second phase of a woman's cycle. See the chapter on vitex in Part 5 for further discussion.

HERBAL PRESCRIPTIONS

- *Vitex agnus-castus*—Dried or liquid preparations delivering 30 to 40 milligrams of the crushed fruit once daily in the morning with some water. Use vitex over a period of several months continuously.
  Actions: Restores normal balance of progesterone and estrogen. Also reduces excess prolactin production in the latter part of the luteal phase.
- Evening primrose oil—3 to 4 grams daily with meals
  Actions: Corrects abnormal essential fatty acid metabolism. Gamma-linolenic acid (GLA) increases the production of hormones known as prostaglandins, which reduce uterine cramping and breast tenderness.
  Note: Remember that EPO is slow acting and probably most effective for breast tenderness and pain associated with your period.

OTHER HERBAL CONSIDERATION

- Dong quai (*Angelica sinensis*)—2 to 3 grams daily in two to three divided doses
  Note: Dong quai may be especially useful if you're having a lot of premenstrual uterine cramping and pain (dysmenorrhea).[1]

NUTRITIONAL SUPPLEMENT CONSIDERATIONS

Note: Dosage recommendations for single nutrients are based on a daily total. These should be adjusted in light of nutrient levels contained in the multiple-vitamin/mineral formulation.

- Multiple-vitamin/mineral supplement—Formulation should be free of allergens and contain adequate amounts of B vitamins (especially vitamin B_6), magnesium, vitamin E, and iron.[2]
- Vitamin B_6—100 milligrams twice daily[3,4]
- Calcium—1,200 milligrams daily[5]
- Magnesium—400 to 600 milligrams daily[6]
- Vitamin E—300 IU daily with meals[7]

DIETARY RECOMMENDATIONS

Dietary modifications are at the heart of any strategy against PMS. The following guidelines should be helpful:

- Reduce or eliminate sugar, salt, and saturated fats from animal sources such as red meat and dairy products. Cut down on simple carbohydrates such as white flour and concentrated carbohydrates, including fruit juices and dried fruits. Avoid junk foods, diet sodas, and caffeine, which is present in coffee, tea, chocolate, and even some over-the-counter drugs. Limiting alcoholic beverages is also recommended.
- Increase your intake of complex carbohydrates and fiber from vegetables, fruits, and grains. Get your protein from sources such as soy and fish.
- Eat small, more frequent meals. This will keep weight down while stabilizing blood sugar.

LIFESTYLE CONSIDERATIONS

An aerobic exercise program is highly recommended. The goal should be four times weekly for 20 to 30 minutes for each session. Relaxation exercises such as yoga or meditation are also recommended. You can also listen to Captain Beefheart singing "Nowadays a Woman's Just Gotta Hit a Man."

VAGINAL YEAST INFECTIONS (RECURRENT)

HERBAL PRESCRIPTIONS

To Reduce Recurrence

- *Echinacea purpurea* or *E. angustifolia*—5 milliliters of the expressed juice or tincture three times daily or one capsule containing 300 milligrams of the dried herb or root three or four times daily for 10 to 14 days

  Action: Helps strengthen the immune response to resist reinfection

- Garlic (standardized garlic powder product containing 1.3% aliin and providing 5,000 to 6,000 micrograms of allicin potential daily)—600 to 900 milligrams daily in two to three divided doses
  Action: Antimicrobial activity against *Candida albicans* and other yeast organisms

Topical Treatments
- Tea tree oil suppository—200 milligrams of oil in a vegetable oil (e.g., coconut oil) base. Insert one suppository in the vagina once daily on alternating days for 7 to 10 days.[1]
  Action: Powerful antiyeast activity
  Warning: Some women may experience a burning sensation with use of tea tree oil intravaginally. Use with caution, and do not exceed the dilution recommended here.
  Note: This is also a potential treatment for bacterial vaginosis.[2]
- Boric acid capsules—Insert one capsule into the vagina twice daily for 2 to 4 weeks.[3]
  Note: This isn't an herbal remedy, but the results in the study were impressive: 98 percent success!

NUTRITIONAL SUPPLEMENT CONSIDERATIONS
- Acidophilus/bifidus probiotic supplement—Use internally one or two times daily. Also effective when used topically either by inserting a gelatin capsule directly into the vagina (don't worry—it will dissolve!) or in a douche.[4] Remember, use probiotics orally when taking antibiotics to reduce the risk of yeast infections.

DIETARY RECOMMENDATIONS
Increase your intake of garlic and yogurt. Try to cut down on sugar in your diet. Consume more complex carbohydrates and fiber from vegetables, fruits, and legumes.

Immune System

RELATED CHAPTERS IN PART 5

- Echinacea
- Eleuthero (Siberian Ginseng)
- Garlic
- Asian Ginseng
- Milk Thistle

CHRONIC FATIGUE IMMUNODEFICIENCY SYNDROME

It has taken the medical world some time to accept chronic fatigue immunodeficiency syndrome (CFIDS). Initially thought to be all in the mind, CFIDS was targeted as the "yuppie flu" and believed to be caused by *Epstein–Barr virus* (the virus causing mononucleosis). It's now an official diagnosis. While we still don't know for sure what causes the condition, new evidence may help unlock the key to successful treatment of CFIDS.

Table 6.2 lists the signs and symptoms for CFIDS. To be diagnosed with CFIDS, a person must meet both the major criteria and eight of the minor symptom criteria, which sounds a bit like trying to figure out who's going to be in the wild card playoffs in football!

I try to address these three major areas with all of my CFIDS patients:

- Regulation of the hypothalamic–pituitary–adrenal (HPA) axis and adrenal function
- Immune function
- Psychological issues

Let's consider these individually.

REGULATION OF THE HPA AXIS AND ADRENAL FUNCTION

Evidence is mounting that CFIDS is a condition caused by dysregulation (poor communication of the HPA axis, resulting in sluggish or ex-

Table 6.2
DIAGNOSTIC CRITERIA FOR CHRONIC FATIGUE
IMMUNODEFICIENCY SYNDROME

Major Criteria

---

1. New onset of persistent or relapsing, debilitating fatigue with no previous history of similar symptoms. Average daily activity reduced or impaired below 50 percent for 6 months.
2. Exclusion of other conditions that may produce similar symptoms.

Minor Symptom Criteria

---

1. Minor fever or chills
2. Sore throat
3. Painful lymph nodes in the neck and underarms
4. Unexplained generalized muscle weakness
5. Muscle tenderness or pain (myalgia)
6. Twenty-four hours of fatigue after exercise that is usually tolerated
7. Generalized headaches, unlike previous headaches
8. Joint pain that moves to different parts of the body
9. Depression and/or anxiety
10. Sleep disturbance (insomnia)
11. Symptoms developing over a few hours to a few days

---

hausted adrenal glands.[1,2] Turn to the chapter "Endocrine System," and review the section on stress and fatigue. Compare the criteria for hypoadrenocorticism (low adrenal function) established by John Tintera back in the late 1940s. They include excessive fatigue and weakness, depression, headaches, insomnia, swollen lymph nodes, and increased allergies; these criteria are remarkably similar to those currently used to describe CFIDS.[3]

A telltale sign of adrenal exhaustion is excessive fatigue following strenuous exercise. This means that the usual rush you get from exercise never comes and your recovery from a workout is slow and drawn out. In other words, exercise makes you feel worse. This shows up in both hypoadrenocorticism and CFIDS.

Low adrenal function upsets blood sugar metabolism, causing hypo-glycemia (low blood sugar). It also hampers the body's ability to fight in-flammation and pain. This is because of the drop-off in production of natural, cortisone-like substances by the adrenals. It's interesting to note that a common condition associated with CFIDS is fibromyalgia (FM). The generalized aches and pains associated with this condition could very well be linked to sluggish adrenal function. In fact, not only does research indicate a huge overlap between persons suffering both FM and CFIDS,[4] but recent studies also suggest that FM is also a result of the endocrine stress center of the body—the HPA axis—functioning improperly.[5]

It's my opinion that CFIDS is the current embodiment of hypoadreno-corticism. By supporting adrenal function through herbs (licorice in the short term and eleuthero or Asian ginseng in the long term), nutrients, diet, and stress reduction, you may be 90 percent of the way toward solv-ing the puzzle of CFIDS.

Immune Function

The immune system of people with CFIDS is also out of balance. Some CFIDS patients show a depressed immune system that resembles the profile seen with HIV (human immunodeficiency virus)-infected pa-tients. Other patients actually have overactive immune systems resem-bling those of people with autoimmune conditions such as lupus.[6,7]

Restoring balance to the immune function is critical. The herbs that work best on the adrenal glands (i.e., eleuthero and Asian ginseng) also promote a balanced immune system. Adaptogens are the perfect starting point for an herbal offensive against CFIDS (see "Adaptogens" in Part 4).

Psychological Issues

While I don't support the premise that most of CFIDS resides in the mind, I do find that many of my CFIDS patients are depressed when they first visit my office. Of course, who wouldn't be with the uncertain nature of CFIDS?

I often use a mild herbal antidepressant such as St. John's wort to counter depression. This is usually short-term because once adrenal function begins to make a comeback, depression will often be one of the first things to go.

HERBAL PRESCRIPTIONS

Short-Term

- Licorice root—5 to 6 grams daily for 6 to 8 weeks[8]

  Actions: Glycyrrhetinic acid in licorice root has been shown to inhibit the enzyme that breaks down cortisol, 11-β-hydroxysteroid dehydrogenase.[9] This means more of those natural cortisonelike substances mentioned earlier are available to the body.

  Note: This is a pretty high dose of licorice root. It's best to use this dose of licorice under the supervision of a qualified health care professional. If your symptoms get worse after a week or two, stop the licorice root. Some people with depression will actually get worse with more cortisol in the body—this may be a sign that your troubles are in that arena and not CFIDS. Also, if you begin to get swelling around your ankles or your blood pressure goes up, it's time to stop the licorice.

Long-Term

Choose one of the following adaptogens:

- Eleuthero (Siberian ginseng)—Standardized, concentrated extract of the root and rhizomes, 300 to 400 milligrams daily; dry, powdered root and rhizomes, 2 to 3 grams daily in two or three divided dosages; alcohol-based extract, 8 to 10 milliliters in two to three divided dosages. Use continuously for 4 to 6 weeks with a 1- to 2-week break before resuming.

  Actions: Promotes and supports normal adrenal function and immune system activity. Eleuthero is my personal favorite for long-term treatment of CFIDS.

- Asian ginseng—100 milligrams twice daily of an extract standardized to contain 5 to 7 percent ginsenosides

  Actions: Promotes and supports normal adrenal function and immune system activity

NUTRITIONAL SUPPLEMENT CONSIDERATIONS

- Magnesium—200 to 300 milligrams twice daily[10]
  Note: It's best to consider magnesium after having your doctor check to see whether you have a deficiency first. Persons with CFIDS and low magnesium will respond best to supplementing this mineral.
- L-Carnitine—1 gram three times daily[11]
- Vitamin B complex—50 to 100 milligrams daily

DIETARY RECOMMENDATIONS

Low adrenal function often leads to low blood sugar (hypoglycemia). A good way to counter low blood sugar is to eat small, frequent meals. In addition to your three major meals, try a midmorning and midafternoon snack. Snacks don't mean a candy bar or diet soda! Try fruit, a salad, or a bag of mixed nuts. Breakfast is an important meal. Don't skip it!

Move your diet away from simple carbohydrates (primarily sweets) and toward the complex carbohydrates and dietary fiber found in vegetables, fruits, and legumes. Keep your protein intake at a normal level by consuming soy, fish, and nuts.

Reports have also indicated that food allergies may play a part in CFIDS.[12] Work with a qualified health care professional to identify and eliminate food allergens.

OTHER CONSIDERATIONS

Be sure your doctor rules out low thyroid function.[13] Follow a good relaxation program. If you also have fibromyalgia, add acupuncture or massage to your treatment plan. You shouldn't stop exercising, as moderate exercise has been shown to help people with CFIDS.[14] Just don't overdo it, as this can lead to significant worsening of your symptoms.

COLDS AND FLU

The common cold is the bane of mainstream medicine. Everybody gets colds, but modern medicine doesn't know how to cure them. A good case of the flu, and you're in the same boat. The best we're offered is decongestants, cough medicines, and acetaminophen to chase away our symptoms. Problem is, none of that stuff makes a difference.

In fact, the aches and fever associated with the flu and the nasal congestion, sore throat, and headache that accompany a cold are really signs that the body is doing its best to end the infection. It's not pleasant while it's occurring, but our immune systems should be applauded for their efforts and not be interfered with.

Herbal medicines also relieve symptoms (see the discussions on coughs, sinus infections, and sore throats in "Ears, Nose, Throat, and Respiratory Tract" and on diarrhea in "Digestive System"). Where they really shine, however, is in their ability to support the immune system. First, they support the immune system in its fight to keep the system infection free. This means that around cold and flu season, the herbal prescriptions listed below are perfect defenses to prevent a cold or flu. Second, they speed the healing process once you've become sick. Your best friend here is echinacea. You may ache and feel lousy, but echinacea will usually shorten your time of suffering.

Last but not least, don't use flu vaccines if you're basically a healthy individual. Flu vaccines may be necessary for the very young and very old as well as those with impaired immune systems, but the rest of us don't need them! Follow the recommendations here—you'll be healthier and your immune system will thank you.

HERBAL PRESCRIPTIONS
Treatment
- *Echinacea purpurea* or *E. angustifolia*—20 to 40 drops of the expressed (i.e., squeezed) juice of the *E. purpurea* herb juice initially; then 20 to 40 drops of the juice every 2 hours throughout the day for 48 hours or until symptom relief is noted. Alternatively, 900 to 1,200 mg of dried herb or root of either *E. purpurea* or *E. angustifolia* or 3 to 5 milliliters of tincture daily may replace the expressed juice product. Limit use to 7 to 10 days.
  Action: May strengthen the immune system response and decrease the duration and severity of symptoms

Note: An alternative is to use Esberitox®, a combination of echinacea, thuja, and wild indigo. Take 3 tablets (you can chew them) three times daily for 7 to 10 days.

- *Andrographis paniculata* extract—400 milligrams three times daily for 5 to 10 days[1]

  Note: Long used for a variety of diseases in traditional Chinese medicine, andrographis is emerging as another interesting herbal approach to decrease the severity and duration of the common cold.

Prevention

- Eleuthero (Siberian ginseng)—Standardized, concentrated extract of the root and rhizomes, 300 to 400 milligrams daily; dry, powdered root and rhizomes, 2 to 3 grams daily in two or three divided doses; alcohol-based extract, 8 to 10 milliliters in two to three divided doses. Use continuously for 4 to 6 weeks with a 1- to 2-week break before resuming.

  Actions: Promotes a healthy immune response and supports normal adrenal function; offers particularly good support for a person under a lot of stress

OTHER HERBAL CONSIDERATION

- Black elderberry extract (Sambucol®)—4 tablespoons per day for adults and 2 tablespoons for children[2]

  Note: While the data to support this product are pretty weak, I've heard some interesting feedback from health care professionals recommending it to patients for the flu. One word of warning: Definitely avoid this stuff if it's offered to you by a couple of old spinster sisters in the form of elderberry wine!

NUTRITIONAL SUPPLEMENT CONSIDERATIONS

- Vitamin C—1 to 2 grams every 3 to 4 hours[3]
- Zinc (gluconate or gluconate-glycine)—One chewable lozenge (15 to 25 milligrams of zinc per lozenge) up to ten times daily[4]

  Note: Great for sore throats, zinc lozenges should be taken at the first sign of a cold and used only for 7 to 10 days.

And from the "because it's good for you, bubeleh" department:

- Rest
- Lots of water
- Chicken soup

HIV Infection/AIDS

As we begin the new millennium, it's becoming apparent that complementary and alternative medicine will play more of a supportive role in the long-term management of HIV infection. With the success of new antiretroviral drug therapies, the focus among practitioners of alternative medicine should be how best to improve the quality of life and promote optimal wellness in their patients with HIV infection. This isn't intended to sound fatalistic, it's just a reality check—a lot of emotion and effort was thrown into trying to figure out the "cure" in the past two decades. I'm just suggesting channeling that energy into an area that is likely to be more productive.

So, with that said, I still like my rant from the first edition of the book. Here we go again!

Excuse me while I vent.

I was reading in the newspaper that Senator Jesse Helms thinks we're spending too much money on research for anti-HIV drugs and treatments for acquired immunodeficiency syndrome (AIDS). Carrying the homophobic banner forward, Senator Helms suggested that those who had AIDS essentially deserved it.

I'd like to suggest that Senator Helms be reminded of the fact that a large part of his financial base comes from the tobacco industry. Ironic that a self-proclaimed "health expert" like Senator Helms has been responsible for shielding an industry that is directly responsible for thousands of deaths yearly.

Thanks, I feel better.

Numerous resources offer a wide range of information about HIV infection. Here are one Web site, three organizations, and a publication I find useful:

The Body
www.thebody.com
The Body is a convenient gateway to almost every key resource for persons with HIV infection. It includes access to the organizations listed here as well as government agencies such as the Food and Drug Administration.

Gay Men's Health Crisis (GMHC)
The Tisch Building
119 West 24 Street
New York, NY 10011
(212) 367-1000
www.gmhc.org
Founded in 1981 by volunteers, GMHC is the world's oldest and largest AIDS service, education, and advocacy organization. It serves thousands of men, women, and children with HIV and AIDS; educates the public about HIV prevention and treatment; and fights for fair and effective AIDS policies at all levels of government. GHMC also produces the publication *Treatment Issues,* a monthly newsletter that provides reliable information on experimental AIDS therapies.

Project Inform
205 13th Street, #2001
San Francisco, CA 94103
(415) 558-8669
www.ProjectInform.org
Project Inform has been at the front lines in the fight against HIV and AIDS since 1985. It was organized to provide vital information on the diagnosis and treatment of HIV disease to HIV-infected individuals, their caregivers, and the health care and services providers. In addition to preparing fact sheets on specific treatments, common infections, and strategies for maintaining health, Project Inform also publishes the *PI Perspective* several times each year.

Seattle Treatment Exchange Project (STEP)
1123 E. John Street
Seattle, WA 98102
(206) 329-4857
step100@aol.com

STEP is an organization of men and women dedicated to bringing treatment information to those infected with HIV or at risk of HIV infection, to health care providers, and to members of HIV service organizations. It produces a publication known as the *STEP Perspective* that covers treatment issues ranging from antiretroviral drugs, supportive therapies for prevention of secondary infections, and alternative therapies. STEP has also produced a set of fact sheets on HIV testing, general treatment strategies, nutrition, and alternative therapies, including some herbal treatments.

AIDS Treatment News
P.O. Box 411256
San Francisco, CA 94141
(415) 255-0588
www.aidsnews.org

AIDS Treatment News is one of the most popular and well-written guides to experimental and complementary as well as standard AIDS treatments. Edited and published by John James, the publication attempts to increase awareness of different treatments and their combinations that may serve to make HIV infection a manageable condition.

As I've already mentioned, it's my opinion that herbs, vitamins and minerals, and other alternative medicines are best viewed as complementary at this point. In other words, use them to help increase your chances of long-term survival. I don't know of any natural therapies that will replace current antiretroviral drug therapies.

Last, make educated choices. Read as many articles, books, and case studies as you can. Talk to long-term survivors and find out what they do. Use the resources listed here. Don't get caught up in the latest "miracle cure." The so-called miracle workers are usually trying to take short cuts based on commercial greed.

Immune-enhancing herbs offer the greatest benefit when started as early as possible in the course of HIV infection. If you start with a helper T lymphocyte (CD4 cell) count over 200, you'll have better odds of a successful response (i.e., an increase in your count). If you're below 200 in your CD4 count, don't expect a significant increase, but don't give up on using adaptogens. Other benefits, including adrenal support and antioxidant activity, are useful at all stages of HIV infection. These herbs can be used safely with standard antiviral drugs.

Herbal prescriptions may also play a role in decreasing your chance of getting certain secondary infections or complications. I regularly recommend garlic as a preventive tool to help the body combat yeast, cytomegalovirus, and *Mycobacterium avium* (the bacterium that causes tuberculosis in AIDS patients) infections.

Herbs may also protect you against the negative consequences of AIDS drugs. I've found that milk thistle extract reduces the side effects caused by some antiretroviral drugs and helps keep the liver functioning optimally. A standardized extract from the sap of an Amazon rain forest tree (*Croton lechleri*) known as SB Normal Stool Formula (Shaman Botanicals.com) may help reduce diarrhea due to AIDS or antiretroviral drugs such as Viracept®.

SUPPORTIVE HERBAL PRESCRIPTIONS
Herbs Affecting the Immune System
- Boxwood (*Buxus sempervirens*) extract (SPV 30)—990 milligrams daily[1]

  Note: The study completed in France with boxwood extract focused on persons with HIV infection who were asymptomatic. The promising results found that delayed progression of the disease to AIDS-related complex (ARC) and the associated secondary infections (e.g., oral leukoplaki and thrush, herpes zoster, etc.). Clearly, more studies need to be completed so we can know more about the role boxwood may play in the management of HIV infection.

- Eleuthero (Siberian ginseng)—Standardized, concentrated extract of the root and rhizomes, 600 to 800 milligrams daily in two divided doses; dried powder of the root and rhizomes, 4 to 6 grams daily in two or three divided dosages; alcohol-based extract (33 percent alcohol), 16 to 20 milliliters in two to three divided doses. Use continuously for 4 to 6 weeks with a 1- to 2-week break before resuming.[2]
- Astragalus—6 to 12 grams daily[3]

  Note: Immunomodulating herbs such as eleuthero or astragalus provide excellent support if you're receiving chemotherapy for Kaposi's sarcoma. They will help the bone marrow bounce back and produce white blood cells following chemotherapy.[4]

OTHER CONSIDERATIONS

- Maitake and shiitake mushroom extracts
- Bitter melon
- Licorice extract

Antimicrobial Herbs and Potential Treatment of Thrush

- Garlic (standardized garlic powder product containing 1.3 percent aliin and providing 5,000 to 6,000 micrograms of allicin potential daily)—600 to 900 milligrams daily in two to three divided doses or chew one clove of garlic daily[5,6,7]
- Tea tree oil mouthwash (do not exceed a 5 percent concentration of tea tree oil)—Swish 15 milliliters in your mouth for 30 to 60 seconds and then spit it out; repeat this four times daily.[8]

  Note: The product used in this very interesting study is called Breath-Away and is sold by Melaleuca, Inc., from Idaho Falls, Idaho. When I called the customer service people at the company to find out more about the product (mainly the concentration of tea tree oil in the mouthwash), I was informed that was proprietary information and they couldn't tell me. In the words of the B-52s, Melaleuca must be "living in their own private Idaho!"

Treatment of Diarrhea

- SB Normal Stool Formula™ (standardized extract of the sap from *Croton lechleri*, a tree found throughout the rain forest of South America)—750 milligrams four times daily[9]

  Note: Developed by Shaman Botanicals.com, the extract is standardized to approximately 70 percent SP-303, a proanthyocynanidin oligomer that has been shown to be effective in treating individuals with AIDS-associated diarrhea.[10] This is a great alternative to standard antidiarrheal drugs and is an excellent adjunct to counter the diarrhea commonly associated with antiretroviral drugs such as Viracept®.

Liver Support

- Milk thistle extract (standardized to 80 percent silymarin)—420 milligrams of silymarin daily in three divided doses

NUTRITIONAL SUPPLEMENT CONSIDERATIONS

Recent research promotes antioxidant nutrients for people with HIV infection. Don't forget flavonoids from herbal and dietary sources! The nutrient recommendations here are total daily amounts. Please remember to factor in how much you're getting from your multiple-vitamin and mineral formula.

- Selenium—200 micrograms daily[11]
- Vitamin E—400 IU daily[12]
- Vitamin A—10,000 IU daily[13]
- Vitamin C—1 gram three to five times daily[14]
- Vitamin B_{12}—1,000 micrograms daily[15]

  Note: I prefer to use an intramuscular injection of 1,000 micrograms (1 milliliter) twice monthly. This should be done by a qualified health care professional.
- Folic acid—800 micrograms daily[16]

OTHER NUTRIENT CONSIDERATIONS

- Vitamin B_1
- Vitamin B_6

- *N*-acetyl cysteine
- Glutamine
- L-carnitine
- Methionine

DIETARY RECOMMENDATIONS

A key consideration if you have HIV infection is your weight—not if you have too much, but if you have too little. Unexplained weight loss is a warning sign that should be shared with your doctor. Also, if you're having diarrhea, see your doctor.

The easy way out would be to recommend a vegetarian diet with a whole-foods focus. Unfortunately, it's not that simple if your immune system is working poorly. Be very cautious of raw produce. Be sure it's washed well before using. Also, avoid consuming raw eggs (found, e.g., in Caesar salad dressing) and raw milk. Use plastic cutting boards—wood harbors bacteria—for preparing meat and fish, and wash them thoroughly with hot soapy water after use. That goes for your hands also. The Food and Drug Administration has a good summary on food safety issues for persons with HIV.

OK, now you can think about the healthy, whole-foods diet. Remember, raw garlic, turmeric, and other recommended spices win favor with your immune system as well as your taste buds.

OTHER LIFESTYLE CONSIDERATIONS

Research continues to show that a large and loving personal support group helps people with HIV infection and AIDS to survive longer. Develop a moderate exercise program and try yoga, meditation, or any other discipline that encourages a healthy mind–body connection.

I recommend acupuncture for most of my HIV-infected patients. Acupressure or massage are other options.

Male Health
Conditions

BALDNESS

I don't have a clue! My glowing pate has defied attempts to save the follicles naturally. If you have any suggestions that warrant sharing with our bald brethren, please drop me a line, and I'll put it in the next edition.

Note for second edition: Hey, thanks for nothing! Not only am I looking progressively more like Yul Brynner, but I'm also going gray! Is there no justice in the world?

BENIGN PROSTATE ENLARGEMENT/PROSTATE CANCER PREVENTION

If you are a male between 40 and 59 years of age, there is a 50 to 60 percent chance that you have benign enlargement of the prostate gland. This condition, known as *benign prostatic hyperplasia* (BPH), begins in many men in their fourth decade. Distressing symptoms usually begin after age 50 years.[1] The cause, which has yet to be discovered, may be related to hormonal changes in middle-aged and elderly men.

Problems with urine flow are the major symptoms of BPH. The symptoms can occur when the enlarged prostate gland impinges on the outlet of the bladder and the urethra (the tube carrying urine from the bladder). However, some men have these lower urinary tract symptoms (lovingly referred to as "LUTS" by urologists) who don't seem to have an enlarged prostate. Listed here are common signs and symptoms of BPH:

- Dysuria—painful urination
- Hesitancy to urinate
- Straining to urinate
- Decreased force and caliber of urinary stream
- Prolonged dribbling after urination
- Sensation of incomplete bladder emptying
- Increased frequency of urination
- Nocturia—frequent urination at night

In addition to these symptoms, complications may arise, including bladder infections, involuntary urination, and bleeding in the urinary tract.

Accurate medical diagnosis is critical to rule out prostate cancer.

HERBAL PRESCRIPTION

- Saw palmetto (liposterolic extract of saw palmetto berries)—320 milligrams daily, taken all at once or in two separate doses
  Actions: Acts locally in the prostate to reduce the binding of dihydro-testosterone in the periurethral area (area of prostate surrounding the urethra—the tube carrying urine from the bladder) and inhibits the production of growth factors that may contribute to BPH. This should be your first choice for long-term treatment of BPH.

OTHER HERBAL CONSIDERATIONS

- Beta-sitosterol—20 milligrams three times daily[2,3]
  Actions: The products used in Europe for BPH are actually a mixture of phytosterols from African star grass (*Hypoxis rooperi*). Sterols have anti-inflammatory properties.[4]
- Pygeum (liposterolic extract of the bark)—100 milligrams daily, taken all at once or in two separate doses
  Actions: Anti-inflammatory and decongestant (antiedema) properties[5]
- Nettle root extract—120 milligrams twice daily
  Actions: Anti-inflammatory and decongestant (antiedema) properties.[6] European extracts are sometimes used in combination with saw palmetto or pygeum.
- Flower pollen extract (Cernilton)—Two capsules (dose per capsule not available) twice daily[7]

NUTRITIONAL SUPPLEMENT CONSIDERATIONS

These are primarily for prevention of prostate cancer:

- Selenium—200 micrograms daily[8]
- Vitamin E—400 IU daily[9]
- Lycopene—7 milligrams daily[10]
- Zinc (monomethionine or citrate)—30 milligrams daily[11]

DIETARY RECOMMENDATIONS

Again, the intent here is prevention of both BPH and prostate cancer.

Keep your intake of saturated fats low. This includes red meat, milk, and fried oils. Include more polyunsaturated fats by eating vegetables and fish, and use olive oil for cooking. A vegetarian diet has been shown to reduce the amount of circulating hormones in the body—this also reduces the risk of BPH as well as prostate cancer.[12,13] A vegetarian diet also adds dietary fiber and antioxidant nutrients. Soy products should be a staple of your vegetarian strategy against BPH and prostate cancer.[14] Also, you can get your lycopene from the diet by eating tomatoes and tomato-based products. Finally, regular consumption of green tea is also good for the health of your prostate.[15]

A BRIEF NOTE ON PROSTATITIS

An affliction of many younger men, prostatitis can be due initially to a bacterial infection. However, some men develop a chronic, inflammatory problem known as chronic, nonbacterial prostatitis. While I've noticed some success using pygeum or saw palmetto for this condition, the best approach is to use a pollen extract from Great Britain known as Cernilton (discussed earlier).[16]

IMPOTENCE (ERECTILE DYSFUNCTION)

It's not uncommon after I give a public lecture for some middle-aged man to linger in the wings until the crowd has thinned out. The usual topic of conversation is impotence.

Male impotence (also known as erectile dysfunction) affects about one-fourth of men over 50 years of age and is estimated to affect some 15 million men in the United States. Awareness and openness about the condition has changed considerably in the past few years with the Viagra™ ads featuring Bob Dole and the amount of public education that seems to follow any major drug introduction.

Male impotence is the inability either to attain or sustain an erection sufficient for intercourse. It can sometimes be due to psychological or emotional problems, as opposed to physiological ones. Seeking counseling either alone or with your partner may be the first step toward solving the problem.

If the problem is not psychological, a thorough medical work-up by a urologist should take place. Diseases such as diabetes, hypothyroidism, and multiple sclerosis can cause impotence. Drugs used to lower blood pressure, tranquilizers, and sedatives (be sure to read the fine print on the drug insert) also can be at fault. Chronic alcohol abuse also is a common cause of impotence.

Contrary to popular belief, your age should have nothing to do with your ability to have a normal erection. In other words, impotence is a preventable condition in many men past 50! The most common cause of impotence in men over 50 is atherosclerosis. Poor blood flow to the erectile tissue of the penis results in an impaired ability to have an erection.

Another common cause of impotence in men over 50 is partial or complete surgical removal of the prostate as part of treatment for prostate cancer. See the dietary recommendations for prevention of prostate cancer in the earlier section "Benign Prostate Enlargement."

HERBAL PRESCRIPTION

- *Ginkgo biloba* extract—240 milligrams daily in two to three divided doses[1,2]

  Action: Improves blood flow to the erectile tissue of the penis

  Note: Remember that ginkgo may be particularly useful if your impotence is secondary to taking antidepressants known as selective serotonin reuptake inhibitors (e.g., Prozac, Zoloft).

OTHER HERBAL CONSIDERATIONS

- Yohimbine—15 to 20 milligrams daily[3]

  Note: This is an approved treatment for male impotence in the United States. Derived from the bark of the West African yohimbe tree, this alkaloid also increases blood flow to erectile tissue. However, unlike ginkgo, it commonly causes side effects such as anxiety, high blood pressure, and headaches. It's particularly unsafe for men with posttraumatic stress disorder to take as it may seriously exacerbate their symptoms.[4] Taking the risk-to-benefit ratio into consideration, you're better off starting with ginkgo.

- Muria puama (*Ptychopetalum olacoides*)—1 to 1.5 grams daily[5]

Note: This Brazilian herb has one very small pilot study to its credit. Its mechanism of action is unknown; neither is its safety with long-term use.

- Asian ginseng (standardized extract containing 5 to 7 percent ginsenosides)—100 to 200 milligrams twice daily. Use continuously for 3 to 4 weeks with a 1- to 2-week break between.
Note: An adaptogenic herb, it has been used for centuries in traditional Chinese medicine as a tonic for impotence.

NUTRITIONAL SUPPLEMENT CONSIDERATIONS

- Dehydroepiandrosterone (DHEA)—50 milligrams daily[6]
Note: It's a good idea to have your doctor measuring levels of DHEA in your blood while you're taking it. High levels may increase risk of prostate cancer.
- L-Arginine—2,800 milligrams daily[7]
Note: Arginine may help dilate blood vessels. Research for its use in impotence should be considered preliminary.

LIFESTYLE CONSIDERATIONS

Follow the dietary recommendations in the section on atherosclerosis. Also, if you smoke, stop. Smoking is a leading cause of impotence. Alcohol abuse is also another common cause of impotence.

INFERTILITY

Infertility is defined as the inability of a couple to achieve conception or to bring a pregnancy to term after a year or more of regular, unprotected intercourse. Subfertility means you're having difficulty conceiving regardless of time. While infertility has been regarded as the primary fault of the woman in the past, actual numbers suggest that males are the responsible party 40 percent of the time and a contributing factor another 20 percent of the time.

Male infertility is commonly due to varicocele (an enlargement of veins of the spermatic cord). However, many cases are listed as "idiopathic"—modern medicine's way of saying, "I don't know." A number of factors may contribute to idiopathic infertility including smoking, alcohol abuse, exposure to heavy metals (Rob Zombie excluded), stress, lack of exercise, and chemotherapy.

Diagnosis of infertility in a man focuses on the quality of his sperm. Factors that are considered include sperm count, concentration, motility (percentage of motile sperm), rapid linear progression, morphology (how mature and normal the sperm look), and ejaculatory volume. While surgery may be needed in some cases of varicocele or obstructive problems, assisted reproductive technologies (e.g., intrauterine insemination) are often used. However, these assisted reproductive techniques can often be very expensive and frustrating for couples wanting to conceive.

Nutritional interventions such as L-carnitine, zinc, selenium, vitamin E, and vitamin C may be the best place for a man to begin improving his sperm quality and likelihood of successful conception.

HERBAL CONSIDERATION
- Asian ginseng—4 grams daily[1]
  Note: Think of ginseng as a back-up or supportive treatment to the two carnitines, zinc and antioxidant nutrients.

NUTRITIONAL SUPPLEMENT CONSIDERATIONS
- L-carnitine/acetyl-L-carnitine—Studies have looked at the two independent of each other.[2] The dosages used were 3 to 4 grams daily. A product combining the two was recently released on the U.S. market (proXeed™, sigma-tau) and is being studied for men with infertility due to poor sperm quality.
  Note: Carnitine is an essential nutrient for both sperm motility as well as maturation. Using the two types of carnitine together are postulated to give a better effect in these areas than the two separately.
- Zinc (citrate or monomethionine)—30 to 60 milligrams daily[3]
  Note: Zinc is another essential nutrient for sperm health. Supplementing zinc is best reserved for men who have a measured deficiency of zinc.

- Vitamin C—1 gram daily[4]

  Note: Some men have a problem with their sperm sticking together. This is called *agglutination*. Vitamin C is very effective in countering this problem.
- Vitamin E—200 to 400 IU daily[5]
- Selenium—100 to 200 micrograms daily[6]

Mouth and Gums

Related Chapters in Part 5

- Chamomile
- Echinacea

CANKER SORES

Canker sores are small ulcers that occur inside the mouth. They are usually harmless but can be painful. Canker sores occur singly or in groups and last from 7 to 21 days, depending on the type.

The most common form of canker sore is the "minor" form, defined as being less than 1 centimeter in diameter. These usually last 10 to 14 days and heal without scarring and occur chiefly in young adults. The less common, "major" form features sores greater than 1 centimeter in diameter. They last weeks to months and usually heal with scarring. These are most common in younger children. Canker sores are usually recurrent.

HERBAL PRESCRIPTIONS

- Deglycyrrhizinated licorice (DGL)—Gargle with mouthwash (200 milligrams of powdered DGL mixed with 200 milliliters of warm water), swish in mouth for 2 to 3 minutes, and then spit out. This should be done morning and evening for 1 week.[1]
  Note: For a discussion on DGL, please see the section on peptic ulcer disease under "Digestive System."
- *Echinacea purpurea* or *E. angustifolia*—Take 5 milliliters of the expressed juice or tincture three times daily. Swish in mouth before swallowing.

OTHER HERBAL CONSIDERATIONS

- Myrrh—Place powder or liquid extract in warm water and use as a mouthwash three to four times daily.

- Chamomile—Same instructions as for myrrh

NUTRITIONAL SUPPLEMENT CONSIDERATIONS
- Vitamin B complex—50 milligrams daily[2,3]
  Note: A higher than normal incidence of B vitamin and iron deficiencies has been noted in persons with canker sores. Before supplementing iron, be sure to have an iron deficiency diagnosed by your doctor.
- Zinc (chewable tablets)—One or two tablets daily (do not exceed 50 milligrams)[4]
- Lactobacillus acidophilus—Chew 3 to 4 tablets of acidophilus daily.[5]

DIETARY RECOMMENDATIONS
Under the supervision of a health care professional, eliminate potential food allergens. Wheat and other gluten-containing grains should be at the top of your list.[6]

LIFESTYLE CONSIDERATIONS
Several reports have incriminated sodium lauryl sulfate (SLS), a component of some toothpastes, as a potential cause of canker sores. People with recurrent canker sores should use an SLS-free toothpaste for several months to see if such a change helps.[7]

Stress is a major factor contributing to recurrent canker sores. Stress reduction should be a therapeutic goal. Relaxation training, guided imagery, and meditation are among some helpful techniques.[8]

COLD SORES

Cold sores, also known as fever blisters, are often caused by the herpes simplex virus (HSV). Herpes can also cause outbreaks on the genitals and sometimes other areas of the body, including the buttocks, thighs, and abdomen. Highly contagious, herpes is often transmitted by physical contact.

A herpes outbreak is usually heralded by tingling and itching. The actual sore is a cluster of blisters that initially contain a honey-colored fluid. Later, they crust over and then disappear.

Herpes is a recurrent disease, and once it establishes residence in your body, it is with you for life. Recurrent HSV outbreaks on the lips or around the mouth (also known as *herpes labialis*) occur in 20 to 40 percent of the population.

If your doctor decides to treat you for herpes, it will usually be for the genital form. The treatment of choice is acyclovir. Herpes on the lips or mouth is usually treated with a host of topical preparations that reduce swelling and itching. Neither of these treatments reduces recurrence.

Note: The recommendations given here are primarily for self-treatment of HSV-related cold sores. Genital herpes may respond to these topical preparations but often requires acyclovir treatment as well.

HERBAL PRESCRIPTION
Topical Options
- Lemon balm (*Melissa officinalis*) concentrated extract cream (1 percent concentration)—At the onset of prodromal symptoms, apply the cream to the affected area four to five times daily. Use for the duration of the outbreak.[1,2]

  Actions: Lemon balm is antiviral and reduces the recurrence of HSV infections. It lessens swelling and discomfort and speeds healing time.

  Product update: The lemon balm cream used in the clinical studies is sold in the United States as Herpilyn® by Enzymatic Therapy.

OTHER HERBAL CONSIDERATIONS
- Glycyrrhizin-containing ointment (5 percent concentration)—At the onset of the prodromal symptoms (itching and tingling before outbreak), begin applying the ointment to the affected area four times daily. Use for the duration of the outbreak.

  Actions: Glycyrrhizin, which is a component of licorice root, is antiviral and reduces the recurrence of HSV infections. It reduces swelling and discomfort and speeds healing time.
- *Echinacea purpurea*—40 drops of the expressed juice three times daily, or one capsule of dried juice extract three or four times daily

Nutritional Supplement Considerations

- L-lysine—1 to 3 grams daily in two to three divided doses. Begin at the onset of the prodromal period and take for the duration of the outbreak. A preventive dose of 500 to 1,000 milligrams is recommended after the infection has resolved (this is not recommended for those with high cholesterol levels).[3]
- Vitamin C with bioflavonoids—2 to 3 grams daily[4]

Dietary Recommendations

Increase your consumption of foods high in the amino acid lysine, and avoid foods high in the amino acid arginine. Lysine-containing foods include legumes, fish, and chicken. Peanuts, almonds, and other nuts, as well as chocolate, have high levels of arginine.

Lifestyle Considerations

Recurrence of herpes is often associated with stress. Reduce stress through the use of a relaxation program of yoga, meditation, or listening to *Monk's Dream* by Thelonius Monk.

Periodontal Disease

Periodontal disease is a common disorder of the gums and teeth. It is normally broken into two categories: gingivitis and periodontitis. Gingivitis represents a swelling of the gums characterized by redness, change of normal contours, recession, and often bleeding. It is often the precursor of the more serious condition, periodontitis. Periodontitis represents a progression of gingivitis to the point at which pockets form between the teeth and gums and the gums lose their attachment to the teeth. The end result is bone loss in the jaw.

The leading cause of periodontal disease is poor dental hygiene, which leads to the buildup of bacterial plaque. This can often be prevented by proper brushing and daily use of dental floss. Periodontal disease, however, may sometimes be part of a more serious condition such as diabetes, an allergic reaction, or vitamin deficiencies involving vitamin C and niacin. Gingivitis traced to hormonal changes is common during puberty and pregnancy. If you have gingivitis, work closely with your dentist to identify the underlying cause and halt the progression.

Goals in treating periodontal disease include (1) controlling plaque and bacterial buildup, (2) assisting with gum healing, (3) decreasing inflammation and free radical (reactive substances in the body that may cause damage to healthy cells) damage, (4) improving collagen (connective tissue) integrity and strength in the gums, and (5) improving immune function to assist with resistance to infection.

Note: The recommendations listed here are intended to support a regular dental hygiene program that includes conscientious brushing and flossing.

HERBAL PRESCRIPTIONS

Use the following herbs in mouthwash prevention and treatment of periodontal disease:

- Sage oil, peppermint oil, mint oil, menthol, chamomile tincture, expressed juice from *Echinacea purpurea* herb, myrrh tincture, clove oil, and caraway oil—In cases of acute gum inflammation, take 0.5 milliliters of the herbal mixture in half a glass of water three times daily. Rinse slowly in the mouth before spitting out. For daily hygiene, use slightly less of the mixture in half a glass of water and repeat only one or two times daily.[1]

   Actions: See Table 6.3 for a listing of each herb's action.

Toothpaste

- Sage oil, peppermint oil, chamomile tincture, expressed juice from *Echinacea purpurea* herb, myrrh tincture, and rhatany tincture[2]

   Action: In addition to the actions listed in Table 6.3, rhatany tincture tightens the gums through its astringent properties.

NUTRITIONAL SUPPLEMENT CONSIDERATIONS

- Folic acid mouthwash (0.1 percent concentration)—Swish 5 milliliters in the mouth for 1 to 5 minutes three times daily.[3]

Table 6.3
ACTION OF HERBS IN MOUTHWASH FOR PERIODONTAL DISEASE

Herb	Actions
Sage oil, peppermint oil, caraway oil, and menthol	Inhibit the growth of microorganisms (e.g., bacteria) that may cause inflammation Prevent bad breath Caraway oil increases blood flow to affected tissue.
Myrrh	Astringent effect on the gums, helping to tighten them, which helps stop bleeding.
Clove oil	Alleviates pain
Echinacea	Increases the body's resistance to infections
Chamomile	Anti-inflammatory actions

- Vitamin C with bioflavonoids—250 milligrams twice daily[4]
- Coenzyme Q_{10}—50 milligrams daily[5]

DIETARY RECOMMENDATIONS

Reduce your simple carbohydrate (including sugar) intake. Eat healthy foods that are high in fiber and complex carbohydrates (vegetables, fruits, and grains). Consumption of foods high in bioflavonoids such as grapes and blueberries is also encouraged. Drinking green tea may also reduce your risk of gum disease as well as cavities.[6]

Musculoskeletal System

RELATED CHAPTERS IN PART 5

- Evening Primrose
- Ginger
- Horse Chestnut

OSTEOARTHRITIS

The term *arthritis* refers to a condition that causes inflammation and tissue damage in the joints of the body. Arthritic conditions include rheumatoid arthritis, osteoarthritis, psoriatic arthritis, juvenile arthritis, and ankylosing spondylitis.

Osteoarthritis (OA), also known as degenerative joint disease, is by far the leading cause of joint disease in the United States. It is estimated that 12 percent of the population between the ages of 25 and 74 years has some evidence of OA. If we move up the scale to persons over 75, the number jumps to 80 percent! Persons with OA are second only to those with heart disease for number of lost workdays in men over the age of 50 years. Among the leading causes of OA are obesity and stress on the joint due to sports or work. Knee replacements are the new boon for orthopedic surgeons. Most of these are due to severe cases of OA.

OA quite simply occurs when the cartilage in the joint wears down due to wear and tear. A vicious cycle ensues wherein the bone begins to build extra layers, becomes weaker, and further contributes to joint destruction. OA is most commonly found in the weight-bearing joints such as the knees and hips. It is also often seen in the spine and hands. One of the telltale signs of OA is morning stiffness in the affected joint that lasts for about 30 minutes. As the disease progresses, the range of motion in the affected joint continues to decline and the ability to use the joint becomes more impaired. The official medical diagnosis takes into consideration the patient's physical movement of the joint and, more importantly, how much degeneration is noted in the joint when X-rayed.

Besides physical therapy, there's not a lot that mainstream medicine has in the way of help for persons with OA. Many people are placed on nonsteroidal anti-inflammatory drugs (NSAIDs) such as ibuprofen and naproxen to alleviate swelling and pain. However, these drugs are associated with stomach and kidney complications when used at large doses for long periods of time.

Nutritional and herbal approaches have much to offer people with OA—particularly those in the earlier stages looking to slow the progression of the disease.

HERBAL PRESCRIPTIONS
- Boswellia extract (standardized to 37.5 to 65 percent boswellic acids)—Take an extract providing 150 milligrams of boswellic acids three times daily.
  Note: While boswellia is typically thought of as a treatment for rheumatoid arthritis, I find it a nice alternative for NSAIDs (e.g., ibuprofen) in persons with OA.
- Capsaicin ointment (0.025 to 0.075 percent concentration)—Apply to affected area four times daily. Be sure to avoid contact with eyes or mouth as this stuff is hot![1]
  Action: Capsaicin is the component of cayenne pepper responsible for its hot taste. It reduces pain by blocking the action of pain fibers and a transmitter chemical known as *substance P*.

OTHER HERBAL CONSIDERATIONS
- Devil's claw root (*Harpagophytum procumbens*)—3 to 4 grams three times daily
- Yucca stalk (*Yucca schidigera*)—1 to 2 grams three times daily

NUTRITIONAL SUPPLEMENT CONSIDERATIONS
- Glucosamine sulfate—500 milligrams three times daily[2,3]

Note: Glucosamine sulfate (GS) should be the cornerstone of any program for OA. Providing an important building block needed for the repair of joint cartilage, GS is the one complementary and alternative medicine that I would place in the "essential" list for persons with OA.

- Chondroitin sulfate—400 milligrams three times daily[4]
  Note: Many dietary supplement formulations combine CS with GS. However, it's been shown to work well by itself.
- S-adenosylmethionine (SAMe)—600 to 1,200 milligrams daily[5]
  Note: The large dosage range for SAMe reflects the fact that different studies have used different doses with varying success. This stuff is expensive! Work with your doctor to find a dose that works best for you.
- Vitamin E—400 to 600 IU daily[6]

OTHER NUTRIENT CONSIDERATIONS

- Nicainamide
- Boron
- Phenylalanine
- Green-lipped mussels (as opposed to the ones with plumbago lipstick)

DIETARY RECOMMENDATIONS

In contrast to rheumatoid arthritis, a direct link to diet has not been as clearly established for OA. There is some evidence that reducing foods in the nightshade family (e.g., tomatoes, white potatoes, all peppers except black pepper, and eggplant) may be helpful in persons with OA.

LIFESTYLE CONSIDERATIONS

Don't stop exercising! Try swimming or another exercise that places less pressure on the joints. If you are overweight, losing a few pounds will make your joints and your cardiovascular system happier.

RHEUMATOID ARTHRITIS

Rheumatoid arthritis (RA) is a very common type of arthritis. Estimates are that 1 to 3 percent of the U.S. population suffers from RA. As opposed to osteoarthritis, which primarily affects an older population, RA most commonly begins around 20 to 40 years of age. Women seem to be more susceptible and have a three times greater incidence of RA than men.

The first appearance of RA is often preceded by a low-grade fever, fatigue, and generalized joint stiffness and pain. Within several weeks, the condition may affect several joints (in some people only one or two joints may be affected), causing swelling and pain. The joints of the hands, feet, wrists, ankles, and knees are most commonly affected. Rheumatoid arthritic joints are often referred to as "hot" because they are red, swollen, and warm to the touch.

Rheumatoid arthritis is usually relapsing. Bouts come and go. After time, however, chronic inflammation causes the joints to become deformed. The goal of any treatment plan should be early intervention to slow progression of joint destruction.

Rheumatoid arthritis is largely believed to be an autoimmune illness. *Autoimmune* refers to the fact that a person's own immune system is attacking a particular part of the body. In the case of RA, the site of action is the joints—specifically, the synovial lining that acts to lubricate the joints and keep them working normally.

What causes RA? Like other autoimmune illnesses, we don't know for sure. Family history of RA may be one predictor. Evidence suggests an infection may trigger the onset of RA.

There's also compelling evidence that diet and the health of our intestinal tract may play a role in RA. As we'll note in the section on dietary recommendations, food allergies and also saturated fats can make RA worse. Without a healthy intestinal tract, allergens from food may pass into the bloodstream and spark an allergic response in the joints. A good diet and the addition of supplements high in healthy bacterial microorganisms (such as members of the *Lactobacillus* and *Bifidobacterium* groups) promote intestinal tract health.

HERBAL PRESCRIPTIONS

Long-Term Treatment

- Boswellia extract (standardized to 37.5 to 65 percent boswellic acids)—Take an extract providing 150 milligrams of boswellic acids three times daily.[1]

  Actions: The resin of this Indian tree contains compounds known as *boswellic acids*. These constituents have anti-inflammatory properties that are similar to those of many NSAIDs (e.g., ibuprofen) but without the side effects seen with those drugs.[2]

- Evening primrose oil (combined with fish oil)—The combination should equal approximately 80 percent evening primrose oil (EPO) and 20 percent fish oil. Take twelve capsules daily with meals in two or three divided doses.[3]

  Action: Evening primrose oil and fish oil provide a balanced supply of essential fatty acids to help the body produce hormones known as *prostaglandins*. These substances help steer the body away from inflammation. Fish oil may work well on its own—please see instructions for use later.

  Note: Borage oil, another source of GLA, has also been used to be treat RA. It may work better in some people than EPO.[4]

Short-Term Relief

- Capsaicin ointment (0.025 to 0.075 percent concentration)—Apply to affected area four times daily. Be sure to avoid contact with eyes or mouth, as this stuff is hot![5]

  Action: See earlier comments under "Osteoarthritis."

OTHER HERBAL CONSIDERATIONS

- Curcumin (from turmeric)—400 milligrams three times daily[6]
- Ginger rhizome powder—2 to 3 grams daily
- Devil's claw root (*Harpagophytum procumbens*)—3 to 4 grams three times daily
- Yucca stalk (*Yucca schidigera*)—1 to 2 grams three times daily

NUTRITIONAL SUPPLEMENT CONSIDERATIONS

Note: Research suggests that people with RA may benefit from the use of antioxidant nutrients.[7] Remember that herbs high in flavonoids are powerful antioxidants (see "Antioxidants" in Part 4).

- Bromelain—See instructions under "Strains and Sprains" later.[8]
- Fish oil (MaxEPA)—10 grams daily with meals in two or three divided doses[9]
- Vitamin E—1,200 to 1,800 international units (IU) daily[10]
  Note: This is a very high dose of vitamin E and may affect bleeding time. Consult with your doctor before using a high dose of vitamin E, particularly if you are taking anticoagulant medications.
- Selenium—200 micrograms daily[11]

OTHER NUTRIENT CONSIDERATIONS
- Pantothenic acid (vitamin B_5)
- Zinc
- Copper
- Boron
- Phenylalanine
- Green-lipped mussels

DIETARY RECOMMENDATIONS

With the guidance of a health care professional trained in nutrition, eliminate potential food allergens from your diet. Recent research promotes a 7- to 10-day therapeutic fast as a powerful tool in the treatment of RA.[12] Fasting not only clears allergens from your system but also gives your intestinal tract a chance to recover and reestablish a normal balance of healthy microorganisms. Remember that fasting should be done only under the guidance of a qualified health care professional. Fasting is not recommended for persons with diabetes or HIV infection or for young children. Be sure your nutritionally trained health care professional rules out any food allergens that may be triggering your arthritis.

Shift your diet in the vegetarian direction.[13] Increase your intake of onions, garlic, and turmeric. Reducing fats from animal sources such as red meat and dairy products is essential. Also, avoid fried foods and reduce your intake of sweets.

LIFESTYLE CONSIDERATIONS

Yoga is an excellent form of exercise for people with RA. I also highly recommend acupuncture or some form of massage as part of your regular treatment program.

SPRAINS AND STRAINS

WHAT MY TRAINER TOLD ME

Immediately after the injury or sprain, apply RICE: rest, ice, compression, and elevation. This decreases circulation to the injured area and lessens swelling. It's good to have some homeopathic arnica around also. Take it internally and also use some arnica gel topically right after the injury. It's great for quickly reducing swelling.

Also, don't forget to see your doctor. Ligament and tendon injuries may need to be stabilized for proper healing.

WHAT MY WIFE TOLD ME

"Oy vey, not another ankle injury!"

HERBAL PRESCRIPTIONS

Topical Considerations

- Horse chestnut extract gel (standardized to contain 2 percent aescin)—Apply a thin layer of the gel over the injured area once or twice daily, and then gently rub it into the skin.[1] Avoid contact with your eyes.

  Action: Widely used in Europe for sports injuries, horse chestnut extract gel contains aescin, which has been proven to reduce inflammation and swelling at the site of the injury.[2]

Supplements for Internal Use

- Bromelain (at least 2,000 MCU [milk-clotting units] per gram)— 1,500 milligrams three times daily between meals[3]

Note: Bromelain is a proteolytic (protein digesting) enzyme from pineapple. Its potency is measured in MCUs. While it may help you digest protein following a meal, you want to take it away from food for it to act as an anti-inflammatory agent. Other proteolytic enzymes that may also help with injury recovery include trypsin and chymotrypsin.

- Curcumin—600 milligrams three times daily[4]
- Manganese—15 milligrams daily
- Vitamin C (with bioflavonoids)—2 to 3 grams daily

  Note: Bromelain and curcumin are excellent for both short- and long-term recovery. Manganese and vitamin C with flavonoids are long-term therapies that will help strengthen injured ligaments or tendons.

PHYSICAL THERAPY CONSIDERATIONS
- Ultrasound
- TENS (transcutaneous electrical nerve stimulation)

Nervous System

RELATED CHAPTERS IN PART 5

- Chamomile
- Evening Primrose
- Feverfew
- *Ginkgo biloba*
- Asian Ginseng
- Kava-Kava
- St. John's Wort
- Valerian

AGE-RELATED COGNITIVE DECLINE AND EARLY-STAGE ALZHEIMER'S DISEASE

Although age-related cognitive decline (also known as *mild cognitive impairment* or *age-associated memory impairment*) and Alzheimer's disease are not necessarily linked, they represent two of the major concerns facing older adults. While this introduction spends more time focusing on Alzheimer's disease, keep in mind that the herbal and nutritional recommendations are possibly best suited for persons with age-related cognitive decline; in other words, these supplements may work better before a person actually gets to full-blown Alzheimer's disease.

Age-related changes in memory have been widely studied. Long-term memory seems to be more adversely affected as we age when compared to short-term memory. Memory tasks that require deliberate recall of information and recognition for verbal visual information often become more difficult. While no one knows for sure why these changes occur, some focus has been placed on physiological processes in the body including blood flow to the brain, changes in normal neurotransmitter levels, and even loss of nerve cells in certain parts of the brain.

Except for cardiovascular disease and cancer, the major health care concern among elderly people in U.S. society is dementia. *Dementia* refers to mental deterioration. The most common form of dementia is Alzheimer's disease. Close to 2 million Americans have Alzheimer's, and the incidence is on the rise.

Alzheimer's disease that starts before age 65 is referred to as "presenile" dementia. After 65, you've got "senile" dementia (I believe people over 65 ought to resist the label "senile"). The condition starts with memory loss and signs of depression, including apathy and social withdrawal. As the brain degenerates, these symptoms progress to problems with speaking, impaired ability to make proper judgments, and personality changes including paranoid thoughts. In the advanced stages of the illness, people usually require full-time supervision to counter confusion and aggressive behavior.

Although medicine really knows very little about the condition and how to prevent or treat it, there are a few findings of interest. Medical research has looked at the brains of people with Alzheimer's after they've died and found key areas destroyed and infiltrated with abnormal protein. Also, the neurotransmitters serotonin and acetylcholine—chemical substances that carry messages in the brain—are either low or don't have proper binding sites in Alzheimer's patients. Lastly, Alzheimer's patients show a 30 percent reduction in normal blood flow to the brain.

All of this makes for wonderful discussion among doctors. What *you* really want to know is how to prevent the condition. Although we're a long way from a clear answer, new information is emerging that indicates prevention may involve reducing free radicals in the brain through the use of antioxidant herbs and nutrients.

Note: The recommendations here should be thought of as options for age-related memory loss. As far as Alzheimer's disease, the recommendations made here address early-stage treatment and possibly prevention. Although I'm not opposed to using these recommendations for patients with moderate to advanced Alzheimer's, it is unrealistic to expect very significant results.

HERBAL PRESCRIPTION

- *Ginkgo biloba* extract—120 to 240 milligrams daily in two to three divided doses

  Actions: Improves blood flow to the brain. Protects the cells of the brain from free radical damage. May increase the number of and normalize serotonin receptors in the brain. Ginkgo is effective for treating age-related memory loss and mild cognitive impairment. Research indicates it should be reserved for mild to moderate cases of Alzheimer's disease.

  Note: In 1999, the National Institutes of Health (NIH) Center for Complementary Medicine announced funding for a 5-year study to assess whether ginkgo prevents the occurrence of dementia and/or cognitive decline in older persons. One of the announced sites for the study is the Alzheimer's Disease Research Center at the University of Pittsburgh. The study is planned to begin in 2000 and will use 240 milligrams of ginkgo extract daily.

OTHER HERBAL CONSIDERATIONS

- Asian ginseng—100 milligrams twice daily of an extract standardized to contain 5 to 7 percent ginsenosides[1]

  Actions: Protects cells of the brain and increases serotonin activity; increases mental alertness.

- Huperizine A—200 to 400 micrograms twice daily[2]

  Action: Huperizine A is an alkaloid from a species of Chinese club moss known as *Huperiza serrata*. According to animal studies, it has very specific acetylcholinesterase-inhibiting properties. While it appears somewhat safer than drugs with similar actions (e.g., Cognex®, Aricept®), long-term safety studies are lacking. I don't agree with this being sold as an over-the-counter dietary supplement and would encourage use only under the supervision of a trained health care professional.

NUTRITIONAL SUPPLEMENT CONSIDERATIONS

- Acetyl-L-carnitine— 2 to 3 grams daily[3,4]
- Phosphatidylserine—100 milligrams three times daily[5]

Note: The research on acetyl-L-carnitine (ALC) and phosphatidylserine (PS) suggests that these substances work better in cases of mild cognitive impairment as opposed to Alzheimer's disease. Because they are extremely expensive supplements, it's better to choose one or the other. While my bias is with ginkgo as the primary focus of any program for mild cognitive impairment, I would probably place ALC second on my priority list ahead of PS. The type of PS used in the majority of clinical studies came from cow brains! This quickly lost popularity with the outbreak of mad-cow disease in England (also known as "Mad Cows and Englishmen"). The effectiveness of the soy-derived source of PS being currently sold in the United States remains to be proven.

- Thiamine (vitamin B_1)—10 to 50 milligrams daily[6]
- Folic acid—400 micrograms daily[7]
- Vitamin B_{12}—Intramuscular injection of 1,000 micrograms once monthly
  Note: This treatment should be performed only by a skilled health care practitioner.[8,9]
- Vitamin E—800 to 2000 international units (IU) daily[10,11]
  Note: These are very high doses of vitamin E, particularly if you are taking anticoagulant medication. The higher end of this dosage range (2,000 IU/day) has only been studied with Alzheimer's disease patients. Lower doses should be considered for age-related memory loss. Please check with your doctor before taking such large doses of vitamin E.

ANXIETY

Anxiety is the most common psychiatric diagnosis in U.S. society today. Five percent of the population is diagnosed with anxiety. It commonly afflicts younger adults.

Stress, feelings of isolation, and internal conflicts can all contribute to anxiety. The most obvious trigger is stress. People push themselves daily, forgetting their body's need to relax and recover. Anxiety is often a sign that body reserves (i.e., adrenal glands) have been exhausted.

Less obvious triggers can also lead to the same point. Repressed internal feelings are another source of anxiety. Modern society has also isolated many people, with the resulting feelings of detachment both physically and emotionally producing anxiety.

Acute anxiety attacks are known as panic attacks. Usually lasting a few minutes to 1 or 2 hours, these attacks can be frightening. Shortness of breath, rapid heart beat, and chest pain sometimes accompany these attacks. Although rarely a medical emergency, acute panic attacks can cause hyperventilation. This condition is dangerous and needs to be monitored by a medical professional.

Persons with chronic anxiety may go unnoticed. If they experience attacks of anxiety, they are usually less severe and last longer. These individuals are often uneasy in public and have uncertainty about the future. They commonly complain about chronic fatigue, insomnia, and a variety of physical problems.

As noted in the chapters on kava and valerian in Part 5, antianxiety drugs are among the most common prescriptions in the United States today. The herbal recommendations made here are alternatives for the treatment of mild to moderate anxiety. I also recommend reviewing the discussion on stress and fatigue in the chapter "Endocrine System." A complete program for treating anxiety should include combating adrenal exhaustion.

HERBAL PRESCRIPTION

- Kava-kava extract (30 to 70 percent kava lactones)—The daily dose should deliver 140 to 240 milligrams of kava lactones in two or three divided doses.
  Action: Relaxing effect on the body without a narcotic-like effect on the mind

OTHER HERBAL CONSIDERATIONS

- Valerian root (concentrated root extract—5:1—containing no less than 0.5 percent volatile oils)—300 to 500 milligrams ½ to 1 hour before bedtime. In the morning, take 300 milligrams.

Note: Valerian is sometimes combined with passion flower or St. John's wort in European herbal products used to treat anxiety. I do not recommend using valerian with kava.

For other herbal, nutritional, and lifestyle recommendations, please see the section on stress and fatigue in the chapter "Endocrine System."

ATTENTION DEFICIT–HYPERACTIVITY DISORDER

One need venture no further than the last few volumes of the American Psychiatric Association's *Diagnostic and Statistical Manual of Mental Disorders* to realize the uncertainty surrounding the diagnosis of attention deficit–hyperactivity disorder (ADHD). The last three or four decades have seen this condition labeled minimal brain damage, minimal brain dysfunction, behavior and learning disorder, hyperkinetic-impulsive disorder, hyperkinetic syndrome, developmental hyperactivity, and, finally, attention deficit–hyperactivity disorder. What is apparent is that ADHD is a collection of symptoms or criteria. The decision to label a child with the diagnosis of ADHD is fraught with the potential for error.

Nowhere is this more evident than in attempts to estimate the number of children with ADHD. Recent estimates place the numbers at 10 percent of boys and 3 percent of girls ranging in age from 4 to 11 years old. The central feature of ADHD is difficulty getting things done, both at home and at school, and trouble getting along with adults and other children. The increased activity and short attention span of the child with ADHD have led to the use of stimulant drugs such as Ritalin to control behavior. Paradoxically, these medications work to "slow down" the ADHD child. While sometimes effective in very serious cases, these medications are potentially harmful and may mask symptoms without getting to the core of the problem.

Early intervention and successful treatment of ADHD have become even more important in light of studies predicting that these children face greater problems as adults. Evidence is mounting that children with ADHD are at higher risk for depression, restlessness, alcoholism, and antisocial behavior as adults.[1]

Note: The recommendations here are based more on my clinical experience than published studies. There's a lot of interest currently on the potential benefits of ginkgo and essential fatty acids for children with ADHD. No data to date, but keep these on the radar screen. Work closely with a health care professional well trained in nutrition and herbal medicine when making treatment choices for your child with ADHD.

NUTRITIONAL SUPPLEMENT CONSIDERATIONS

- Vitamin B_6—50 to 100 milligrams daily[2]
- Magnesium—200 milligrams daily[3]
  Note: Be aware of the potential for diarrhea at this dose of magnesium.
- Chromium—100 to 200 micrograms daily[4]
- Docosahexanoic acid (DHA)—200 milligrams daily
  Note: Based on some pilot work in Great Britain with evening primrose oil,[5] there's been a lot of interest in the role that essential fatty acids (EFAs) may play in the management of ADHD. Interest in the past few years has begun to shift from EPO to DHA, an EFA that is found in high concentrations in the brain and critical for neurological development in infants. Researchers have speculated that children with ADHD may be deficient in this EFA. Studies looking at 200 milligrams of DHA daily in children with ADHD are currently under way.

DIETARY RECOMMENDATIONS

Encourage a whole-foods diet, high in protein and complex carbohydrates. Cut down on sugar and other simple carbohydrates.[6] Cut back on processed junk foods high in additives and food colorings. The Hyperactive Children's Support Group of Great Britain recommends that the following food additives be avoided:

Tartrazine	Quinoline Yellow	Caramel
Sunset Yellow	FCF	Cochineal
Benzoic acid	Carmoiic acid	Sodium benzoate
Amaranth	Sulfur dioxide	Sodium nitrate

Red 2G	Potassium nitrate	BHA
Brilliant Blue FCF	BHT	Indigo
Carmine		

Try to avoid foods, such as the following, with high salicylate content:[7]

Plums (canned)	Prunes (canned)
Raspberries (fresh)	Strawberries (fresh)
Peppers	Tomatoes
Almonds	Peanuts
Peppermint tea	Honey

Many spices should be avoided, too: cardamom, cinnamon, cloves, curry, oregano, paprika, pepper, rosemary, sage, turmeric. Lowering the intake of cow's milk, soy, eggs, wheat, citrus, and other potential allergenic foods may be helpful until your child's behavior improves.[8] Identification and elimination of food allergens should be done under the supervision of a trained health care practitioner.

LIFESTYLE CONSIDERATIONS

- Limit TV watching and video games.
- Work with a counselor to discover whether any family relationship problems may be triggering ADHD behaviors.
- Children with ADHD living in urban areas should be tested for possible lead poisoning.

DEPRESSION

The diagnosis of depression includes the presence, for at least 2 weeks, of at least four of the following signs and symptoms:

Poor appetite or significant weight loss
Either lack of sleep or abnormally long periods of sleep
Mental agitation or slowing of mental functioning
Loss of interest in usual activities, including decreased sex drive
Loss of energy and fatigue

Low self-esteem and feelings of worthlessness or self-reproach
Complaints or evidence of decreased ability to concentrate or think clearly
Recurrent thoughts of death or talk of suicide or actual suicide attempts

Depression is a broad definition and can range from mild, situational depression to more serious states requiring medication and possible hospitalization. The depressed individual should be under the supervision of a health care professional. Treatment of depression is usually complicated and requires the input of many different medical specialties.

Older people with mild cognitive decline are susceptible to depression. Depression often occurs with memory loss and, sometimes, irritability. It's ironic that this form of depression is often described as "resistant" because it does not respond well to many prescription antidepressants. As noted in the chapter on ginkgo in Part 5, older people who don't respond to prescription antidepressants may be candidates for ginkgo.

HERBAL PRESCRIPTIONS
Mild to Moderate Depression
- St. John's wort extract—300 to 350 milligrams of a standardized extract three times per day. Higher doses may work for more severe depression, but this treatment should only be attempted after consultation with your doctor. Expect results within 2 to 4 weeks.
  Action: Although shown only in test tube studies to date, St. John's wort may inhibit the reuptake of the neurotransmitters serotonin, norepinephrine, and dopamine.
  Note: Recent studies indicate that St. John's wort may be effective for seasonal affective disorder, a type of depression that hits people during the winter months.[1] The dosage used in the studies is the same as listed above for mild to moderate depression.

Older Individuals with "Resistant" Depression
- *Ginkgo biloba* extract—120 to 240 milligrams daily in two to three divided doses

NUTRITIONAL SUPPLEMENT RECOMMENDATIONS

- Vitamin B complex—50 milligrams once to twice daily[2]
- Folic acid—400 micrograms daily[3]
- Vitamin B_{12}—Intramuscular injection of 1,000 micrograms (1 milliliter) once monthly[4,5]

  Note: The vitamin B_{12} treatment should be performed only by a skilled health care practitioner.
- Vitamin B_6—100 milligrams daily

  Note: Women who have used oral birth control pills and have depression should consider a trial of vitamin B_6. Birth control pills can deplete vitamin B_6.[6] Also, a combination of vitamin B_6, B_{12}, and folic acid helps counter the formation of homocysteine. This substance has been linked to atherosclerosis, as well as depression and dementia, in the elderly.[7] These three nutrients should be paired with ginkgo in elderly depressed individuals.

DIETARY RECOMMENDATIONS

Identify and eliminate food allergens under the supervision of a trained health care practitioner. A trial elimination of wheat and cow's milk may prove beneficial. Small, frequent meals high in protein and complex carbohydrates help regulate blood sugar. Avoid excessive consumption of sugar and other simple carbohydrates.

OTHER CONSIDERATIONS

- Dehydroepiandrosterone (DHEA)—50 to 90 milligrams daily or as directed by your doctor[8]

  Note: Research has suggested that some people with depression may be deficient in DHEA, particularly elderly persons. Use of this hormone should only be done under the supervision of a trained health care professional and continue only as long as your blood tests indicate that DHEA is low.
- Also, be sure your doctor checks for anemia and low thyroid function.

Insomnia

More than one-third of the adult population has trouble sleeping. Stress is a major culprit. However, if stress is affecting your sleep and loss of sleep is making you a wreck the next day, the last thing you want to hear is a lecture on stress reduction. So, let's look at some approaches to help you sleep, and when you're rested, you can read the section on fatigue and stress in the chapter "Endocrine System."

HERBAL PRESCRIPTION

- Valerian root extract—Concentrated root extract (5:1) containing no less than 0.5 percent volatile oils—300 to 500 milligrams ½ to 1 hour before bedtime. Children 6 to 12 years old may respond to half the adult dose.
  Action: Mild central nervous system sedative. Helps you get to sleep quicker and enjoy a deeper sleep. Valerian is not addictive and doesn't cause the "morning hangover" common to many sleep aids.

OTHER HERBAL CONSIDERATIONS

- Chamomile—2 to 3 milliliters of a liquid extract in warm water before bed. Chamomile is a mild sedative and best reserved for infants or young children with restlessness caused by colic or teething.
- Passion flower (concentrated extract)—200 to 300 milligrams 1 hour before bedtime. Liquid preparations should be taken at a dose of 4 to 6 milliliters.[1]
  Action: Mild central nervous system sedative
- Other mild herbal sedatives include scullcap (that's an herb, not a yarmulke!), hops, and corydalis.

OTHER CONSIDERATIONS

- Melatonin—0.5 to 3 milligrams 1½ to 2 hours before bedtime[2]
  Note: I prefer starting with valerian for insomnia. More is known about its effects when used on a regular basis. Melatonin may be more effective for older individuals with insomnia. Personally, I'm

a huge fan of using 1 to 2 milligrams to counter jet lag on trips to Europe.

- Acupuncture—Some clinical studies indicate that acupuncture may be of benefit for people with insomnia.[3]

MIGRAINE HEADACHE

Migraine headaches are characterized by throbbing pain on one or both sides of the head, occasionally accompanied by nausea, vomiting, and sensitivity to light. Approximately 80 percent of migraine headaches are classified as "common" migraines. These migraines last from 1 to 3 days and seldom have any warning signals beforehand.

Other migraine sufferers report symptoms that precede their headaches, including "auras"—blurring or bright spots around certain objects. This may be accompanied by disturbed thinking, anxiety, fatigue, and numbness or tingling on one side of the body. These are referred to as "classic" migraines and may last from 2 to 6 hours. This type of migraine is usually localized to one side of the head and accounts for approximately 10 percent of migraines. The remaining 10 percent come from migraine-like headaches known as *cluster headaches*.

HERBAL PRESCRIPTION
- Feverfew—Dried leaf extract with a standardized parthenolide content of at least 250 micrograms per daily dose; continuous use is recommended for the treatment and prevention of migraine headaches.
  Actions: May inhibit serotonin and inflammatory mediator release from platelets. Improves blood vessel tone in affected area.

OTHER HERBAL CONSIDERATIONS
- Ginger rhizome powder—1 to 2 grams daily
- *Ginkgo biloba* extract—120 to 240 milligrams daily in two to three divided doses[1]

NUTRITIONAL SUPPLEMENT CONSIDERATIONS

- Magnesium—200 to 300 milligrams twice daily[2,3]
  Note: Be aware of the potential for diarrhea at this dose of magnesium.
- Riboflavin (vitamin B_2)—400 milligrams daily[4]
  Note: For the past few years, I've been recommending that persons with migraines consider taking a combination of feverfew, magnesium, and riboflavin. The results have been fabulous!
- MaxEPA (fish oil)—3 to 4 grams daily with meals[5]
- 5-hydroxytryptophan (5-HTP)—200 to 600 milligrams daily[6]
  Note: Although this trytophan-precursor snuck on the market in the last few years and avoided the current ban on over-the-counter tryptophan, I'm nervous about its potential to cause eosinophilia–myalgia syndrome—the dangerous condition attributed to tryptophan before it was banned. So, if you choose to use it, inform your doctor of that choice.

DIETARY RECOMMENDATIONS

Ban foods high in vasoactive amines from your diet. Key among these are aged cheeses, red wine, chocolate, and pickled herring (my wife would divorce me if I banned these!). Identify and eliminate food allergens under the supervision of a health care practitioner.[7] Drop aspartame-containing beverages and foods from your diet.

MISCELLANEOUS CONSIDERATIONS

Relaxation and stress reduction are critical to the long-term success of any program for migraines. Biofeedback, massage, and meditation are methods you can use to reduce stress. Acupuncture has been shown to be a good long-term consideration for treatment of migraines.[8]

NEUROPATHY (DIABETIC)

Diabetic neuropathy is a common complication of diabetes. Affecting approximately 28.5 percent of all diabetics, it's a progressive disorder of the nerves that leads to an initial sensation of "pins and needles" in the soles of the feet and palms of the hands.

Neuropathy can advance to a point at which sufferers have difficulty differentiating temperature and pressure changes in their extremities. This condition can lead to an inability to know when a burn or cut on the foot, for example, has occurred.

HERBAL PRESCRIPTIONS

- Evening primrose oil—4 to 6 grams daily with meals
  Action: Supplies essential fatty acids, such as gamma-linolenic acid (GLA), that are improperly metabolized by diabetics. GLA and other essential fatty acid metabolites increase the levels of protective hormonelike substances known as prostaglandins.
- Capsaicin ointment (0.075 percent concentration)—Apply topically to painful areas four times daily.[1]
  Note: Capsaicin is the pungent (hot) constituent in cayenne pepper. The ointment reduces pain associated with neuropathy. Use cautiously, and be sure not to get it in your eyes or mouth.

OTHER HERBAL CONSIDERATION

- *Ginkgo biloba* extract—120 to 240 milligrams daily in two to three divided doses

NUTRITIONAL SUPPLEMENT CONSIDERATIONS

- Alpha-lipoic acid—800 milligrams daily[2]
- Vitamin B_6—50 to 100 milligrams twice daily[3]
- Vitamin B_{12}—15 to 30 micrograms daily for 7 to 14 days and then one to two times weekly (best delivered by intramuscular injection by a trained health care professional)[4]

DIETARY RECOMMENDATIONS

Please see the recommendations listed for diabetes in the chapter "Endocrine System."

Skin Conditions

RELATED CHAPTERS IN PART 5

- Chamomile
- Evening Primrose
- Milk Thistle
- St. John's Wort
- *Vitex agnus-castus*

ACNE

Acne is a complex skin problem that involves interactions among hormones, hair, sebaceous (oil-secreting) glands (collectively known as *pilosebaceous glands*), and bacteria. Teenagers, both male and female, are more susceptible to acne around the onset of puberty. This is attributed to an outburst in production of the hormone testosterone. Boys produce more testosterone than girls, which probably accounts for the increased incidence of acne in teenage males (one of the "testosterone curses"—male pattern baldness is another).

Acne vulgaris is characterized by open *comedones* (blackheads) or closed comedones (whiteheads). Blocked pilosebaceous glands may also lead to the growth of the bacteria *Propionibacterium acnes*. This can lead to deeper lesions, known as *acne conglobata*, which will often result in scarring.

Some women will experience acne right before their menstrual period. This condition is sometimes referred to as *premenstrual acne*.

Acne rosacea is a form of acne most common in middle-aged to older adults with a history of alcohol abuse. We will not cover it here, but remember to read about milk thistle extract (in Part 5) and digestive bitters (in Part 4).

HERBAL PRESCRIPTIONS

Topical Use

- Tea tree oil (5 to 15 percent solution)—Apply topically to acne lesions three to four times daily.[1]

  Actions: Anti-inflammatory, antibacterial, and cleansing actions. Tea tree oil is a good alternative to benzoyl peroxide.

  Note: Use at the recommended dilution. Stronger concentrations may irritate the skin. Avoid contact with the eyes.

Internal Use

- *Vitex agnus-castus*—Dried or liquid preparations delivering 30 to 40 milligrams of the crushed fruit daily

  Action: Like vitamin B_6, vitex is useful for women experiencing premenstrual acne.

OTHER HERBAL CONSIDERATION

- Burdock root—2 to 3 grams daily in two to three divided doses

NUTRITIONAL SUPPLEMENT CONSIDERATIONS

- Zinc (citrate or monomethionine forms)—60 to 90 milligrams daily for 2 to 3 months and then 30 milligrams daily thereafter[2,3]

  Note: Be sure your copper intake is sufficient when taking this much zinc.
- Vitamin E—400 IU daily with meals
- Selenium—200 micrograms daily[4]
- Vitamin B_6—50 to 100 milligrams daily (useful for premenstrual acne flare-ups)[5]

DIETARY RECOMMENDATIONS

Cut down on simple carbohydrates, meat, dairy products, fried foods, and soda pop (sorry, McDonald's). Adopt a whole-foods diet high in complex carbohydrates and fiber from vegetables, grains, and fruits. Consumption of cold-water fish such as salmon is also recommended.

ECZEMA

Also known as *atopic dermatitis,* eczema is a chronic, itching, inflammatory condition of the skin. Eczema that begins in infancy is characterized by red, weeping, crusted lesions on the face, scalp, and extremities. Older children and adults are more likely to suffer dry, thick, localized patches. The incidence of eczema is estimated at 2 to 7 percent of the population.

Atopic dermatitis involves an allergic reaction. Two-thirds of children with eczema have a positive history of allergic disease in their family. Children whose mothers have allergies have an even greater chance of developing eczema (see "Evening Primrose" in Part 5). Eczema often occurs with other allergy-associated diseases such as asthma and hay fever.

HERBAL PRESCRIPTIONS
Internal Use

- Evening primrose oil—For adults, 4 to 6 grams daily with meals (this includes breast-feeding mothers with a history of allergic disease). For children 1 to 12 years old, 2 to 4 grams daily with meals.
  Note: Remember that children are probably going to respond best, but even then you're looking at approximately 2 to 3 months to see results.
- Chinese herbal combination (Zemaphyte™)—One or two packets of the combination in hot water daily[1, 2]
  Note: This product was created in England and currently bears a patent for use with eczema. It's not yet available in the United States. However, among the ten herbal ingredients in the product is licorice root—probably the key ingredient. I recommend that you consult a specialist well versed in traditional Chinese medicine before you try to put this herbal combination together.

External Use
Apply each of the following topically to the affected area three to four times daily:

- Chamomile cream or ointment—Compared to low-potency, topical (0.25 percent) hydrocortisone in one study[3]

- Witch hazel extract cream (with phosphatidylcholine)[3,4]
- Glycyrrhetinic acid (5-percent concentration; from licorice root)[5]
  Note: I highly recommend the use of glycyrrhetinic acid–containing topical creams or ointments if you are using topical cortisone. Glycyrrhetinic acid has been shown to focus the topical anti-inflammatory action of cortisone and reduce its potential systemic side effects.[6]

OTHER HERBAL CONSIDERATIONS
- Chickweed ointment
- Calendula ointment

DIETARY RECOMMENDATIONS
For children with eczema, the best dietary move is to eliminate food allergens.[7] This is most easily done under the supervision of a health care practitioner well versed in nutrition. Cow's milk, eggs, wheat, and tomatoes are among the leading food triggers of eczema. Food additives and colorings should be reduced also.[8] Mothers with a history of allergies who decide to breast-feed should reduce allergenic foods in their diet. Dietary planning should also include the reduction of saturated fats, particularly those from animal sources. Consume more cold-water fish unless you have an identified allergy to them.

PSORIASIS

Psoriasis is a chronic and recurrent skin disease affecting 2 to 4 percent of the population in the United States. Characterized by well-defined, dry, silvery, and scaling lesions, it can appear on the scalp, the elbows and knees, the back, and the buttocks. Psoriasis may cause pitting in the nails and sometimes is associated with arthritis.

The root problem in psoriasis appears to be accelerated growth of skin cells. The skin cells of psoriasis patients divide approximately 1,000 times faster than normal skin cells!

Other factors contributing to psoriasis are abnormal bowel function, poor protein digestion, and sluggish liver function. All of these boost the levels of toxins in the body. Psoriasis sufferers may have a problem with increased permeability of the bowel, allowing endotoxins to cross more freely across the bowel walls and into the circulation. Certainly, maintaining normal bowel health is important in managing psoriasis.

HERBAL PRESCRIPTIONS
Topical
- Capsaicin ointment (0.025 percent concentration)—Apply to the affected area four times daily. Be sure to avoid contact with your eyes or mouth, because this stuff is hot![1,2]

  Action: Capsaicin is the component that gives cayenne pepper its hot taste. Topically, it relieves the pain and itching that occurs in cases of moderate to severe psoriasis.
- *Aloe vera* cream (0.5 percent concentration)—Apply to the affected area three to four times daily.[3]
- Oregon grape (*Mahonia aquifolium*); 10 percent concentration)—Apply to the affected area three to four times daily.[4]

OTHER HERBAL CONSIDERATIONS
- Milk thistle extract (standardized to 80 percent silymarin)—420 milligrams of silymarin in three divided doses

  Action: Supports and promotes normal liver function. Milk thistle is particularly useful for persons with psoriasis who have a history of alcohol abuse.[5]
- Psyllium husk powder—Mix one rounded teaspoonful in an 8-ounce glass of water or juice and down the hatch! Repeat this two to three times daily for 7 to 10 days.

  Actions: Helps cleanse the bowel and encourages normal elimination
- Burdock root—2 to 3 grams daily in two to three divided doses

DIETARY SUPPLEMENT RECOMMENDATIONS
- MaxEPA (fish oil)—8 to 10 grams daily with meals[6,7]
- Zinc (citrate or monomethionine)—30 milligrams daily[8]
- Selenium—200 micrograms daily[9]
- Folic acid—500 micrograms daily[10]

Dietary Recommendations

Reduce alcohol consumption, junk foods, and animal fats. Follow a whole-foods diet, high in complex carbohydrates and fiber (lots of vegetables and fruits), combined with cold-water fish. Some people may respond to a gluten-free diet, which means eliminating grains such as wheat, oats, rye, and barley.

Vitiligo

Vitiligo is a skin disease that causes patches of skin to lose their normal pigment. It usually appears around the mouth, eyes, and nose as well as the bony prominences of the elbows, knees, and hands.

Vitiligo is caused by an absence of pigment-producing cells called *melanocytes*. Although the exact reason is still unknown, it is widely believed that these cells are destroyed by the body's immune system.

Note: None of the following treatments works rapidly. Allow 6 to 9 months of initial use before making a final evaluation.

Herbal Prescriptions

- St. John's wort extract (standardized 0.3 percent hypericin)—Enough extract to provide 3 to 4 milligrams of hypericin daily
  Action: Hypericin makes the skin more sensitive to ultraviolet light from the sun and other sources, which may serve to activate surviving melanocytes. Be careful, however; vitiligo lesions can burn easily with overexposure to the sun.
- Khella extract (*Ammi visnaga*)—A daily dose of the extract should provide approximately 100 milligrams of the active constituent khellin.[1]
  Action: Like psoralen drugs, khellin stimulates the repigmentation of the skin in some individuals with vitiligo. Higher doses of 120 to 160 milligrams of khellin can cause nausea, insomnia, and an increase in liver enzymes. Your doctor should monitor you closely if you take khella for vitiligo.

NUTRITIONAL SUPPLEMENT CONSIDERATIONS

- Folic acid—2 milligrams twice daily
- Vitamin C—500 milligrams twice daily
- Vitamin B_{12}—1,000 micrograms by intramuscular injection every 2 weeks. This should be performed only by a trained health care professional.

  Note: One study found combining these three nutrients successful in treating 8 of 15 people with vitiligo.[2] Another study found success in 52 of 100 persons with vitiligo using oral supplementation of folic acid (10 milligrams per day) and vitamin B_{12} (2,000 micrograms per day).[3]

- L-phenylalanine—50 to 100 milligrams per kilogram of body weight (e.g. 3,500 to 7,000 milligrams for a 154-pound person)[4]

  Note: Most clinical studies using L-phenylalanine have combined it with ultraviolet (UVA) radiation therapy. One study also used a 10 percent L-phenylalanine gel topically prior to people with vitiligo receiving their UVA treatments.[5]

DIETARY CONSIDERATIONS

Some people with vitiligo have been found to produce less than normal amounts of stomach acid.[6] This leads to poor digestion of many nutrients, including vitamin B_{12}. Try adding herbal digestive bitters before each meal (see the discussion in Part 4).

OTHER SKIN CONDITIONS

ATHLETE'S FOOT (*TINEA PEDIS*)

- Tea tree oil cream (10 to 15 percent concentration)—Apply topically to the affected area two to three times daily.[1]

FUNGAL INFECTION OF THE NAILS (ONYCHOMYCOSIS)

- Tea tree oil—Apply full strength to the affected nail twice daily. Trimming the nail back as much as possible will help with optimal delivery of the tea tree oil.[1]

SHINGLES (*HERPES ZOSTER*)

Apply one of these topical preparations to affected areas four times daily:

- Capsaicin ointment (0.025 percent concentration)—Be sure to avoid contact with eyes or mouth, as this stuff is hot! Capsaicin reduces the nerve pain (neuralgia) that often follows an outbreak of shingles.[1,2]
- Licorice root ointment or gel—May help speed the healing of lesions[3]

Urinary Tract

RELATED CHAPTERS IN PART 5

- Cranberry
- Echinacea
- *Ginkgo biloba*

RECURRENT URINARY TRACT INFECTIONS

Attempting to decide what constitutes "recurrent" with regard to urinary tract infections (UTIs) is not easy.[1] The textbook *General Urology* gets right to the point by stating, "Chronic cystitis [urinary tract infection] is confusing because it means different things to different people: some physicians use the term exclusively to mean unresolved or persistent bladder infections, whereas others use it to mean three or more bouts of bladder infection occurring in the course of one year."[2]

While the definition for recurrent UTIs is somewhat elusive, the hard facts of women suffering from the condition are not. Women suffering from UTIs account for approximately 5.2 million visits to physicians' offices each year. One of five women in the United States will suffer a UTI at some time in her life; of these, 3 percent will experience recurrent disease. Finally, 20 percent of women treated for a simple UTI will suffer a repeat bout.

Two common symptoms of UTI are burning, painful urination and frequent urination. However, recurrent UTIs pose more serious health risks, including scarring of the bladder wall. Pregnant women suffering from UTI run an increased risk of kidney infection due to anatomical pressure on the bladder.[3]

As was noted under "Cranberry" in Part 5, the guilty party in the majority of bacterial-induced UTIs is *Escherichia coli* (called *E. coli* for short), a common inhabitant of the gastrointestinal tract. Most recurrent UTIs can be linked to this organism.

Note: Remember the focus here is on recurrent, and not acute, UTIs. While many traditional herbal approaches are available for treating an acute UTI, it's best to make that choice under the supervision of a physician trained in herbal medicine.

HERBAL PRESCRIPTION

- Cranberry juice extract—400 milligrams of an encapsulated, concentrated extract in the morning and evening. Ample intake of water throughout the day is also recommended.
  Actions: Inhibits the adherence of *E. coli* to the lining of the bladder and helps clear the bacteria from the urine

OTHER HERBAL CONSIDERATIONS

- *Echinacea purpurea* (expressed juice of the herb or encapsulated dried juice)—40 drops of the juice three times daily, or one capsule of the dried juice three or four times daily for 10 to 14 days
  Action: Helps restore healthy immune function in individuals with recurrent infections, especially those who have taken antibiotics for long periods of time
- Goldenseal root—500 milligrams two to three times daily for 10 to 14 days
  Action: Weak antimicrobial activity without the side effects of antibiotics. Action may complement the inhibitory action of cranberry against *E. coli*.[4]
- Marshmallow root—900 milligrams two to three times daily
  Action: Soothing effect (demulcent) on irritated tissue

NUTRITIONAL SUPPLEMENT CONSIDERATIONS

- Vitamin C—1 to 2 grams daily
- Acidophilus/bifidus capsules or powder—Recommended for both oral and vaginal applications[5]

DIETARY RECOMMENDATIONS

Drink four to five 8-ounce servings of water daily. Decrease simple carbohydrates (refined sugar) and artificial sweeteners. Get on an anti–diet soda crusade!

Acupuncture might be of some benefit for women with recurrent UTIs.[6]

SUPPORT FOR KIDNEY FUNCTION
WHILE TAKING IMMUNE-SUPPRESSIVE DRUGS

People who have had kidney transplants are often in a Catch-22 situation. To prevent the body's immune system from rejecting the transplanted kidney, they are given a drug that suppresses the immune system. The most common choice is cyclosporin. Cyclosporin does its job effectively on the immune system, but it has a negative trade-off—it impairs kidney function over time. Two natural medicines may counter this side effect.

- *Ginkgo biloba* extract—120 to 240 milligrams daily in two to three divided doses[1]
- MaxEPA (fish oil)—6 grams daily with meals[2]

Herbal Medicine Resources

WITH the vast array of herbal products currently available, health care consumers and professionals are clamoring to find credible information to further their education in this area. Since many of these herbal supplements are being used for conditions requiring careful medical monitoring, finding a physician with training or experience in the use of herbs is also important.

ORGANIZATIONS OFFERING HERBAL MEDICINE INFORMATION

American Botanical Council
P.O. Box 144345
Austin, TX 78714-4345
(512) 926-4900; fax (512) 926-2345
Web site: www.herbalgram.org

Headed by Mark Blumenthal, the hardest-working man in the herb world, the American Botanical Council produces educational materials for both the public and professionals. They copublish *HerbalGram* with the Herb Research Foundation. They're also responsible for creating the first English translation of the German Commission E monographs. The American Botanical Council also has an excellent list of books on herbal medicine.

Herb Research Foundation
1007 Pearl Street, Suite 200
Boulder, CO 80302
(303) 449-2265; fax (303) 449-7849
Web site: www.herbs.org

This nonprofit organization is dedicated to the dissemination of reliable information on herbs. The Herb Research Foundation offers published summaries on specific herbs and also herbal approaches to certain health conditions.

ONE STOP SHOPPING FOR HERBAL AND ALTERNATIVE MEDICINE INFORMATION

Healthnotes, Inc.
1505 SE Gideon, Suite 200
Portland, OR 97202
(503) 234-4092; fax (503) 234-4052
Web site: www.healthnotes.com

HEALTH CARE PROFESSIONAL REFERRAL

American Association of Naturopathic Physicians
601 Valley Street, Suite 105
Seattle, WA 98109-4229
(206) 298-0126; fax (206) 298-0129
Web site: www.naturopathic.org

Want to know if there's a naturopathic physician in your area? The American Association of Naturopathic Physicians is the place to call. Their referral line will give you a local listing of naturopaths who have graduated from credible postgraduate institutes such as the ones listed here (professional schools teaching herbal medicine). These physicians not only have been extensively trained in the clinical use and safety of herbal medicines but have had to complete state licensing boards that demonstrate competency in this area.

American Holistic Medical Association
4101 Lake Boone Trail, #201
Raleigh, NC 26707
(919) 787-5146

An eclectic collection of medical doctors, osteopathic physicians, naturopathic physicians, and nurses, the American Holistic Medical Association promotes the use of alternative and complementary therapies in medical practice. Its former president is that well-known Prima author Alan Gaby.

PROFESSIONAL SCHOOLS TEACHING HERBAL MEDICINE

Bastyr University
14500 Juanita Drive NE
Kenmore, WA 98028
(425) 823-1200
Web site: www.bastyr.edu

National College of Naturopathic Medicine
049 SW Porter
Portland, OR 97201
(503) 499-4343
Web site: www.ncnm.edu

Southwest College of Naturopathic Medicine and Health Sciences
2140 East Broadway Road
Tempe, AZ 85282
(602) 858-9100

University of Bridgeport College of Naturopathic Medicine
60 Lafayette Street
Bridgeport, CT 06601
(203) 576-4109
Web site: www.bridgeport.edu/naturopathy

The Canadian College of Naturopathic Medicine
2300 Yonge Street, 18th Floor
Box 2431
Toronto, Ontario, Canada M4P 1E4
(416) 486-8584

MY FAVORITE BOOKS ON HERBAL MEDICINE

Weiss RF: *Herbal Medicine.* Ab Arcanum, Gothenberg, Sweden, 1988.

Robbers JE, and Tyler VE: *Tyler's Herbs of Choice: The Therapeutic Use of Phytomedicinals.* Haworth Herbal Press, Binghamton, New York, 1999.

Blumenthal M, ed.: *Herbal Medicine: Expanded Commission E Monographs.* Integrative Medical Communications, Newton, Massachusetts, 2000.

McCaleb RS, Leigh E, and Morien K: *The Encyclopedia of Popular Herbs.* Prima Health, Roseville, California, 2000.

Werbach MR and Murray MT: *Botanical Influences on Illness: A Sourcebook of Clinical Research.* Third Line Press, Tarzana, California, 2000.

Foster S: *101 Medicinal Herbs: An Illustrated Guide.* Interweave Press, Loveland, Colorado, 1998.

Foster S and Chongxi Y: *Herbal Emissaries: Bringing Chinese Herbs to the West.* Healing Arts Press, Rochester, Vermont, 1993.

Hoffman D: *The Herbal Handbook: A User's Guide to Medical Herbalism.* Healing Arts Press, Rochester, Vermont, 1998.

My Favorite Books on Alternative and Complementary Medicine

For which I'm a coauthor:

Lininger S, Wright J, Austin S, Brown D, and Gaby A: *The Natural Pharmacy.* Prima Publishing, Roseville, California, 1999.

Lininger S, Gaby A, Austin S, Batz F, Yarnell Y, Brown D, and Constantine G: *A–Z Guide to Drug–Herb–Vitamin Interactions.* Prima Publishing, Roseville, California, 1999.

For which I'm not:

Hudson T: *Women's Encyclopedia of Natural Medicine.* Keats Publishing, Lincolnwood, Illinois, 1999.

Favorite Nonherb Books

One Hundred Years of Solitude, Gabriel Garcia Marquez
In the Skin of a Lion, Michael Ondaatje
Mama Day, Gloria Naylor
Geek Love, Katherine Dunn
Beloved, Toni Morrison
To the Wedding, John Berger
The Crossing, Cormac McCarthy
Very Old Bones, William Kennedy
Paris Trout, Pete Dexter
The Book of Laughter and Forgetting, Milan Kundera
Middle Passage, Charles Johnson
Postcards, E. Annie Proulx
World's End, T. C. Boyle
Music for Torching, A. M. Homes
Sharpshooter Blues, Lewis Nordan
American Pastoral, Philip Roth
Texaco, Patrick Chamoiseau

FAVORITE CDS TO TAKE HERBS BY

Kind of Blue, Miles Davis
In a Silent Way, Miles Davis
Good Guys, Art Ensemble of Chicago
Impressions, John Coltrane
Shape of Jazz to Come, Ornette Coleman
Music from Big Pink, The Band
Charms of the Night Sky, Dave Douglas
Funkify Your Life, The Meters
Bringing It All Back Home, Bob Dylan
Nine Below Zero, Wayne Horvitz
Gone, Just Like a Train, Bill Frisell
Monk's Dream, Thelonius Monk
Blues and Roots, Charles Mingus
There's a Riot Goin' On, Sly and the Family Stone
Where's Your Cup, Henry Threadgill
Rain Dogs, Tom Waits
Kiko, Los Lobos
The Chess Box Set, Muddy Waters

References

INTRODUCTION

1. Industry overview 1999. *Nutrition Business Journal* 4:1–5, 1999.
2. Wetzel MS, Eisenberg DM, and Kaptchuk TJ: Course involving complementary and alternative medicine at US schools. *JAMA* 280:784–787, 1998.
3. Jancin B: Alternative care coverage will placate consumers. *Internal Medicine News* December 1, 1999, p. 46.
4. Eisenberg DM, Kessler RC, et al.: Unconventional medicine in the United States. *New Engl J Med* 328:246–252, 1993.
5. Eisenberg DM, Davis RB, et al.: Trends in alternative medicine use in the United States, 1990–1997. *JAMA* 280:1569–1575, 1998.
6. Brody J: Herbal remedies tied to pregnancy risks. *New York Times* March 9, 1999.
7. Ondrizek RR, Chan PJ, et al.: An alternative medicine study of herbal effects on the penetration of zona-free hamster oocytes and the integrity of sperm deoxyribonucleic acid. *Fertil Steril* 71:517–522, 1999.
8. Agarwal A: Do herbal supplements impair male fertility? An expert responds to the Loma Linda studies. *Healthnotes Rev Complementary Integrative Med* 6:74–75, 1999.
9. Coverage of alternative medicine in journals. *Modern Medicine* October, 1999.
10. Stolberg SG: Alternative care gains a foothold. *New York Times* January 31, 2000.
11. Angell M and Kassirer JP: Alternative medicine—the risks of untested and unregulated remedies [Editorial]. *New Engl J Med* 339:839–841, 1998.
12. Brown D and Petrich C: Louis–Harris poll finds high patient demand and growing mainstream professional interest in herbal supplements. *Healthnotes Rev Complementary Integrative Med* 6:52–53, 1999.

PART 2: QUESTIONS COMMONLY ASKED ABOUT HERBAL SUPPLEMENTS

1. Farnsworth NR, Akerele O, et al.: Medicinal plants in therapy. *Bulletin World Health Organization* 63:965–981, 1985.
2. Eisenberg DM, Davis RB, et al.: Trends in alternative medicine use in the United States, 1990–1997. *JAMA* 280:1569–1575, 1998.
3. Stolberg SG: Alternative care gains a foothold. *New York Times* January 31, 2000.

4. Stolberg SG: Alternative care gains a foothold. *New York Times* January 31, 2000.
5. Eisenberg DM, Davis RB, et al.: Trends in alternative medicine use in the United States, 1990–1997. *JAMA* 280:1569–1575, 1998.

PART 3: PHYTOTHERAPY: A RATIONAL MODEL FOR HERBAL MEDICINE IN THE UNITED STATES

1. Schilcher H: The significance of phytotherapy in Europe: An interdisciplinary and comparative study. *Zeits Phtyother* 14:132–139, 1993.
2. Gruenwald J: The emerging role of herbal medicine in health care in Europe. *Drug Information J* 32:151–153, 1998.
3. Blumenthal M, ed.: *Herbal Medicine: Expanded Commission E Monographs.* Integrative Medicine Communications, Newton, Massachusetts, 2000, pp. 481–483.
4. Blumenthal M, ed.: *Herbal Medicine: Expanded Commission E Monographs.* Integrative Medicine Communications, Newton, Massachusetts, 2000, p. 475.

PART 4: CATEGORIES OF HERBAL MEDICINES

1. Brekhman II and Dardymov IV: New substances of plant origin which increase nonspecific resistance. *Annu Rev Pharmacol* 9:419–430, 1969.
2. Wagner H, Nörr H, and Winterhoff H: Plant adaptogens. *Phytomedicine* 1:63–76, 1994.
3. Harman D: Free radicals in aging. *Molecular Cell Biochem* 84:155–161, 1988.
4. Diplock AT: Antioxidant nutrients and disease prevention: An overview. *Am J Clin Nutr* 53(Suppl.):373–379, 1991.
5. Bindoli A, Cavallini L, and Sliprandi N: Inhibitory action of silymarin on lipid peroxide formation in rat liver mitochondria and microsomes. *Biochem Pharmacol* 26:2405–2409, 1977.
6. Frankel EN, Kramer J, et al.: Inhibition of oxidation of human low-density lipoprotein by phenolic substances in red wine. *Lancet* 341:454–457, 1993.
7. Hertog MG, Feskens EJ, et al.: Dietary antioxidant flavonoids and risk of coronary heart disease: The Zutphen elderly study. *Lancet* 342:1007–1011, 1993.
8. Bushman JL: Green tea and cancer in humans: A review of the literature. *Nutr Cancer* 31:151–159, 1998.
9. Robbers JE, Tyler VE: *Tyler's Herbs of Choice: The Therapeutic Use of Phytomedicinals.* Haworth Herbal Press, Binghamton, New York, 1999, pp. 66–72.
10. Weiss RF: *Herbal Medicine.* Ab Arcanum, Gothenburg, Sweden, 1988, pp. 75–78.
11. Hoffman D: *The Herbal Handbook: A User's Guide to Medical Herbalism.* Healing Arts Press, Rochester, Vermont, 1998, pp. 54–57.
12. Ridker PM and McDermott WV: Comfrey herb tea and hepatic veno-occlusive disease. *Lancet* ii:657–658, 1989.
13. Robbers JE, Tyler VE: *Tyler's Herbs of Choice: The Therapeutic Use of Phytomedicinals.* Haworth Herbal Press, Binghamton, New York, 1999, pp. 220–222.
14. Lien EJ and Gao H: Higher plant polysaccharides and their pharmacological activities. *International Journal of Oriental Medicine* 15:123–140, 1990.
15. Pastors JG, Blaidsell PW, et al.: Psyllium fiber reduces rise in postprandial glucose and insulin concentrations in patients with non-insulin-dependent diabetes. *Am J Clin Nutr* 53:1431–1435, 1991.

References

380

16. Passmore AP, Wilson-Davies K, et al.: Chronic constipation in long stay elderly patients: A comparison of lactulose and a senna–fiber combination. *Br Med J* 307:769–771, 1993.

PART 5: COMMONLY PRESCRIBED HERBAL MEDICINES

BILBERRY

1. Cunio L: *Vaccinium myrtillus. Aust J Med Herbalism* 5:81–85, 1993.
2. Robbers JE, Tyler VE: *Tyler's Herbs of Choice: The Therapeutic Use of Phytomedicinals.* Haworth Herbal Press, Binghamton, New York, 1999, p. 65.
3. Baj A, Bombardelli E, et al.: Qualitative and quantitative evaluation of *Vaccinium myrtillus* anthocyanins by high-resolution gas chromatography and high-performance liquid chromatography. *J Chromatography* 279:365–372, 1983.
4. Pizzorno JE and Murray MT: *A Textbook of Natural Medicine.* Churchill Livingstone, London, 1999, pp. 991–996.
5. Bonati A: How and why should we standardize phytopharmaceutical drugs for clinical validation? *J Ethnopharmacol* 32:195–197, 1991.
6. Yarnell E: Review of clinical trials on oligomeric proanthocyanidins. *Healthnotes Rev Alternative Complementary Med* 6:92–94, 1999.
7. Alfieri R and Sole P: Influence des anthocyanosides administrés par voie parenterale sur l'adaptoelectroretinogramme du lapin. *CR Soc Biol* 158:2338, 1964.
8. Vaughan D and Asbury T: *General Ophthalmology.* Lange Medical Publications, Los Altos, California, pp. 163–164.
9. Salvayre R, Braquet P, et al.: Comparison of the scavenger effect of bilberry anthocyanosides with various flavonoids. *Proceed Int Bioflavonoid Symposium,* Munich, 1981, pp. 437–442.
10. Lietti A and Forni G: Studies on *Vaccinium myrtillus* anthocyanosides. I. Vasoprotective and anti-inflammatory activity. *Arzneim-Forsch Drug Res* 26:829–832, 1976.
11. Mian E, Curri SB, et al.: Anthocyanosides and the walls of microvessels: Further aspects of the mechanism of action of their protective effect in syndromes due to abnormal capillary fragility. *Minerva Med* 68:3565–3581, 1977.
12. Colantuoni A, Bertuglia S, et al.: Effects of *Vaccinium myrtillus* anthocyanosides on arterial vasomotion. *Arzneim-Forsch Drug Res* 41:905–909, 1991.
13. Pulliero G, Montin S, et al.: *Ex vivo* study of the inhibitory effects of *Vaccinium myrtillus* anthocyanosides on human platelet aggregation. *Fitoterapia* 60:69–75, 1989.
14. Monbiosse JC, Braquest P, et al.: Non-enzymatic degradation of acid-soluble calf skin collagen by superoxide ion: Protective effect of flavonoids. *Biochem Pharmacol* 32:53–58, 1983.
15. Rao CN, Rao VH, and Steinman B: Influence of bioflavonoids on the collagen metabolism in rats with adjuvant induced arthritis. *Ital J Biochem* 30:54–62, 1981.
16. Terrase J and Moinade S: Premiers resultats obtenus avec un nouveau facteur vitamonique P, les anthocyanosides, extraits du *Vaccinium myrtillus. Presse Med* 72:397–400, 1964.
17. Sala D, Rolando M, et al.: Effect of anthocyanosides on visual performance at low illumination. *Minerva Oftalmol* 21:283–285, 1979.
18. Muth ER, Laurent JM, and Jasper P: The effect of bilberry nutritional supplementation on night visual acuity and contrast sensitivity. *Altern Med Rev* 5:164–173, 2000.
19. Gandolfo E: Perimetric follow-up of myopic patients treated with anthocyanosides and beta-carotene. *Boll Ocul* 69:57–71, 1990.

References

20. Scharrer A and Ober M: Anthocyanosides in the treatment of retinopathies. *Klin Monatsbl Augenheilkd Beih* 178:386–389, 1981.

21. Perossini M, Guidi G, et al.: Diabetic and hypertensive retinopathy therapy with *Vaccinium myrtillus* (Tegens®). Double-blind, placebo-controlled clinical trial. *Ann Ottamol Clin Ocul* 113:1173, 1987.

22. Bravetti G: Preventive medical treatment of senile cataracts with vitamin E and anthocyanosides: clinical evaluation. *Annals Ottamol Clin Ocul* 115:109, 1989.

23. Werbach MR and Murray MT: *Botanical Influences on Illness*. Third Line Press, Tarzana, California, 1994, pp. 271–272.

24. Grismond GL: Treatment of pregnancy-induced phlebopathies. *Minerva Gynecol* 33:221–230, 1981.

25. Boniface R, Miskulin M, et al.: Pharmacological properties of *Vaccinium myrtillus* anthocyanosides: Correlation with results of treatment of diabetic microangiopathy. In: *Flavonoids and Bioflavonoids* (Farka L, Gábor M, Kállay F, eds.). Elsevier, Berlin, 1985, pp. 293–301.

BLACK COHOSH

1. Schulz V, Hänsel R, Tyler VE: *Rational Phytotherapy: A Physicians' Guide to Herbal Medicine*. Springer-Verlag, Berlin, 1998, pp. 288–292.

2. Foster S: Black cohosh (*Cimicifuga racemosa*): A literature review. *HerbalGram* 45:33–49, 1999.

3. Hand W: *The House Surgeon and Physician*. Peter B. Cleason & Company, Hartford, Connecticut, 1818, p. 169.

4. Blumenthal M, Busse WR, et al., eds.: *The Complete Commission E Monographs*. Integrative Medicine Communications, Boston, Massachusetts, 1998, p. 90.

5. Gruenwald J: Standardized black cohosh (*Cimicifuga*) extract clinical monograph. *Quart Rev Natural Med* Summer: 117–125, 1998.

6. Jarry H, Harnischfeger G, Düker E: Studies on endocrine effects of the contents of *Cimicifuga racemosa*. 2. In vitro binding of compounds to estrogen receptors. *Planta Medica* 51:316–319, 1985.

7. Jarry H, Harnischfeger G: Studies on endocrine effects of the contents of *Cimicifuga racemosa*. 1. Influence on the serum concentration of pituitary hormones in ovariectomized rats. *Planta Medica* 51:46–49, 1985.

8. Düker EM, Kopanski L, et al.: Effects of extracts from *Cimicifuga racemosa* on gonadotropin release in menopausal women and ovariectomized rats. *Planta Medica* 57:420–424, 1991.

9. Einer-Jensen N, Zhao J, et al.: *Cimicifuga* and *Melbrosia* lack estrogenic effects in mice and rats. *Maturitas* 25:149–153, 1996.

10. Liske E, Wüstenberg P, Boblitz N: Human pharmacological investigations during treatment of climacteric complaints with *Cimicifuga racemosa* (Remifemin®): No estrogen-like effects [Poster presentation]. 2nd International Congress on Phytomedicine, London, October 15–16, 1998.

11. Lieberman S: A review of the effectiveness of *Cimicifuga racemosa* (black cohosh) for the symptoms of menopause. *J Women's Health* 7:525–529, 1998.

12. Liske E: Therapeutic efficacy and safety of *Cimicifuga racemosa* for gynecological disorders. *Advances Therapy* 15:45–53, 1998.

13. Stoll W. Phytomedicine influences atrophic vaginal epithelium: Double-blind study of cimicifuga versus estrogenic substance. *Therapeuticon* 1:23–31, 1987.

14. Warnecke G: Using phyto-treatment to influence menopause symptoms. *Med Welt* 36:871–874, 1985.

15. Stolze H: The other way to treat symptoms of menopause. *Gyne* 1:14–16, 1982.
16. Liske E, Wüstenberg P: Therapy of climacteric complaints with *Cimicifuga racemosa:* A herbal medicine with clinically proven evidence [Poster presentation]. 9th Annual Meeting, the North American Menopause Society, Toronto, September 16–19, 1998.
17. Blumenthal M, Busse WR, et al., eds.: *The Complete Commission E Monographs.* Integrative Medicine Communications, Boston, Massachusetts, 1998, p. 90.

CHAMOMILE

1. Mann C and Staba EJ: The chemistry, pharmacology, and commercial formulations of chamomile. In: *Herbs, Spices, and Medicinal Plants: Recent Advances in Botany, Horticulture, and Pharmacology,* Vol. 1 (Craker LE and Simon JE, eds.). Oryx Press, Phoenix, Arizona, 1986, pp. 235–280.
2. Robbers JE, Tyler VE: *Tyler's Herbs of Choice: The Therapeutic Use of Phytomedicinals.* Haworth Herbal Press, Binghamton, New York, 1999, pp. 69–71.
3. Foster S: *Herbal Renaissance.* Gibbs-Smith Publisher, Salt Lake City, Utah, 1994, pp. 64–67.
4. Grieve M: *A Modern Herbal.* Dover Publications, New York, 1971, pp. 185–188.
5. Foster S, Tyler VE: *Tyler's Honest Herbal.* Haworth Herbal Press, Binghamton New York, 1999, pp. 105–108.
6. Wichtl M: *Herbal Drugs and Phytopharmaceuticals.* CRC Press, Boca Raton, Florida, 1994, pp. 322–325.
7. Jakolev V, Isaac O, et al.: Pharmacological investigations with compounds of chamomile. II. New investigations on the antiphlogistic effects of (–)-α-bisabolol and bisabolol oxides. *Planta Med* 35:125–140, 1979.
8. Jakolev V, Isaac O, and Flaskamp E: Pharmacological investigations with compounds of chamomile. VI. Investigations on the antiphlogistic effects of chamazulene and matricine. *Planta Med* 49:67–73, 1983.
9. Della Loggia R, Tubaro A, et al.: The role of flavonoids in the antiinflammatory activity of *Chamomilla recutita.* In: *Plant Flavonoids in Biology and Medicine: Biochemical, Pharmacological, and Structure–Activity Relationships* (Cody V, Middleton E, and Harborne JB, eds.). Alan R. Liss, New York, pp. 481–484, 1986.
10. Achterrath-Tuckerman U, Kunde R, et al.: Pharmacological investigations with compounds of chamomile. V. Investigations on the spasmolytic effect of compounds of chamomile and Kamillosan® on the isolated guinea pig ileum. *Planta Med* 39:38–50, 1980.
11. Beil W, Birkholz C, Sewing KF: Effects of flavonoids on parietal cell acid secretion, gastric mucosal prostaglandin production and *Helicobacter pylori* growth. *Arzneim-Forsch Drug Res* 45:697–700, 1995.
12. Weiss RF: *Herbal Medicine.* Ab Arcanum, Gothenberg, Sweden, 1988, pp. 1–11.
13. Tyler VE: Phytomedicines in Western Europe: Their potential impact on herbal medicine in the United States. *HerbalGram* 30:24–30, 67–68, 1994.
14. *Matricaria flos.* European Scientific Cooperative on Phytotherapy (ESCOP) Monograph, October 1990.
15. Weizman Z, Alkrinawi S, et al.: Efficacy of herbal tea preparation in infantile colic. *J Pediatrics* 122:650–652, 1993.
16. Mills SY: *Out of the Earth: The Essential Book of Herbal Medicine.* Viking Press, London, 1991, pp. 448–451.
17. Nasemann T: Kamillosan® therapy in dermatology. *Z Allg Med* 25:1105–1106, 1975.

18. Aggag ME and Yousef RT: Study of the antimicrobial activity of chamomile oil. *Planta Med* 22:140–144, 1972.
19. Bradley PR, ed.: Matricaria flower. In: *British Herbal Compendium,* Vol. 1. British Herbal Medicine Association, Bournemouth, Dorset, England 1992, pp. 154–157.
20. Glowania HJ, Raulin C, and Swoboda M: The effect of chamomile on wound healing—a controlled, clinical, experimental double-blind trial. *Z Hautkr* 62:1262–1271, 1987.
21. Albring M, Albrecht H, et al.: The measuring of the antiinflammatory effect of a chamomile compound on the skin of volunteers. *Meth Find Exp Clin Pharmacol* 5:75–77, 1983.
22. Aergeerts P, Albring M, et al.: Vergleichende Prüfung von Kamillosan®-crème gegenüber steroidalen (0.25% hydrocortisone, 0.75% flucotinbutylester) and nichsteroidsalen (5% bufexamac) Externa in der Erhaltungstherapie von Ekzemerkrankungen. *Z Hautkr* 60: 270–277, 1985.
23. Blumenthal M, Busse WR, et al., eds.: *The Complete Commission E Monographs.* Integrative Medicine Communications, Boston, Massachusetts, 1998, p. 107.
24. Mann C and Staba EJ: The chemistry, pharmacology, and commercial formulations of chamomile. In: *Herbs, Spices, and Medicinal Plants: Recent Advances in Botany, Horticulture, and Pharmacology,* Vol. 1 (Craker LE and Simon JE, eds.). Oryx Press, Phoenix, Arizona, 1986, pp. 235–280.
25. Jensen-Jarolim E, Reider N, et al.: Fatal outcome of anaphylaxis to chamomile-containing enema during labor: A case study. *J Allergy Clin Immunol* 102:1041–1042, 1998.

CRANBERRY

1. Blatherwick NR and Long ML: Studies on urinary acidity. II. The increased acidity produced by eating prunes and cranberries. *J Biol Chem* 57:815, 1923.
2. Bodel PT, Cotran R, and Kass EH: Cranberry juice and the antibacterial action of hippuric acid. *J Lab Clin Med* 54:881–888, 1959.
3. Moen DV: Observations on the effectiveness of cranberry juice in urinary tract infections. *Wis Med J* 61:282–283, 1962.
4. Papas PN, Brusch CA, and Ceresia GC: Cranberry juice in the treatment of urinary tract infections. *Southwest Med* 47:17–20, 1966.
5. Schaefer AJ: Recurrent urinary tract infection in the female patient. *Urology* 32(Suppl):12–15, 1988.
6. Bettman LR: Pathogenesis of urinary tract infections: Host susceptibility and bacterial virulence factors. *Urology* 32(Suppl):9–11, 1988.
7. Sobota AE: Inhibition of bacterial adherence by cranberry juice: Potential use for the treatment of urinary tract infections. *J Urol* 131:1013–1016, 1984.
8. Schmidt DR and Sobota AE: An examination of the anti-adherence activity of cranberry juice on urinary and nonurinary bacterial isolates. *Microbios* 55:173–181, 1988.
9. Zafiri D, Ofek I, et al.: Inhibitory activity of cranberry juice on adherence of type 1 and type P fimbriated *Escherichia coli* to eucaryotic cells. *Antimicrob Agents Chemother* 33:92–98, 1989.
10. Ofek I, Goldhar J, et al.: Anti-*Escherichia coli* adhesion activity of cranberry and blueberry juices. *New Engl J Med* 324:1599, 1991.
11. Howell AB, Vorsa N, et al.: Inhibition of the adherence of P-fimbriated *Escherichia coli* to uroepithelial-cell surfaces by proanthocyanidin extracts from cranberry [Letter]. *New England J Med* 339:1085–1086, 1998.
12. Walker EB, Barney DP, et al.: Cranberry concentrate: UTI prophylaxis [Letter]. *J Family Pract* 45:167–168, 1997.

13. Avorn J, Monane M, et al.: Reduction of bacteriuria and pyuria after ingestion of cranberry juice. *JAMA* 271:751–754, 1994.
14. Gibson L, Pike L, and Kilbourn JP: Effectiveness of cranberry juice in preventing urinary tract infections in long-term care facility patients. *J Naturopath Med* 2:45–47, 1991.
15. Leaver RB: Cranberry juice. *Professional Nurse* 11:525–526, 1996.
16. Saltzman JR, Kemp JA, et al.: Effect of hypochlorhydria due to omeprazole treatment or atrophic gastritis on protein-bound vitamin B12 absorption. *J Am Coll Nutr* 13: 584–591, 1994.

ECHINACEA

1. Melchart D, Linde K, et al.: Immunomodulation with echinacea—a systemic review of controlled clinical trials. *Phytomedicine* 1:245–254, 1994.
2. Brevoort P: The booming U.S. botanical market: A new overview. *HerbalGram* 144:33–48, 1998.
3. Hobbs C: Echinacea: A literature review. *HerbalGram* 30:33–48, 1994.
4. Foster S: Echinacea Education Monograph. *Quart Rev Nat Med* Winter:19–28, 1993.
5. Foster S: *Echinacea, Nature's Immune Enhancer*. Healing Arts Press, Rochester, Vermont, 1991.
6. Bauer R: *Echinacea*: Biological effects and active principles. In: *Phytomedicines of Europe: Chemistry and Biological Activity* (Lawson LD, Bauer R, eds.). American Chemical Society, Washington, D.C., 1998, pp. 140–157.
7. Stimpel M, Proksch A, et al.: Macrophage activation and induction of macrophage cytotoxicity by purified polysaccharide fractions from the plant *Echinacea purpurea. Infect Immunity* 46:845–849, 1984.
8. Leuttig B, Steinmüller C, et al.: Macrophage activation by the polysaccharide arabinogalactan isolated from plant cell cultures of *Echinacea purpurea. J Natl Cancer Inst* 81:669–675, 1989.
9. Kuhn O: Echinacin® and phagocyte reaction. *Arzneim-Forsch Drug Res* 3:194–200, 1953.
10. Wagner H and Proksch A: Immunomodulatory drugs of fungi and higher plants. In: *Economic and Medicinal Plant Research*, Vol. 1 (Farnsworth N, Hikino H, and Wagner H, eds.). Academic Press, Orlando, Florida, 1985, pp. 113–155.
11. Gaisbauer M, Schleich T, et al.: Phagocytic activity of granulocytes using chemiluminescence measurement. *Arzneim-Forsch Drug Res* 40:594–598, 1990.
12. Hoheisel O, Sandberg M, et al.: Echinagard treatment shortens the course of the common cold: a double-blind, placebo-controlled clinical trial. *Eur J Clin Res* 9:261–268, 1997.
13. Brikenborn RM, Shah DV: Degenring Echinaforce® and other *Echinacea* fresh plant preparations in the treatment of the common cold: A randomized, placebo-controlled, double-blind clinical trial. *Phytomedicine* 6:1–5, 1999.
14. Dorn M, Knick E, Lewith G: Placebo-controlled, double-blind study of *Echinacea pallida* radix in upper respiratory tract infections. *Comp Therapy Med* 5:40–42, 1997.
15. Henneicke-von Zepelin HH, Hentschel C, et al.: Efficacy and safety of a fixed combination phytomedicine in the treatment of the common cold (acute viral respiratory infection): Results of a randomized, double-blind, placebo-controlled, multicenter study. *Current Med Res Opinion* 15:214–227, 1999.
16. Melchart D, Walther E, et al.: Echinacea root extracts for the prevention of upper respiratory tract infections: A double-blind, placebo-controlled randomized trial. *Arch Family Med* 7:541–545, 1998.

17. Grimm W, Müller HH. A randomized controlled trial of the effect of fluid extract of *Echinacea purpurea* on the incidence and severity of colds and respiratory infections. *Am J Med* 106:138–143, 1999.

18. Calabrese C: Personal communication, November, 1998.

19. Braunig B, Dorn M, et al.: *Echinacea purpurea* root for strengthening the immune response in flu-like infections. *Zeitschrift Phytother* 13:7–13, 1992.

20. Coeugniet E and Kühnast R: Recurrent candidiasis: Adjuvant immunotherapy with different formulations of Echinacin®. *Therapiewoche* 36:3352–3358, 1986.

21. Blumenthal M, Busse WR, et al., eds.: *The Complete Commission E Monographs.* Integrative Medicine Communications, Boston, Massachusetts, 1998, pp. 122–123.

ELEUTHERO

1. Baranov AI: Medicinal uses of ginseng and related plants in the Soviet Union: Recent trends in the Soviet literature. *J Ethnopharmacol* 6:339–353, 1982.

2. Foster S and Chingxi Y: *Herbal Emissaries.* Healing Arts Press, Rochester, Vermont, 1992, pp. 73–79.

3. Brekhman II and Dardymov IV: New substances of plant origin which increase non-specific resistance. *Annu Rev Pharmacol* 4:419–430, 1969.

4. Brekhman II: *Man and Biologically Active Substances.* Pergamon Press, Oxford, 1980.

5. Collisson RJ: Siberian ginseng (*Eleutherococcus senticosus*). *Br J Phytother* 2:61–71, 1991.

6. Farnsworth NR, Kinghorn AD, Soejarto DD, and Waller DP: Siberian ginseng (*Eleutherococcus senticosus*): Current status as an adaptogen. In: *Economic and Medicinal Plant Research,* Vol. 1 (Wagner H, Hikino HZ, and Farnsworth NR, eds.). Academic Press, London, 1985, pp. 155–215.

7. Hikino H, Takahashi M, et al.: Isolation and hypoglycemic activity of eleutherans A, B, C, D, E, F and G: Glycans of *Eleutherococcus senticosus* roots. *J Nat Prod* 49:293–297, 1986.

8. Tintera JW: The hypoadrenocortical state and its management. *NY State J Med* 55:1869–1876, 1955.

9. Wagner H, Nörr H, and Winterhoff H: Plant adaptogens. *Phytomedicine* 1:63–76, 1994.

10. Farnsworth NR, Kinghorn AD, Soejarto DD, and Waller DP: Siberian ginseng (*Eleutherococcus senticosus*): Current status as an adaptogen. In: *Economic and Medicinal Plant Research,* Vol. 1 (Wagner H, Hikino HZ, and Farnsworth NR, eds.). Academic Press, London, 1985, pp. 155–215.

11. Fulder S: The drug that builds Russians. *New Sci* 21:576–579, 1980.

12. Asano K, Takahashi T, et al.: Effect of *Eleutherococcus senticosus* extract on human working capacity. *Planta Med* 37:175–177, 1986.

13. McNaughton L: A comparison of Chinese and Russian ginseng as ergogenic aids to improve various facets of physical fitness. *Int Clin Nutr Rev* 9: 32–35, 1989.

14. Dowling EA, Redondo DR, et al.: Effect of *Eleutherococcus senticosus* on submaximal and maximal exercise performance. *Med Sci Sports Exer* 28:482–489, 1996.

15. Gubchenko PP and Fruentov NK: Comparative study of the effectiveness of *Eleutherococcus* and other plant adaptogens as remedies for increasing the work capacity of flight personnel. In: *New Data on Eleutherococcus: Proceedings of the Second International Symposium on Eleutherococcus,* Moscow, 1984, pp. 240–251.

16. Collisson RJ: Siberian ginseng (*Eleutherococcus senticosus*). *Br J Phytother* 2:61–71, 1991.

17. Ben-Hur E and Fulder S: Effect of *P. ginseng* saponins and *Eleutherococcus* S. on survival of cultured mammalian cells after ionizing radiation. *Am J Chin Med* 9:48–56, 1981.

18. Bohn B, Nebe CT, and Birr C: Flow-cytometric studies with *Eleutherococcus senticosus* extract as an immunomodulating agent. *Arzneim-Forsch Drug Res* 37:1193–1196, 1987.

19. Brekhman II: Eleutherococcus: 20 Years of Research and Clinical Applications. Presentation at the 1st International Symposium on Eleutherococcus, Hamburg, Germany, May 29, 1980.

20. Zykov MP and Protasova SF: Prospects of immunostimulating vaccination against influenza including the use of *Eleutherococcus* and other preparations of plants. In: *New Data on Eleutherococcus: Proceedings of the Second International Symposium on Eleutherococcus,* Moscow, 1984, pp. 164–169.

21. Yarameko KV: The main aspects of the use of *Eleutherococcus* extract in oncology. In: *New Data on Eleutherococcus and Other Adaptogens.* The Far Eastern Scientific Center, USSR Academy of Sciences, Vladivostok, USSR, 1981, pp. 75–78.

22. Institute of Oncology, Ministry of Health, Georgia, USSR. Reported in: Brekhman II: *Eleutherococcus: Clinical Data.* USSR Foreign Trade Publication, Medexport, USSR, 1970.

23. Kupin VI, Polevaya EB, and Sorokin AM: Increased immunologic reactivity of lymphocytes in oncologic patients treated with *Eleutherococcus* extract. In: *New Data on Eleutherococcus: Proceedings of the Second International Symposium on Eleutherococcus,* Moscow, 1984, pp. 294–300.

24. Sutton F: Personal communication, 1994.

25. McRae S: Elevated serum digoxin levels in a patient taking digoxin and Siberian ginseng. *Canadian Med Assoc J* 155:293–295, 1996.

EVENING PRIMROSE

1. Kesteloot H, Lesaffre E, and Joossens JV: Dairy fat, saturated animal fat, and cancer risk. *Prevent Med* 20:226–236, 1991.

2. Erasmus E: *Fats and Oils.* Alive Books, Vancouver, British Columbia, Canada, 1986, pp. 34–44.

3. Horrobin DF and Manku MS: Clinical biochemistry of essential fatty acids. In: *Omega-6 Essential Fatty Acids: Pathophysiology and Roles in Clinical Medicine.* Alan R. Liss, New York, 1990, pp. 21–54.

4. Horrobin DF: Gamma linolenic acid: An intermediate in essential fatty acid metabolism with potential as an ethical pharmaceutical and as a food. *Rev Contemp Pharmacother* 1:1–45, 1990.

5. Tilvis RS and Miettinen TA: Fatty acid composition of serum lipids, erythrocytes and platelets in insulin-dependent women. *J Clin Endocrinol Metab* 61:741–745, 1985.

6. Gibson RA and Rassias G: Infant nutrition and human milk. In: *Omega-6 Essential Fatty Acids: Pathophysiology and Roles in Clinical Medicine.* Alan R. Liss, New York, 1990, pp. 283–293.

7. Oil of evening primrose. *Lawrence Review of Natural Products.* November, 1993.

8. Jenkins DK, Mitchell JC, et al.: Effects of different sources of gamma-linolenic acid on the formation of essential fatty acid and prostanoid metabolism. *Med Sci Res* 16:525–526, 1988.

9. Barre DE, Holub BJ, and Chapkin RS: The effect of borage oil supplementation on human platelet aggregation, thromboxane B2, prostaglandin E1, and E2 formation. *Nutr Res* 13:739–751, 1993.

10. Horrobin DF: Nutritional and medical importance of gamma-linolenic acid. *Prog Lipid Res* 31:163–194, 1992.

11. Manku MS, Horrobin DF, et al.: Essential fatty acids in the plasma phospholipids of patients with atopic eczema. *Br J Dermatol* 110:643–648, 1984.

12. Grulee CG and Sanford HH: The influence of breast and artificial feeding on infantile eczema. *J Pediatr* 9:223–225, 1936.

13. Businco L, Ioppi M, et al.: Breast milk from mothers of children with newly developed eczema has low levels of long chain polyunsaturated fatty acids. *J Allergy Clin Immunol* 91:1134–1139, 1993.

14. Cant A, Shay J, and Horrobin DF: The effect of maternal supplementation with linoleic and gamma-linolenic acids on the fat composition and content of human milk: A placebo-controlled trial. *J Nutr Sci Vitaminol* 37:573–579, 1991.

15. Morse PF, Horrobin DF, et al.: Meta-analysis of placebo-controlled studies of the efficacy of Epogam in the treatment of atopic eczema. Relationship between plasma essential fatty acid changes and clinical response. *Br J Dermatol* 121:75–90, 1989.

16. Bordoni A, Biagi PL, et al.: Evening primrose oil (Efamol) in the treatment of children with atopic eczema. *Drugs Exp Clin Res* 14:291–297, 1987.

17. Berth-Jones J and Graham-Brown RAC: Placebo-controlled trial of essential fatty acid supplementation in atopic dermatitis. *Lancet* 341:1557–1560, 1993.

18. Horrobin DF and Morse PF: Evening primrose oil and atopic eczema [Letter to the Editor]. *Lancet* 345:260–261, 1995.

19. Whitaker DK, Cilliers J, de Beer C: Evening primrose oil (Epogam®) in the treatment of chronic hand dermatitis: disappointing therapeutic results. *Dermatology* 193:115–120, 1996.

20. Janossy IM, Raguz JM, et al.: Effects of a cream containing 12.5% evening primrose oil on atopic disposition. *H & G Journal* 70:498–502, 1995.

21. Reichert RG: Evening primrose oil and diabetic neuropathy. *Quart Rev Nat Med* Summer:141–145, 1995.

22. Jamal GA and Charmichael H: The effect of gamma-linolenic acid on human diabetic peripheral neuropathy: A double-blind placebo-controlled trial. *Diabetic Med* 7:319–323, 1990.

23. Keen H, Payan J, et al.: Treatment of diabetic neuropathy with gamma-linolenic acid. *Diabetes Care* 16:8–15, 1993.

24. Brush MG, Watson SJ, et al.: Abnormal essential fatty acid levels in plasma of women with premenstrual syndrome. *Am J Obstet Gynecol* 150:363–366, 1984.

25. Horrobin DF, Manku MS, et al.: Abnormalities in plasma essential fatty acid levels in women with premenstrual syndrome and with nonmalignant breast disease. *J Nutr Med* 2:259–264, 1991.

26. McFayden IJ, Forest AP, et al.: Cyclical breast pain—some observations and the difficulties in treatment. *Brit J Clinical Practice* 46:161–164, 1992.

27. Gateley CA, Niers M, et al.: Drug treatments for mastalgia: 17-year experience in the Cardiff mastalgia clinic. *J R Soc Med* 85:12–15, 1992.

28. Pye JK, Mansel RE, and Hughes LE: Clinical experience of drug treatment for mastalgia. *Lancet* ii:373–377, 1985.

29. Cyclical breast pain—what works and what doesn't. *Drug Therapeut Bull* 30:1–3, 1992.

30. Collins A, Cerin A, et al.: Essential fatty acids in the treatment of premenstrual syndrome. *Obstet Gynecol* 81:93–98, 1993.

31. O'Brien PM and Massil H: Premenstrual syndrome: Clinical studies on essential fatty acids. In: *Omega-6 Essential Fatty Acids: Pathophysiology and Roles in Clinical Medicine.* Alan R. Liss, New York, 1990, pp. 523–545.

32. Brenner RR: Nutritional and hormonal factors influencing desaturation of essential fatty acids. *Prog Lipid Res* 20:41–48, 1982.

References

388

FEVERFEW

1. Feverfew. *Lawrence Review of Natural Products*. September, 1994.
2. Hobbs C: Feverfew (*Tanacetum parthenium*). *HerbalGram* 20:26–35, 1989.
3. Awang DVC: Herbal medicine, feverfew. *Canadian Pharm J* 122:266–270, 1989.
4. Hepinstall S, Awang DVC, et al.: Parthenolide content and bioactivity of feverfew (*Tanacetum parthenium*). Estimation of commercial and authenticated feverfew products. *J Pharm Pharmacol* 44:391–395, 1992.
5. Awang DVC: Parthenolide: The demise of a facile theory of feverfew activity. *J Herbs Spices Medicinal Plants* 5:95–98, 1998.
6. Hannington E: Migraine: The platelet hypothesis after 10 years. *Biomed Pharmacother* 43:719–726, 1989.
7. Hepinstall S, White A, et al.: Extracts of feverfew inhibit granule secretion in blood platelets and polymorphonuclear leukocytes. *Lancet* i:1071–1074, 1985.
8. Makheja AN and Bailery JM: A platelet phospholipase inhibitor from the medicinal herb feverfew (*Tanacetum parthenium*). *Prostaglandins, Leukotrienes Med* 8:653–660, 1982.
9. Pugh WJ and Sambo K: Prostaglandin synthetase inhibitors in feverfew. *J Pharm Pharmacol* 40:743–745, 1988.
10. Sumner H, Salan U, et al.: Inhibition of 5-lipoxygenase and cyclo-oxygenase in leukocytes by feverfew. *Biochem Pharmacol* 43:2313–2320, 1992.
11. Pattrick M, Hepinstall S, and Doherty M: Feverfew in rheumatoid arthritis: A double blind, placebo controlled study. *Ann Rheum Dis* 48:547–549, 1989.
12. Johnson ES, Kadam NP, et al.: Efficacy of feverfew as prophylactic treatment of migraine. *Br Med J* 291:569–573, 1985.
13. Murphy JJ, Hepinstall S, and Mitchell JR: Randomized double-blind placebo-controlled trial of feverfew in migraine prevention. *Lancet* ii:189–192, 1988.
14. Palevitch D, Earon G, Carasso R: Feverfew (*Tanacetum parthenium*) as a prophylactic treatment for migraine: A double-blind, placebo-controlled study. *Phytotherapy Res* 11:508–511, 1997.
15. De Weerdt CJ, Bootsma HPR, Hendriks H: Herbal medicines in migraine prevention. *Phytomedicine* 3:225–230, 1996.

GARLIC

1. Foster S and Chongxi Y: *Herbal Emissaries: Bringing Chinese Herbs to the West.* Healing Arts Press, Rochester, Vermont, 1992, pp. 86–92.
2. Fulder S and Blackwood J: *Garlic: Nature's Original Remedy.* Healing Arts Press, Rochester, Vermont, 1991, pp. 15–25.
3. Leung AY, Foster S: *Encyclopedia of Common Natural Ingredients Used in Food, Drugs and Cosmetics.* John Wiley & Sons, New York, 1996, pp. 260–264.
4. Lawson LD, Wang ZJ, and Hughes BG: Identification and HPLC quantitation of the sulfides and dialk(en)yl thiosulfinates in commercial garlic products. *Planta Med* 57:363–370, 1991.
5. Hughes BG and Lawson LD: Antimicrobial effects of *Allium sativum* L. (garlic), *Allium ampeloprasum* L. (elephant garlic), and *Allium cepa* L. (onion), garlic compounds and commercial garlic supplement products. *Phytother Res* 5:154–158, 1991.
6. Lawson LD and Hughes BG: Characterization of the formation of allicin and other thiosulfinates from garlic. *Planta Med* 58:345–350, 1992.
7. Robbers JE, Tyler VE: *Tyler's Herbs of Choice: The Therapeutic Use of Phytomedicinals.* Haworth Herbal Press, Binghamton, New York, 1999, pp. 132–137.

8. Kieswetter H, Jung F, et al.: Effect of garlic on thrombocyte aggregation, microcirculation, and other risk factors. *Int J Clin Pharmacol Ther Toxicol* 29:151–155, 1991.

9. Breithaupt-Grögler K, Ling M, et al.: Protective effect of chronic garlic intake on elastic properties of the aorta in the elderly. *Circulation* 96:2649–2655, 1997.

10. Josling P, Walerpa A, and Grunwald J, eds.: The action of garlic in the pathogenesis of atherosclerosis: Selected abstracts from the 4th and International Congress on Phytotherapy. *Eur J Clin Res* 3A:1–12, 1992.

11. Kleijnen J, Knipschild P, and Ter Riet G: Garlic, onion and cardiovascular risk factors. A review of the evidence from human experiments with emphasis on commercially available preparations. *Br J Clin Pharmacol* 28:535–544, 1989.

12. Gebhardt R: Multiple inhibitory effects of garlic extracts on cholesterol biosynthesis in hepatocytes. *Lipids* 28:613–619, 1993.

13. Gebhardt R, Beck H, and Wagner KG: Inhibition of cholesterol biosynthesis by allicin and ajoene in rat hepatocytes and HepG2 cells. *Biochim Biophys Acta* 1213:57–62, 1994.

14. Orekhov AN, Pivovarova EM, Tertov VV: Garlic powder tablets reduce atherogenicity of low density lipoprotein. A placebo-controlled double-blind study. *Nutr Metab Cardiovascular Dis* 6:21–31, 1996.

15. Munday JS, James KA, et al.: Daily supplementation with aged garlic extract, but not raw garlic, protects low-density lipoprotein against in vitro oxidation. *Atherosclerosis* 143:399–404, 1999.

16. Reuter HD: Garlic (*Allium sativum* L.) in the prevention and treatment of atherosclerosis. *Br J Phytother* 3:3–9, 1993/1994.

17. Legnani C, Frascaro M, et al.: Effects of a dried garlic preparation on fibrinolysis and platelet aggregation in healthy subjects. *Arzneim-Forsch Drug Res* 43:119–122, 1993.

18. Apitz-Castro R, Badimon JJ, and Badimon L: Effect of ajoene, the major antiplatelet compound from garlic, on platelet thrombus formation. *Thromb Res* 68:145–155, 1992.

19. Pareddy SR and Rosenberg JM: Does garlic have useful medicinal purposes? *Hosp Pharm Rep* 8:27, 1993.

20. Weber ND, Anderson DO, et al.: *In vitro* virucidal effects of *Allium sativum* (garlic) extract and compounds. *Planta Med* 58:417–423, 1992.

21. Nai-lan G, Dao-pei L, et al.: Demonstrations of the anti-viral activity of garlic extract against human cytomegalovirus in vitro. *Chin Med J* 106:93–96, 1993.

22. Shoji S, Furuishi K, et al.: Allyl compounds selectively killed human immunodeficiency virus (type-1) infected cells. *Biochem Biophys Res Commun* 194:610–621, 1993.

23. Ghannoum MA: Studies on the anticandidal mode of action of *Allium sativum* (garlic). *J Gen Microbiol* 134:2917–2924, 1988.

24. Hughes BG and Lawson LD: Antimicrobial effects of *Allium sativum* L. (garlic), *Allium ampeloprasum* L. (elephant garlic), and *Allium cepa* L. (onion), garlic compounds and commercial garlic supplement products. *Phytother Res* 5:154–158, 1991.

25. Lin XY, Liu JZ, and Milner JA: Dietary garlic suppresses DNA adducts caused by N-nitroso compounds. *Carcinogenesis* 15: 349–352, 1994.

26. Ip C, Lisk DJ, and Stoewsand GS: Mammary cancer prevention by regular garlic and selenium-enriched garlic. *Nutr Cancer* 17:279–286, 1992.

27. Dwivedi C, Rohlfs S, et al.: Chemoprevention of chemically induced skin tumor development by diallyl sulfide and diallyl disulfide. *Pharmaceutical Res* 9:1668–1670, 1992.

28. Koscielny J, Klüssebdorf D, et al.: The antiatherosclerotic effect of *Allium sativum*. *Atherosclerosis* 144:237–249, 1999.

References

29. Mader FH: Treatment of hyperlipidemia with garlic-powder tablets. *Arzneim-Forsch Drug Res* 40:1111–1116, 1990.
30. Vorberg G and Schneider B: Therapy with garlic: Results of a placebo-controlled, double-blind study. *Br J Clin Pract* 44(Suppl. 69):7–11, 1990.
31. Jain AK, Vargas R, et al.: Can garlic reduce serum lipids? A controlled clinical study. *Am J Med* 94:632–635, 1993.
32. Holzgartner H, Schmidt U, and Kuhn U: Comparison of the efficacy and tolerance of a garlic preparation vs. bezafibrate. *Arzneim-Forsch Drug Res* 42:1473–1477, 1992.
33. Silagy C and Neil A: Garlic as a lipid lowering agent—a meta-analysis. *J R Coll Physicians London* 28:39–45, 1994.
34. Warshafsky S, Kramer RS, and Sivak SL: Effect of garlic on total serum cholesterol. *Ann Int Med* 119:599–605, 1993.
35. Isaachson JL, Moser M, et al.: Garlic powder and plasma lipids and lipoproteins. *Arch Internal Med* 158:1189–1194.
36 Neil HAW, Silagy SA, et al.: Garlic powder in the treatment of moderate hyperlipidemia: a controlled trial and meta-analysis. *J Royal College Physicians London* 30:329–334, 1996.
37. Simons LA, Blasubramaniam S, et al.: On the effect of garlic on plasma lipids and lipoproteins in mild hypercholesterolemia. *Atherosclerosis* 113:219–225, 1995.
38. McCrindle BW, Helden E, Conner WT: Garlic extract therapy in children with hypercholesterolemia. *Arch Pediatr Adolesc Med* 152:1089–1094, 1998.
39. Berthold HK, Sudhop T, von Bergmann K: Effect of a garlic preparation on serum lipoproteins and cholesterol metabolism. *JAMA* 279:1900–1902, 1998.
40. Lawson L: Garlic powder for hyperlipidemia—Analysis of recent negative results. *Quart Rev Natural Med* Fall:187–188, 1998.
41. Silagy C and Neil AW: A meta-analysis of the effect of garlic on blood pressure. *J Hypertens* 12:463–468, 1994.
42. Kieswatter H, Jung F, et al.: Effects of garlic coated tablets in peripheral arterial occlusive disease. *Clin Invest* 71:383–386, 1993.
43. Despande RG, Khan MB, et al.: Inhibition of *Mycobacterium avium* complex isolates from AIDS patients by garlic (*Allium sativum*). *J Antimicrob Chemother* 32:623–626, 1993.
44. Davis LE, Shen J, and Royer RE: *In vitro* synergism of concentrated *Allium sativum* extract and amphotericin B against *Cryptococcus neoformans*. *Planta Med* 60:546–549, 1994.
45. Steinmetz KA, Kushi LH, et al.: Vegetables, fruit, and colon cancer in the Iowa women's health study. *Am J Epidemiol* 139:1–5, 1994.
46. Dorant E, vander Brandt PA, et al.: Garlic and its significance for the prevention of cancer in humans: A critical view. *Br J Cancer* 67:424–429, 1993.
47. Mennella JA and Beauchamp GK: The effects of repeated exposure to garlic-flavored milk on the nursling's behavior. *Pediatr Res* 34:805–808, 1993.

GINGER

1. Awang DVC: Ginger. *Can Pharm J* 125:309–311, 1992.
2. Foster S and Chongxi Y: *Herbal Emissaries: Bringing Chinese Herbs to the West.* Healing Arts Press, Rochester, Vermont, 1992, pp. 92–102.
3. Foster S and Chongxi Y: *Herbal Emissaries: Bringing Chinese Herbs to the West.* Healing Arts Press, Rochester, Vermont, 1992, pp. 92–102.
4. Hikino H: Research on oriental medicinal plants. In: *Economic and Medicinal Plant Research,* Vol. 1 (Wagner H, Hikino H, and Farnsworth N, eds.). Academic Press, New York, 1985.

5. Robbers JE, Tyler VE: *Tyler's Herbs of Choice: The Therapeutic Use of Phytomedicinals*. Haworth Herbal Press, Binghamton, New York, 1999, pp. 47–51.

6. Bradley PR, ed.: *British Herbal Compendium*, Vol. 1. British Herbal Medicine Association, Bournemouth, Dorset, England, 1992, pp. 112–114.

7. Yamahara J, Huang Q, et al.: Gastrointestinal motility enhancing effect of ginger and its active constituents. *Chem Pharm Bull* 38:430–431, 1990.

8. Yamahara J, Miki K, et al.: Cholagogic effect of ginger and its active constituents. *J Ethnopharmacol* 13:217–225, 1985.

9. Al-Yahya MA, Rafatullah S, et al.: Gastroprotective activity of ginger in albino rats. *Am J Chin Med* 17:51–56, 1989.

10. Goso Y, Ogata Y, et al: Effects of traditional herbal medicine on gastric mucin against ethanol-induced gastric injury in rats. *Comp Biochem Physiol* 113C:17–21, 1996.

11. Kawai T, Kinoshita K, et al.: Anti-emetic principles of *Magnolia obovata* bark and *Zingiber officinale* rhizome. *Planta Med* 60:17–20, 1994.

12. Suekawa M, Ishige A, et al.: Pharmacological studies on ginger. I. Pharmacological actions of pungent constituents, (6)-gingerol and (6)-shogaol. *J Pharmacobio Dyn* 7:836–848, 1984.

13. Sharma SS, Kochupillai V, et al: Antiemetic efficacy of ginger (*Zingiber officinale*) against cisplatin-induced emesis in dogs. *J Ethnopharmacol* 57:93–96, 1997.

14. Holtmann S, Clarke AH, et al.: The anti-motion sickness mechanism of ginger. *Acta Oto-Laryngol* 108:168–174, 1989.

15. Backon J: Ginger: Inhibition of thromboxane synthetase and stimulation of prostacyclin. Relevance for medicine and psychiatry. *Med Hypotheses* 20:271–278, 1986.

16. Verma SK, Singh J, et al.: Effect of ginger on platelet aggregation in man. *Indian J Med Res* 98:240–242, 1994.

17. Kuchi F, Iwakami S, et al.: Inhibition of prostaglandin and leukotriene biosynthesis by gingerols and diarylheptanoids. *Chem Pharm Bull* 40:387–391, 1992.

18. Onogi T, Minami M, et al.: Capsaicin-like effect of (6)-shogaol on substance P-containing primary afferents of rats: A possible mechanism of its analgesic action. *Neuropharmacology* 31:1165–1169, 1992.

19. Mowrey DB and Clayson DE: Motion sickness, ginger, and psychophysics. *Lancet* i:655–657, 1982.

20. Grontved A, Brask T, et al.: Ginger root against seasickness. *Acta Oto-Laryngol* 105:45–49, 1988.

21. Riebenfeld D, Borzone L: Randomized double-blind study comparing ginger (Zintona®) and dimenhydrinate in motion sickness. *Healthnotes Rev Comp Integrative Med* 6:98–101, 1999.

22. Carredu P: Motion sickness in children: Results of a double-blind study with ginger (Zintona®) and dimenhydrinate. *Healthnotes Rev Comp Integrative Med* 6:102–107, 1999.

23. Schmid R, Schick T, et al: Comparison of seven commonly used agents for prophylaxis of seasickness. *J Travel Med* 1:203–206, 1994.

24. Stewart JJ, Wood MJ, et al.: Effects of ginger on motion sickness susceptibility and gastric function. *Pharmacology* 42:111–120, 1991.

25. Blumenthal M, Busse WR, et al., eds.: *The Complete Commission E Monographs*. Integrative Medicine Communications, Boston, Massachusetts, 1998, pp. 135–136.

26. Fulder S, Tenne M: Ginger as an anti-nausea remedy in pregnancy and the issue of safety. *HerbalGram* 38:47–50, 1996.

27. Fischer-Rasmussen W, Kjaer SK, et al.: Ginger treatment of hyperemesis gravidarum. *Eur J Obstet Gynecol Reprod Biol* 38:19–24, 1990.

References

28. Phillips S, Ruggier R, and Hutchison SE: *Zingiber officinale* (ginger)—an antiemetic for day case surgery. *Anaesthesia* 48:715–717, 1993.

29. Bone ME and Wilkinson DJ: Ginger root—a new antiemetic. *Anaesthesia* 45:669–671, 1990.

30. Arfeen Z, Owen H, et al: A double-blind, randomized controlled trial of ginger for the prevention of postoperative nausea and vomiting. *Anaesthesia Intensive Care* 23:449–452, 1995.

31. Srivastava KC and Mustafa T: Ginger (*Zingiber officinale*) in rheumatism and musculoskeletal disorders. *Med Hypotheses* 39:342–348, 1992.

32. Mustafa T and Srivastava KC: Ginger (*Zingiber officinale*) in migraine headache. *J Ethnopharmacol* 29:267–273, 1990.

33. Pace JC: Oral ingestion of encapsulated ginger and reported self-care actions for the relief of chemotherapy-associated nausea and vomiting. *Dissertation Abstr International* 8:3297, 1987.

34. Meyer K, Schwartz J, et al: *Zingiber officinale* (ginger) used to prevent 8-MOP associated nausea. *Dermatol Nursing* 7:242–244, 1995.

35. Blumenthal M, Busse WR, et al., eds.: *The Complete Commission E Monographs.* Integrative Medicine Communications, Boston, Massachusetts, 1998, pp. 135–136.

36. Lininger SW, Gaby A, et al: *The A–Z Guide to Drug–Herb–Vitamin Interactions.* Prima Publishing, Rocklin, CA, 1999, pp. 248–249.

GINKGO BILOBA

1. Blumenthal M, ed.: *Herbal Medicine: Expanded Commission E Monographs.* Integrative Medicine Communications, Newton, Massachusetts, 2000, pp. 160–169.

2. Blumenthal M: Herb market levels after five years of boom. *HerbalGram* 47:64–65, 1999.

3. Foster S, Tyler VE: *Tyler's Honest Herbal.* Haworth Herbal Press, Binghamton, New York, 1999.

4. Schulz V, Hänsel R, Tyler VE: *Rational Phytotherapy: A Physicians' Guide to Herbal Medicine.* Springer-Verlag, Berlin, 1998, pp. 38–50.

5. Busse W: History and chemistry of *Ginkgo biloba. Rev Bras Neurol* 30(Suppl. 1):3S–6S, 1994.

6. DeFeudis FV: *Ginkgo biloba Extract (ECb 761): From Chemistry to the Clinic.* Ullstein Medical, Wiesbaden, Germany, 1998, pp. 1–3.

7. Drieu K: Preparation and definition of *Ginkgo biloba* extract. In: *Rokan* (Ginkgo biloba): *Recent Results in Pharmacology and Clinic* (Fünfgeld EW, ed.). Springer-Verlag, Berlin, 1988, pp. 32–36.

8. *Ginkgolides: Chemistry, Biology, Pharmacology and Clinical Perspectives,* Vol. 1 (Braquet P, ed.). JR Prous Science Publishers, Barcelona, 1989.

9. *Ginkgolides: Chemistry, Biology, Pharmacology and Clinical Perspectives,* Vol. 2 (Braquet P, ed.). JR Prous Science Publishers, Barcelona, 1989.

10. Krieglstein J: Neuroprotective properties of *Ginkgo biloba*—constituents. *Z Phytother* 15:92–96, 1994.

11. Bruno C, Cuppini R, et al.: Regeneration of motor nerves in bilobalide-treated rats. *Planta Med* 59:302–307, 1993.

12. Clostre F: From the body to the cellular membranes: The different levels of pharmacological action of *Ginkgo biloba* extract. In: *Rokan* (Ginkgo biloba): *Recent Results in Pharmacology and Clinic* (Fünfgeld EW, ed.). Springer-Verlag, Berlin, 1988, pp. 180–198.

13. Jung F, Mrowietz C, et al.: Effect of *Ginkgo biloba* on fluidity of blood and peripheral microcirculation in volunteers. *Arzneim-Forsch Drug Res* 40:589–593, 1990.

14. Heiss WD and Zeiler K: The influence of drugs on cerebral blood flow. *Pharmakotherapie* 1:137–144, 1978.

15. Kleijnen J and Knipschild P: *Ginkgo biloba* for cerebral insufficiency. *Br J Clin Pharmacol* 34:352–358, 1992.

16. Harman D: Free radicals in aging. *Mol Cell Biochem* 84:155–161, 1988.

17. Droy-Lefaix MT: Effect of the antioxidant action of *Ginkgo biloba* extract (EGb 761) on aging and oxidative stress. *Age* 20:141–149, 1997.

18. Ferrandini C, Droy-Lefaix MT, and Christen Y, eds.: Ginkgo biloba *Extract (EGb 761) as a Free Radical Scavenger.* Elsevier, Paris, 1993.

19. Harman D: Free radical theory of aging: A hypothesis on pathogenesis of senile dementia of the Alzheimer's type. *Age* 16:23–30, 1993.

20. Lamant V, Mauco G, et al.: Inhibition of the metabolism of platelet activating factor (PAF-acether) by three specific antagonists from *Ginkgo biloba. Biochem Pharmacol* 36:2749–2752, 1987.

21. Kroegel C: The potential pathophysiological role of platelet-activating factor in human disease. *Klin Wochenschr* 66:373–378, 1988.

22. Kroegel C, Kortsik C, et al.: The pathophysiological role and therapeutic implications of platelet activating factor in diseases of aging. *Drugs Aging* 2:345–355, 1992.

23. Krieglstein J: Neuroprotective properties of *Ginkgo biloba*—constituents. *Z Phytother* 15:92–96, 1994.

24. Stein DG and Hoffman SW: Chronic administration of *Ginkgo biloba* extract (EGb 761) can enhance recovery from traumatic brain injury. In: *Effects of* Ginkgo biloba *Extract (EGb 761) on the Central Nervous System* (Christen Y, Costentin J, and Lacour M, eds.). Elsevier, Paris, 1992, pp. 95–104.

25. Rigney U, Kimber S, and Hindmarch I: The effect of acute doses of standardized *Ginkgo biloba* extract on memory and psychomotor performance. *Phytotherapy Res* 13:408–415, 1999.

26. Itil TM, Eralp E, et al.: Central nervous system effects of *Ginkgo biloba,* a plant extract. *Am J Therapeutics* 3:63–73, 1996.

27. Luthringer R, D'Arbringy P, and Macher JP: *Ginkgo biloba* extract (EGb 761) and event-related potentials mapping profile. In: *Effects of* Ginkgo biloba *Extract (EGb 761) on Aging and Age-Related Disorders* (Christen Y, Courtis Y, Droy-Lefaix MT, eds.). Elsevier, Paris, 1995, pp. 107–118.

28. Le Bars P: Personal communication, 1999.

29. Itil TM, Ahmed I, et al.: The pharmacological effects of *Ginkgo biloba,* a plant extract, on the brain in comparison to tacrine. Abstract of a presentation at the Annual NCDEU Meeting of the National Institutes of Mental Health, May 28–31, 1996.

30. Kleijnen J and Knipschild P: *Ginkgo biloba* for cerebral insufficiency. *British J Clin Pharmacol* 34:352–358, 1992.

31. Hopfenmüller W: Proof of the therapeutic effectiveness of a *Ginkgo biloba* special extract: Meta-analysis of 11 clinical trials in aged patients with cerebral insufficiency [in German]. *Arzneim-Forsch Drug Res* 44:1005–1013, 1994.

32. Wesnes K, Simmons D, and Rook M: A double-blind placebo-controlled trial of Tanakan in the treatment of idiopathic impairment in the elderly. *Human Psychopharmacol* 2:159–169, 1987.

33. Israel L, Dell'Accio E, et al.: *Ginkgo biloba* extract and memory training programs—comparative assessment on elderly outpatients. *Psychologie Médicale* 19:1431–1439, 1987.

34. Gräbel E: The influence of *Ginkgo biloba* extract (EGb 761) on mental performance: A double-blind study under computerized measurement conditions in patients with cerebral insufficiency. *Fortschr Med* 110:73–76, 1992.

References

35. Vesper J and Hänsgen KD: Efficacy of *Ginkgo biloba* in 90 outpatients with cerebral insufficiency caused by old age. *Phytomedicine* 1:9–16, 1994.

36. Winther K, Randløv, et al.: Effect of *Ginkgo biloba* extract on cognitive function and blood pressure in elderly subjects. *Current Ther Res* 59:881–888, 1998.

37. Oken BS, Storzbach DM, and Kaye JA: The efficacy of *Ginkgo biloba* on cognitive function in Alzheimer's disease. *Arch Neurol* 55:1409–1415, 1998.

38. Le Bars PL, Katz MM, et al.: A placebo-controlled, double-blind, randomized trial of an extract of *Ginkgo biloba* for dementia. *JAMA* 278:1327–1332, 1997.

39. Winkler MA: Aging: A global issue [Editorial]. *JAMA* 278:1378, 1997.

40. Kanowski S, Herrmann WM, et al.: Proof of efficacy of the *Ginkgo biloba* special extract EGb 761 in outpatients suffering from mild to moderate primary degenerative dementia of the Alzheimer type or multi-infarct dementia. *Pharmacopsychiatry* 29:47–56, 1996.

41. Maurer K, Ihl R, et al.: Clinical efficacy of *Ginkgo biloba* special extract EGb 761 in dementia of the Alzheimer's type. *J Psychiatr Res* 31:645–655, 1997.

42. Hofferberth B: The efficacy of EGb 761 in patients with senile dementia of the Alzheimer type—a double-blind, placebo-controlled study on different levels of investigation. *Human Psychopharmacopsychiatry* 9:215–222, 1994.

43. Lesser IM, Mena I, et al.: Reduction in cerebral blood flow in older depressed patients. *Arch Gen Psychiatr* 51:677–686, 1994.

44. Schubert H and Halama P: Depressive episode primarily unresponsive to therapy in elderly patients: Efficacy of *Ginkgo biloba* extract (EGb 761) in combination with antidepressants. *Geriatr Forsch* 3:45–53, 1993.

45. Cohen AJ and Bartlik B: *Ginkgo biloba* for antidepressant-induced sexual dysfunction. *J Sex Marital Therapy* 24:139–145, 1998.

46. Ellison JM and DeLuca P: Fluoxetine-induced genital anesthesia relieved by *Ginkgo biloba* extract [Letter]. *J Clin Psychiatry* 59:199–200, 1998.

47. Schneider B: *Ginkgo biloba* extract in peripheral arterial disease: Meta-analysis of controlled clinical trials. *Arzneim-Forsch Drug Res* 42:428–436, 1992.

48. Blume J, Kieser M, and Hölscher U: Placebo-controlled, double-blind study on the efficacy of *Ginkgo biloba* special extract EGb 761 in maximum-level trained patients with intermittent claudication. *VASA* 25:265–274, 1996.

49. Peters H, Kieser M, Hölscher U: Demonstration of the efficacy of *Ginkgo biloba* special extract EGb 761® on intermittent claudication—a placebo-controlled, double-blind multicenter trial. *VASA* 27:106–110, 1998.

50. Schweizer J, Hautmann C: Comparison of two dosages of *Ginkgo biloba* extract EGb 761 in patients with peripheral arterial occlusive disease Fontaine's stage IIb. *Arzneim-Forsch Drug Res* 49:900–904, 1999.

51. Meyer B: A multicenter, randomized study of *Ginkgo biloba* extract versus placebo in the treatment of tinnitus. In: *Rokan* (Ginkgo biloba): *Recent Results in Pharmacology and Clinic* (Fünfgeld EW, ed.). Springer-Verlag, Berlin, 1988, pp. 245–250.

52. Morgenstern C and Biermann E: *Ginkgo biloba* special extract EGb 761 in the treatment of tinnitus aurium: Results of a randomized, double-blind, placebo-controlled study. *Fortschr Med* 115:7–11, 1997.

53. Holgers K, Axelsson A, and Pringle I: *Ginkgo biloba* extract for the treatment of tinnitus. *Audiology* 33:85–92, 1994.

54. Sohn M and Sikora R: *Ginkgo biloba* extract in the therapy of erectile dysfunction. *J Sex Educ Ther* 17:53–61, 1991.

References

55. Roncin JP, Schwartz F, D'Arbringy P: EGb 761 in control of acute mountain sickness and vascular reactivity to cold exposure. *Aviat Space Environ Med* 67:445–452, 1996.

56. DeFeudis FV: Ginkgo biloba *Extract (EGb 761): From Chemistry to the Clinic*. Ullstein Medical, Wiesbaden, Germany, 1998, pp. 198–201.

57. Blumenthal M, Busse WR, et al., eds.: *The Complete Commission E Monographs*. Integrative Medicine Communications, Boston, Massachusetts, 1998, pp. 136–138.

58. Matthews MK: Association of *Ginkgo biloba* with intracerebral hemorrhage [Letter]. *Neurology* 50:1933–1934, 1998.

59. Rosenblatt M and Mindell J: Spontaneous hyphema associated with ingestion of *Ginkgo biloba* extract [Letter]. *New Engl J Med* 336:1108, 1997.

60. Rowin J and Lewis SL: Spontaneous bilateral subdural hematomas associated with chronic *Ginkgo biloba* ingestion [Letter]. *Neurology* 46:1775–1776,

61. Gilbert GJ: *Ginkgo biloba* [Letter]. *Neurology* 48:1137, 1997.

ASIAN GINSENG

1. Foster S: Three ginsengs: Asian, American, and Siberian. *Herb Companion* June/July:75–77, 1995.

2. Duke JA: *Ginseng: A Concise Handbook*. Reference Publications, Algonac, Michigan, 1989.

3. Foster S and Chongxi Y: *Herbal Emissaries: Bringing Chinese Herbs to the West*. Healing Arts Press, Rochester, Vermont, 1992, pp. 102–112.

4. Hu SY: Knowledge of ginseng from Chinese records. *J Chin Univ Hong Kong* 4:283–305, 1977.

5. Hu SY: The genus *Panax* (ginseng) in Chinese medicine. *Econ Bot* 30:11–28, 1976.

6. Foster S and Chongxi Y: *Herbal Emissaries: Bringing Chinese Herbs to the West*. Healing Arts Press, Rochester, Vermont, 1992.

7. Hikino H: Traditional remedies and modern assessment: The case of ginseng. In: *The Medicinal Plant Industry* (Wijeskera R, ed.). CRC Press, Boca Raton, Florida, 1991, pp. 149–166.

8 Shibata S, Tanaka O, et al.: Chemistry and pharmacology of *Panax*. In: *Economic and Medicinal Plant Research*, Vol. 1 (Wagner H, Hikino H, and Farnsworth NR, eds.). Academic Press, London, 1985, pp. 217–284.

9. Mowrey DB: Understanding standardized ginseng extracts. *Townsend Lett Doctors* October: 505–509, 1989.

10. Tomoda M, Hirabayashi K, et al.: Characterization of two novel polysaccharides having immunological activities from the root of *Panax ginseng*. *Biol Pharm Bull* 16:1087–1090, 1993.

11. Brekhman II and Dardymov IV: New substances of plant origin which increase non-specific resistance. *Ann Rev Pharmacol* 4:419–430, 1969.

12. Wagner H, Nörr H, and Winterhoff H: Plant adaptogens. *Phytomedicine* 1:63–76, 1994.

13. Hiai S, Yokoyama H, et al.: Stimulation of pituitary–adrenocortical system by ginseng saponin. *Endocrinol Jpn* 26:661–665, 1979.

14. Fulder SJ: Ginseng and the hypothalamic–pituitary control of stress. *Am J Chin Med* 9:112–118, 1981.

15. Le Gal M, Cathebras P, and Strüby K: Pharmaton capsules in the treatment of functional fatigue: A double-blind study versus placebo evaluated by a new methodology. *Phytotherapy Res* 10:49–53.

16. Petkov VD and Mosharrof AH: Age- and individual-related specificities in the effects of standardized ginseng extract on learning and memory (experiments in rats). *Phytother Res* 1:80–84, 1987.

17. D'Angelo L, Grimaldi R, et al.: A double-blind, placebo-controlled clinical study of a standardized ginseng extract on psychomotor performance in healthy volunteers. *J Ethnopharmacol* 16:15–22, 1986.

18. Medvedev MA: The effect of ginseng on the working performance of radio operators. In: *Papers on the Study of Ginseng and Other Medicinal Plants of the Far East*, Vol. 5. Primorskoe Knizhone Izdatelsvo, Vladivostok, USSR, 1963.

19. Owen RT: Ginseng—a pharmacological profile. *Drugs Today* 17:343–351, 1981.

20. Wesnes KA, Faleni RA, et al.: The cognitive, subjective, and physical effects of a *Ginkgo biloba/Panax ginseng* combination in healthy volunteers with neurasthenic complaints. *Psychopharmacol Bulletin* 33:677–683, 1997.

21. Forgo I: The duration of effect of the standardized ginseng extract G115 in healthy competitive athletes. *Notabene Medici* 15:636–640, 1985.

22. McNaughton L: A comparison of Chinese and Russian ginseng as ergogenic aids to improve various facets of physical fitness. *Int Clin Nutr Rev* 9:32–35, 1989.

23. Pieralisi G, Rapari P, and Vecchiet L: Effects of a standardized ginseng extract combined with dimethylaminoethanol bitartrate, vitamins, minerals, and trace elements on physical performance during exercise. *Clin Ther* 13:372–382, 1991.

24. Avakia EV and Evonuk E: Effects of *Panax ginseng* extract on tissue glycogen and adrenal cholesterol depletion during prolonged exercise. *Planta Med* 36:43–48, 1979.

25. Allen JD, McLung J, et al.: Ginseng supplementation does not enhance healthy young adults' peak aerobic exercise performance. *J Am Coll Nutr* 17:462–466, 1998.

26. Slavati G, Genovesi G, et al.: Effects of *Panax ginseng* C.A. Meyer saponins on male infertility. *Panmineva Med* 38:249–254, 1996.

27. Zhang T, Hoshino M, et al.: Ginseng root: Evidence for numerous regulatory peptides and insulinotropic activity. *Biomed Res* 11:49–54, 1990.

28. Suzuki Y and Hikino H: Mechanisms of hypoglycemic activity of panaxans A and B, glycans of *Panax ginseng* roots: Effects on plasma levels, secretion, sensitivity and binding of insulin in mice. *Phytother Res* 3:20–24, 1989.

29. Waki I, Kyo H, et al.: Effects of a hypoglycemic component of ginseng radix on insulin biosynthesis in normal and diabetic animals. *J Pharmacobio Dyn* 5:547–554, 1982.

30. Sotaniemi EA, Haapakoski E, and Rautino A: Ginseng therapy in non-insulin-dependent diabetic patients. *Diabetes Care* 18:1373–1375, 1995.

31. Ben-Hur E and Fulder S: Effect of *Panax ginseng* saponins and *Eleutherococcus senticosus* on survival of cultured mammalian cells after ionizing radiation. *Am J Chin Med* 9:48–56, 1981.

32. Kim HS, Jang CG, and Lee MK: Antinarcotic effects of the standardized ginseng extract G115 on morphine. *Planta Med* 56:158–163, 1990.

33. Voskresensky ON, Devayathina TA, et al.: Effect of *Eleutherococcus* and ginseng on the development of free radical pathology. In: *New Data on Eleutherococcus, Proceedings of the 2nd International Symposium on Eleutherococcus*. Moscow, 1984, pp. 141–145.

34. Kim H, Chen X, and Gillis CN: Ginsenosides protect pulmonary vascular endothelium against free radical-induced injury. *Biochem Biophys Res Commun* 189:670–676, 1992.

35. Yamamoto M, Uemura T, et al.: Serum HDL-cholesterol-increasing and fatty liver-improving actions of *Panax ginseng* in high cholesterol diet-fed rats with clinical effect on hyperlipidemia in man. *Am J Chin Med* 11:1–4, 1983.

36. Yun TK and Choi SY: A case-control study of ginseng intake and cancer. *Int J Epidemiol* 19:871–876, 1990.

References

37. Yun TK and Choi SY: Non-organ specific cancer prevention of ginseng: A prospective study in Korea. *Int J Epidemiol* 27:359–364, 1998.

38. Tode T, Kikuchi Y, et al.: Inhibitory effects by oral administration of ginsenoside Rh2 on the growth of human ovarian cancer cells in nude mice. *J Cancer Res Clin Oncol* 120:24–26, 1993.

39. Hau DM and You ZS: Therapeutic effects of ginseng and mitomycin C on experimental liver tumors. *Int J Oriental Med* 15:10–14, 1990.

40. Yun YS, Lee YS, et al.: Inhibition of autochthonous tumor by ethanol insoluble fraction from *Panax ginseng* as an immunomodulator. *Planta Med* 59:521–524, 1993.

41. Scaglione F, Ferrara F, et al.: Immunomodulatory effects of two extracts of *Panax ginseng* C.A. Meyer. *Drugs Exp Clin Res* 16:537–542, 1990.

42. Scaglione F, Cattaneo G, et al.: Efficacy and safety of the standardized ginseng extract G 115 for potentiating vaccination against common cold and/or influenza syndrome. *Drugs Exptl Clin Res* 22:65–72, 1996.

43. Tyler V: The quality of herbal products in the United States today. *Healthnotes Rev Comp Integrative Med* 6:178–181, 1999.

44. Siegel RK: Ginseng abuse syndrome. *JAMA* 241:1614–1615, 1979.

45. Robbers JE, Tyler VE: *Tyler's Herbs of Choice: The Therapeutic Use of Phytomedicinals.* Haworth Herbal Press, Binghamton, New York, 1999, pp. 236–239.

46. Blumenthal M, Busse WR, et al., eds.: *The Complete Commission E Monographs.* Integrative Medicine Communications, Boston, Massachusetts, 1998, pp. 138–139.

47. Janetzy K and Morreale AP: Probable interaction between warfarin and ginseng. *Am J Health System Pharm* 54:692–693, 1997.

48. Hopkins MP, Androff L, and Benninghoff AS: Ginseng face cream and unexplained vaginal bleeding. *Am J Obstet Gynecol* 159:1121-1122, 1988.

49. Greenspan EM: Ginseng and vaginal bleeding. *JAMA* 249:2018, 1983.

HAWTHORN

1. Hamon NW: Hawthorns: The genus *Crataegus. Can Pharm J* 121:708–709, 724, 1988.

2. Wichtl M: *Herbal Drugs and Phytopharmaceuticals.* CRC Press, Boca Raton, Florida, pp. 161–166.

3. Grieve M: *A Modern Herbal.* Dover Publications, New York, 1971, pp. 385–386.

4. Loew D: Pharmacological and clinical results with *Crataegus* special extracts in cardiac insufficiency. *European Scientific Cooperative on Phytotherapy Phytotelegram* 6:20–26, 1994.

5. Rewerski VW, Piechocki T, et al.: Some pharmacological properties of oligomeric procyanidin isolated from hawthorn (*Crataegus oxyacantha*). *Arzneim-Forsch Drug Res* 17:490–491, 1967.

6. Weiss RF: *Herbal Medicine.* Ab Arcanum, Gothenberg, Sweden, 1988, pp. 162–169.

7. Maevers VW and Hensel H: Changes in local myocardial blood flow following oral administration of a *Crataegus* extract to non-anesthetized dogs. *Arzneim-Forsch Drug Res* 24:783–785, 1974.

8. Ammon HP and Handel M: *Crataegus:* Toxicology and pharmacology. *Planta Med* 43:101–120, 1981.

9. Wagner H and Grevel J: Cardiotonic drugs. IV. Cardiotonic amines from *Crataegus oxyacantha. Planta Med* 45:98–101, 1982.

10. Nasa Y, Hashizume H, et al.: Protective effect of *Crataegus* extract on the cardiac mechanical dysfunction in isolated perfused working rat heart. *Arzneim-Forsch Drug Res* 43:945–949, 1993.

11. Weikl A and Noh HS: The influence of *Crataegus* on global cardiac insufficiency. *Herz Gefäße* 11:516–524, 1993.

12. Schlegelmilch R and Heywood R: Toxicity of *Crataegus* (hawthorn) extract (WS 1442). *J Am Coll Toxicol* 13:103–111, 1994.
13. Blesken VR: Use of *Crataegus* in cardiology. *Fortschr Med* 15:290–292, 1992.
14. Leuchtgens H: *Crataegus* special extract (WS 1442) in cardiac insufficiency. *Fortschr Med* 111:352–354, 1993.
15. Weikl A, Assmus KD, et al.: Crataegus special extract WS 1442: Objective proof of efficacy in patients with cardiac insufficiency (NYHA II). *Fortschr Med* 114:291–296, 1996.
16. Schmidt U, Kuhn U, et al.: Efficacy of the hawthorn (*Crataegus*) preparation LI 132 in 78 patients with chronic congestive heart failure defined as NYHA functional class II. *Phytomedicine* 1:17–24, 1994.
17. Tauchert M, Ploch M, and Hubner WD: Effectiveness of hawthorn extract LI 132 compared with the ACE inhibitor Captopril: Multicenter double-blind study with 132 NYHA stage II. *Muench Med Wochenschr* 136(Suppl):S27–S33, 1994.
18. Hanack T and Bruckel MH: The treatment of mild stable forms of angina pectoris using Crategutt® novo. *Therapiewoche* 33:4331–4333, 1983.
19. Nasa Y, Hashizume H, et al.: Protective effect of *Crataegus* extract on the cardiac mechanical dysfunction in isolated perfused working rat heart. *Arzneim-Forsch Drug Res* 43:945–949, 1993.
20. Bahorun T, Trotin F, et al.: Antioxidant activities of *Crataegus monogyna* extracts. *Planta Med* 60:323–328, 1994.
21. Trunzler VG, Schuler E.: Vergleichende Studien über Wirkungen eines *Crataegus*-extraktes, ven Digitoxin, Digoxin, und Γ-Strophanthin am isolierten Warmblüterherzen. *Arzneim-Forsch Drug Res* 12:198, 1962.
22. Blumenthal M, Busse WR, et al., eds.: *The Complete Commission E Monographs*. Integrative Medicine Communications, Boston, Massachusetts, 1998, pp. 142–144.
23. Upton R, ed.: *Hawthorn leaf with flower*. American Herbal Pharmcopoeia, Santa Cruz, California, 1999.

Horse Chestnut

1. Callam M: Prevalence of chronic leg ulceration and severe chronic venous disease in western countries. *Phlebologie* 7(Suppl):6–12, 1992.
2. Wren RC: *Potter's New Cyclopedia of Botanical Drugs and Preparations*. CW Daniel Co, Saffron Walden, Essex, England, 1985, p. 147.
3. Grieve M: *A Modern Herbal*, vol. 1. Dover Publications, New York, 1971, p.192.
4. Robbers JE, Tyler VE: *Tyler's Herbs of Choice: The Therapeutic Use of Phytomedicinals*. Haworth Herbal Press, Binghamton, New York, 1999, pp. 147–149.
5. Schulz V, Hänsel R, Tyler VE: *Rational Phytotherapy: A Physicians' Guide to Herbal Medicine*. Springer-Verlag, Berlin, 1998, pp. 129–136.
6. Yoshikawa M, Murakami T, et al.: Bioactive saponins and glycosides. III. Horse chestnut. (1): The structures, inhibitory effects on ethanol absorption, and hypoglycemic activity of escins Ia, Iib, IIa, Iib, IIIa from the seeds of *Aesculus hippocastinum* L. *Chem Pharmaceut Bull* 844:1454–1464, 1996.
7. Guillaume M, Padioleau F: Veinotonic effect, vascular protection, anti-inflammatory and free radical scavenging properties of horse chestnut seed extract. *Arzneim-Forsch Drug Res* 44:25–35, 1994.
8. Kreysel HW, Nissen HP, Enghofer E: A possible role of lysosomal enzymes in the pathogenesis of varicosis and the reduction in their serum activity by Venostasin®. *VASA* 12:377–382, 1983.

References

399

9. Facino RM, Carini M, et al.: Anti-elastase and anti-hyaluronidase activities of saponins and sapogenins from *Hedera helix, Aesculus hippocastinum,* and *Ruscus aculeatus*: Factors contributing to their efficacy in the treatment of venous insufficiency. *Archives Pharmazie* 328:720–724, 1995.

10. Calabrese C, Preston P: Report of the results of a double-blind, randomized, single dose trial of a topical 2% escin gel versus placebo in the acute treatment of experimentally induced hematoma in volunteers. *Planta Med* 59:394–397, 1993.

11. Pittler MH, Ernst E: Horse-chestnut seed extract for chronic venous insufficiency: A criteria-based systematic review. *Arch Dermatol* 134:1356–1360, 1998.

12. Friederich HC, Vogelsberg H, Neiss A: A report on the internal usefulness of venous pharmaceuticals. *Z Hautkr* 53:369–374, 1978.

13. Rudofsky G, Neiss A, et al.: Edema protective effect and clinical efficacy of horse chestnut extract in a double-blind study. *Phlebol Proktol* 15:47–54, 1986.

14. Diehm C, Trampisch HJ, et al.: Comparison of leg compression stocking and oral horse-chestnut seed extract therapy in patients with chronic venous insufficiency. *Lancet* 347: 292–294, 1996.

15. Blumenthal M, Busse WR, et al., eds.: *The Complete Commission E Monographs.* Integrative Medicine Communications, Boston, Massachusetts, 1998, pp. 148–149.

16. Pittler MH, Ernst E: Horse-chestnut seed extract for chronic venous insufficiency: A criteria-based systematic review. *Arch Dermatol* 134:1356–1360, 1998.

17. Hellberg K, Ruschewski W, de Vivie R: Drug induced acute renal failure after heart surgery. *Thoraxchirurgie Vaskulare Chirurgie* 23:396–399, 1975.

18. Wilhelm K, Feldmeir C: The prevention and treatment of post-operative and post-traumatic edema. Chemical laboratory tests on the renal tolerance of beta-aescin (Reparil®). *Medizinische Klinik* 70:2079–2083, 1975.

19. Escribano MM, Munoz-Bellido FJ, et al.: Contact urticaria due to aescin. *Contact Dermatitis* 37:233, 1997.

20. Blumenthal M, Busse WR, et al., eds.: *The Complete Commission E Monographs.* Integrative Medicine Communications, Boston, Massachusetts, 1998, pp. 148–149.

21. Brinker F: *Herb Contraindications and Drug Interactions.* Eclectic Medical Publishers, Sandy, Oregon, 1997, p. 54.

KAVA-KAVA

1. Singh YN: Kava: An overview. *J Ethnopharmacol* 37:13–45, 1992.

2. Newell WH: The kava ceremony in Tonga. *J Polynesian Soc* 56:364–417, 1947.

3. Singh YN: *Kava: A Bibliography.* Pacific Information Center, University of the South Pacific, Suva, Fiji, 1986.

4. Lebot V, Merlin M, and Lindstrom L: *Kava: The Pacific Drug.* Yale University Press, New Haven, Connecticut, 1992.

5. Murray MT: Natural anxiolytics—kava and L.72 anti-anxiety formula. *Am J Nat Med* 1:10–14, 1994.

6. Weiss RF: *Herbal Medicine.* Ab Arcanum, Gothenberg, Sweden, 1988, p. 298.

7. Lewin L: *Uber* Piper methysticum *(Kawa).* A. Hirschwald, Berlin, 1886.

8. Meyer HJ: Pharmacology of kava. In: *Ethnopharmacological Search for Psychoactive Drugs* (Efron DH, Holmstedt B, and Kline NS, eds.). Raven Press, New York, 1979, pp. 133–140.

9. Bone K: Kava—a safe herbal treatment for anxiety. *Br J Phytother* 3:145–153, 1994.

References

10. Buckley JP, Furgiulel AR, and O'Hara MJ: Pharmacology of kava. In: *Ethnopharmacological Search for Psychoactive Drugs* (Efron DH, Holmstedt B, and Kline NS, eds.). Raven Press, New York, 1979, pp. 141–151.

11. Davies LP, Drew CA, et al.: Kava pyrones and resin: Studies on GABA$_A$, GABA$_B$, and benzodiazepine binding sites in rodent brain. *Pharmacol Toxicol* 71:120–126, 1992.

12. Holm E, Staedt U, et al.: Studies on the profile of the neurophysiological effects of D,L-kavain: Cerebral sites of action and sleep–wakefulness–rhythm in animals. *Arzneim-Forsch Drug Res* 41:673–683, 1991.

13. Jamieson DD and Duffield PH: The antinociceptive actions of kava components in mice. *Clin Exp Pharmacol Physiol* 17:495–508, 1990.

14. Kretzschmar R and Meyer HJ: Vergleichende Unterschungen über die Antikonvulsive Wirksamkeit der Pyronverbindungen aus *Piper methysticum* Forst. *Arch Int Pharmacodyn Ther* 177:261–277, 1969.

15. Backhauß and Krieglstein J: Extract of kava (*Piper methysticum*) and its methysticin constituents protect brain tissue against ischemic damage to rodents. *Eur J Pharmacol* 215: 265–269, 1992.

16. Johnson D, Frauendorf A, et al.: Neurophysiological active profile and tolerance of kava extract WS 1490. *Therapiewoche Neurologie Psychiatr* 5:349–354, 1991.

17. Saletu B, Grünberger J, et al.: EEG-brain mapping, psychometric and psychophysiological studies on the central effects of kavain—a kava plant derivative. *Hum Psychopharmacol* 4:169–190, 1989.

18. Munte TF, Heinze HJ, et al.: Effects of oxazepam and an extract of kava roots (*Piper methysticum*) on event-related potentials in a word-recognition task. *Pharmacoelectroencephalography* 27:46–53, 1993.

19. Kinzler E, Krömer J, and Lehmann E: Efficacy of kava special extract in patients with conditions of anxiety, tension and excitation of non-psychotic origin. *Arzneim-Forsch Drug Res* 41:584–588, 1991.

20. Volz HP, Kieser M: Kava-kava extract WS 1490 versus placebo in anxiety disorders—a randomized placebo-controlled 25-week outpatient trial. *Pharmacopsychiatry* 30:1–5, 1997.

21. Warnecke G: Psychosomatic disorders in the female climacterium: Clinical efficacy and tolerance of kava extract WS 1490. *Fortsch Med* 109:119–122, 1991.

22. Woelk H, Kapoula O, et al.: A comparison of kava special extract WS 1490 and benzodiazepines in patients with anxiety. *Zeits Allg Med* 69:271–277, 1993.

23. Singh NN, Ellis CR, et al.: Randomized, double-blind, placebo-controlled study on the effectiveness and safety of Kavatrol™ in a non-clinical sample of adults with daily stress and anxiety. Unpublished manuscript, 1998.

24. Jappe U, Franke I, et al.: Sebotropic drug reaction resulting from kava-kava therapy: A new entity? *J Amer Acad Dermatol* 38:104–106, 1998.

25. Herberg KW: Driving ability after intake of kava special extract WS 1490. *Zeits Allgemeinmed* 69:271–277, 1993.

26. Blumenthal M, Busse WR, et al., eds.: *The Complete Commission E Monographs*. Integrative Medicine Communications, Boston, Massachusetts, 1998, pp. 156–157.

27. Almeida JC, Grimsely EW. Coma from the health food store: Interaction between kava and alprazolam. *Arch Internal Med* 125:940–941, 1996.

28. Herberg KW: Effect of special extract WS 1490 combined with ethyl alcohol on safety-relevant performance parameters. *Blutalkohol* 30:96–105, 1993.

References

MILK THISTLE

1. Foster S, and Tyler VE: *Tyler's Honest Herbal.* Haworth Herbal Press, Binghamton, New York, 1999, pp. 253–255.

2. Culpepper N: *The English Physician Enlarged.* H. Colbert, London, 1787.

3. Felter HW and Lloyd JU: *King's American Dispensary.* Original printing 1898; reprint by Eclectic Medical Publications, Portland, Oregon, 1983.

4. Wagner H, Horhammer L, and Munster R: The chemistry of silymarin (silybin), the active principle of the fruits of *Silybum marianum* (L.) Gaertn. *Arzneim-Forsch Drug Res* 18:688–696, 1968.

5. Pelter A and Hansel R: The structure of silibinin (*Silybum* substance E6)—the first flavonolignan. *Tetrahedron Lett* 25:2911–2916, 1968.

6. Hikino H, Kiso Y, et al.: Antihepatotoxic actions of flavonolignans from *Silybum marianum* fruits. *Planta Med* 50:248–250, 1984.

7. Faulstich H, Jahn W, and Wieland T: Silibinin inhibition of amatoxin uptake in the perfused rat liver. *Arzneim-Forsch Drug Res* 30:452–454, 1980.

8. Tuchweber B, Sieck R, and Trost W: Prevention by silibinin of phalloidin induced hepatotoxicity. *Toxicol Appl Pharmacol* 51:265–275, 1979.

9. Shear NH, Malkiewicz IM, et al.: Acetaminophen-induced toxicity to human epidermal cell line A431 and hepatoblastoma cell line Hep G2, in vitro, is diminished by silymarin. *Skin Pharmacol* 8:279–291, 1995.

10. Palasicano G, Portinacasa P, et al.: The effect of silymarin on plasma levels of malondialdehyde in patients receiving long-term treatment with psychotropic drugs. *Curr Ther Res* 55:537–545, 1994.

11. Campos R, Garrido A, et al.: Silibinin dihemisuccinate protects against glutathione depletion and lipid peroxidation induced by acetaminophen on rat liver. *Planta Med* 55:417–419, 1989.

12. Feher J, Lang I, et al.: Free radicals in tissue damage in liver diseases and therapeutic approach. *Tokai J Exp Clin Med* 11:121–134, 1986.

13. Valenzuela A, Aspillaga M, et al.: Selectivity of silymarin on the increase of the glutathione content in different tissues of the rat. *Planta Med* 55:420–422, 1989.

14. Muzes G, Deak G, et al.: Effect of the bioflavonoid silymarin on the in vitro activity and expression of superoxide dismutase (SOD) enzyme. *Acta Physiol Hung* 78:3–9, 1991.

15. Maguilo E, Scevola D, and Carosi GP: Studies on the regenerative capacity of the liver in rats subjected to partial hepatectomy and treated with silymarin. *Arzneim-Forsch Drug Res* 23:161–167, 1973.

16. Sonnenbichler J and Zetl I: Stimulating influence of a flavonolignan derivative on proliferation, RNA synthesis and protein synthesis in liver cells. In: *Assessment and Management of Hepatobiliary Disease* (Okolicsanyi L, Csomos G, and Crepaldi G, eds.). Springer-Verlag, Berlin, 1987, pp. 265–272.

17. Sonnenbichler J, Goldberg M, et al.: Stimulating effects of silibinin on the DNA-synthesis in partially hepatectomized rat livers: Non-response in hepatoma and other malignant cell lines. *Biochem Pharmacol* 35:538–541, 1986.

18. Boigk G, Stroedter L, et al.: Silymarin retards collagen accumulation in early and advanced biliary fibrosis secondary to complete bile duct obliteration in rats. *Hepatology* 26:643–649, 1997.

19. Schuppan D, Strösser W: Legalon® lessens fibrosing activity in patients with chronic liver disease. *Zeits Allgemeinmed* 74:577–584, 1998.

20. Albrecht M, Frerick H, et al.: Therapy of toxic liver pathologies with Legalon®. *Z Klin Med* 47:87–92, 1992.

21. Leng-Peschlow E: Alcohol-related liver diseases—use of Legalon® for therapy. *Pharmedicum* 2:22–27, 1994.
22. Salmi HA and Sama S: Effect of silymarin on chemical, functional and morphological alterations of the liver. *Scand J Gastroenterol* 17:517–521, 1982.
23. DiMario FR, Farini L, et al.: The effects of silymarin on the liver function parameters of patients with alcohol-induced liver disease: A double-blind study. In: *Der Toxisch-metabolische Leberschaden* (De Ritis F, Csomos G, and Braatz R, eds.). Hans. Verl-Kontor, Lubeck, Germany, 1981, pp. 54–58.
24. Feher J, Derk G, et al.: The hepatoprotective effect of treatment with silymarin in patients with chronic alcoholic liver disease. *Orvosi Hetilap* 130:2723–2727, 1989.
25. Ferenci R, Dragosics B, et al.: Randomized controlled trial of silymarin treatment in patients with cirrhosis of the liver. *J Hepatol* 9:105–113, 1989.
26. Velussi M, Cernogoi AM, et al.: Long-term (12 months) treatment with an antioxidant drug (silymarin) is effective on hyperinsulinemia, exogenous insulin need and malondialdehyde levels in cirrhotic diabetic patients. *J Hepatology* 26:871–879, 1997.
27. Pares A, Planas R, et al.: Effects of silymarin in alcoholic patients with cirrhosis of the liver: results of a controlled, double-blind, randomized and multicenter trial. *J Hepatology* 28:615–621, 1998.
28. Berenguer J and Carrasco D: Double-blind trial of silymarin versus placebo in the treatment of chronic hepatitis. *Muench Med Wochenschr* 119:240–260, 1977.
29. Poser G: Experience in the treatment of chronic hepatopathies with silymarin. *Arzneim-Forsch Drug Res* 21:1209–1212, 1971.
30. Vailati A, Aristia L, et al.: Randomized open study of the dose–effect relationship of a short course of IdB 1016 in patients with viral or alcoholic hepatitis. *Fitoterapia* 64:219–227, 1993.
31. Buzzelli G, Moscarella S, et al.: A pilot study on the liver protective effect of silybinphosphatidylcholined complex (IdB 1016) in chronic active hepatitis. *Int J Clin Pharmacol Ther Toxicol* 31:456–460, 1993.
32. Palasciano G, Portincasa P, et al.: The effect of silymarin on plasma levels of malondialdehyde in patients receiving long-term treatment with psychotropic drugs. *Curr Ther Res* 55:537–545, 1994.
33. Invernizzi R, Bernuzzi S, et al.: Silymarin during maintenance therapy of acute promyelocytic leukemia [Letter]. *Haematologica* 78:340–341, 1993.
34. Allain H, Schück S, et al.: Aminotransferase levels and silymarin in de novo tacrine-treated patients with Alzheimer's disease. *Dementia Geriatr Cogn Disorders* 10:181–185, 1999.

ST. JOHN'S WORT

1. Wichtl M: *Herbal Drugs and Phytopharmaceuticals.* CRC Press, Boca Raton, Florida, 1994, pp. 273–275.
2. Blumenthal M, ed.: *Herbal Medicine: Expanded Commission E Monographs.* Integrative Medicine Communications, Newton, Massachusetts, 2000, pp. 359–366.
3. Hobbs C: St. John's wort, *Hypericum perforatum* L. *HerbalGram* 18/19:24–33, 1989.
4. Schulz V, Hänsel R, Tyler VE: *Rational Phytotherapy: A Physician's Guide to Herbal Medicine.* Springer-Verlag, Berlin, 1998, pp. 50–65.
5. Blumenthal M, ed.: *Herbal Medicine: Expanded Commission E Monographs.* Integrative Medicine Communications, Newton, Massachusetts, 2000, pp. 359–366.
6. Gruenwald J: Standardized St. John's wort clinical monograph. *Quart Rev Natural Med* Winter:289–299, 1997.

7. Müller WE, Singer A, et al.: Hyperforin represents the neurotransmitter reuptake inhibiting constituent of *Hypericum* extract. *Pharmacopsychiatry* 31(Suppl 1):16–21, 1998.

8. Reichert RG: St. John's wort for depression. *Quart Rev Nat Med* Spring:17–18, 1994.

9. Müller WE, Rolli M, et al.: Effects of Hypericum extract (LI 160) in biochemical models of antidepressant activity. *Pharmacopsychiatry* 30(Suppl):102–107, 1997.

10. Lenoir S, Degenring FH, Saller R: A double-blind randomized trial to investigate three different concentrations of a standardized fresh plant extract obtained from the shoot tips of *Hypericum perforatum*. *Phytomedicine* 6:141–146, 1999.

11. Müller WE, Singer A, et al.: Hyperforin represents the neurotransmitter reuptake inhibiting constituent of *Hypericum* extract. *Pharmacopsychiatry* 31(Suppl 1):16–21, 1998.

12. Lavie D: Antiviral pharmaceutical compositions containing hypericin or pseudohypericin. European Patent Application No. 87111467.4, filed August 8, 1987, European Patent Office, Publ. No. 0 256 A 2:175–177, 1987.

13. Someya H: Effect of a constituent of *Hypericum erectum* on infection and multiplication of Epstein–Barr virus. *J Tokyo Med Coll* 43:815–826, 1985.

14. Moraleda G, Wu TT, et al.: Inhibition of duck hepatitis B virus replication by hypericin. *Antiviral Res* 20:235–247, 1993.

15. Meruelo D, Lavie G, and Lavie D: Therapeutic agents with dramatic antiretroviral activity and little toxicity at effective doses: Aromatic polycyclic diones hypericin and pseudohypericin. *Proc Natl Acad Sci USA* 85:5230–5234, 1988.

16. Lavie G, Valentine F, et al.: Studies of the mechanism of action of the antiretroviral agents hypericin and pseudohypericin. *Proc Natl Acad Sci USA* 86:5963–5967, 1989.

17. Hudson JB, Harris L, and Towers GHN: The importance of light in the anti-HIV effect of hypericin. *Antiviral Res* 20:173–178, 1993.

18. James J: Hypericum: Common herb shows antiretroviral activity. *AIDS Treatment News* 63:1–5, 1988.

19. James J: Hypericin/St. John's wort: Experience so far. *AIDS Treatment News* 74:1–6, 1989.

20. Payne DL: Unpublished observations. Fall, 1989.

21. James J: Hypericin results: Community Research Alliance Study. *AIDS Treatment News* 96:2–4, 1990.

22. Gulick RM, McAuliffe V, et al.: Phase I studies of hypericin, the active component in St. John's wort, as an antiretroviral agent in HIV-infected adults. *Annals Inter Med* 130:510–514, 1999.

23. Gurummadhva R, Udupa AL, et al.: Calendula and hypericum: Two homeopathic drugs promoting wound healing in rats. *Fitoterapia* 62:508–510, 1991.

24. Sakar MK and Tamer AU: Antimicrobial activity of different extracts from some *Hypericum* species. *Fitoterapia* 61:464–466, 1990.

25. Linde K, Ramirez G, et al.: St. John's wort for depression—an overview and meta-analysis of randomized clinical trials. *BMJ* 313:253–258, 1996.

26. Sommer H, Harrer G: Placebo-controlled double-blind study examining the effectiveness of an Hypericum preparation in 105 mildly depressed patients. *J Geriatric Psychiatry Neurol* 7(Suppl 1):S9–S11, 1994.

27. Hänsgen KD, Vesper J, Ploch M: Multicenter double-blind study examining the antidepressant effectiveness of the Hypericum extract LI 160. *J Geriatric Psychiatry Neurol* 7(Suppl 1): S15–S18, 1994.

28. Vorbach EU, Hübner WD, Arnoldt KH: Effectiveness and tolerance of the Hypericum extract LI 160 in comparison with imipramine: Randomized double-blind study with 135 outpatients. *J Geriatric Psychiatry Neurol* 7(Suppl 1):S19–S23, 1994.

References

29. Vorbach EU, Arnoldt KH, Hübner WD: Efficacy and tolerability of St. John's wort extract LI 160 versus imipramine in patients with severe depressive episodes according to ICD-10. *Pharmacopsychiatry* 30(Suppl):81–85, 1997.

30. Philipp M, Kohnen R, Hiller KO: Hypericum extract versus imipramine or placebo in patients with moderate depression: randomized multicenter study of treatment of eight weeks. *BMJ* 319:1534–1539, 1999.

31. Wheatley D: LI 160, an extract of St. John's wort versus amitriptyline in mildly to moderately depressed outpatients—controlled six week clinical trial. *Pharmacopsychiatry* 30(Suppl):77–80, 1997.

32. Harrer G, Hübner WD, Pouduzweit H: Effectiveness and tolerance of the Hypericum extract LI 160 compared to maprotiline: A multicenter double-blind study. *J Geriatric Psychiatry Neurol* 7(Suppl 1):S24–S28, 1994.

33. Harrer G, Schmidt U, et al.: Comparison of equivalence between the St. John's wort extract Lo-HYP-57 and fluoxetine. *Arzneim-Forsch Drug Res* 49:289–296, 1999.

34. Laakman G, Dienel A, Kieser M: Clinical significance of hyperforin for the efficacy of Hypericum extracts on depressive disorders of different severities. *Phytomedicine* 5:435–442, 1998.

35. Monograph, *Hyperici herba* (St. John's wort). *European Scientific Cooperative for Phytotherapy,* March, 1996.

36. Woelk H, Burkhard G, Gruenwald J: Benefits and risks of Hypericum extract LI 160: Drug monitoring study with 3250 people. *J Geriatric Psychiatry Neurol* 7(Suppl 1):S34–S38, 1994.

37. Araya OS and Ford EJ: An investigation of the type of photosensitization caused by the ingestion of St. John's wort (*Hypericum perforatum*) by calves. *J Comp Pathol Ther* 91:135–141, 1981.

38. Brockmöller J, Reum T, et al.: Hypericin and pseudohypericin: Pharmacokinetics and effects on photosensitivity in humans. *Pharmacopsychiatry* 30(Suppl):94–101, 1997.

39. Blumenthal M, Busse WR, et al., eds.: *The Complete Commission E Monographs.* Integrative Medicine Communications, Boston, Massachusetts, 1998, pp. 214–2   15.

40. Demott K: St. John's wort tied to serotonin syndrome. *Clinical Psychiatry News* 26:28, 1998.

41. Gordon JB: SSRIs and St. John's wort: Possible toxicity? *American Family Physician* 57:950, 1998.

42. Johne A, Brockmöller J, et al.: Pharmacokinetic interaction of digoxin with an herbal extract from St. John's wort (*Hypericum perforatum*). *Clin Pharmacol Ther* 66:338–345, 1999.

43. Nebel A, Schneider BJ, et al.: Potential metabolic interaction between St. John's wort and theophylline [Letter]. *Ann Pharmacother* 33:502, 1999.

44. Maurer A, Johne A, et al.: Interaction of St. John's wort extract with phenprocoumon [Abstract]. *Eur J Clin Pharmacol* 55:A22, 1999.

45. Mai I, Schmider J, et al.: Unpublished results, May, 1999. Reported in: Johne A, Brockmöller J, Bauer S, et al.: Pharmacokinetic interaction of digoxin with an herbal extract from St. John's wort (*Hypericum perforatum*). *Clin Pharmacol Ther* 66:338–345, 1999.

46. Piscitelli SC, Burstein AH, et al.: Indinavir concentrations and St. John's wort [Letter]. *Lancet* 355:547–548, 2000.

47. Ruschitzka F, Meier P, et al.: Acute transplant rejection due to Saint John's wort [Letter]. *Lancet* 355:548–549, 2000.

SAW PALMETTO

1. Leung AY, Foster S: *Encyclopedia of Common Natural Ingredients Used in Foods, Drugs, and Cosmetics.* John Wiley & Sons, New York, 1996, pp. 467–469.

2. Foster S: *101 Medicinal Herbs.* Interweave Press, Loveland, Colorado, 1998, pp. 180–181.

3. Robbers JE, Tyler VE: *Tyler's Herbs of Choice: The Therapeutic Use of Phytomedicinals.* Haworth Press, New York, 1999, pp. 103–105.

4. Schulz V, Hänsel R, Tyler VE: *Rational Phytotherapy: A Physician's Guide to Herbal Medicine.* Springer-Verlag, Berlin, 1998, pp. 226–228.

5. Di Silverio F, Flammia GP, et al.: Plant extracts in BPH. *Minerva Urol Nefrol* 45:143–149, 1993.

6. Geller J: Overview of benign prostatic hypertrophy. *Urology* 34(Suppl.):57–68, 1989.

7. Bartsch W, Klein H, et al.: Enzymes of androgen formation and degradation in the human prostate. *Ann NY Acad Sci* 595:53–66, 1990.

8. Tenover JS: Prostates, pates, and pimples. The potential medical uses of steroid 5-α-reductase inhibitors. *Endocrinol Metab Clin North Am* 20:893–903, 1991.

9. Schulz V, Hänsel R, Tyler VE: *Rational Phytotherapy: A Physician's Guide to Herbal Medicine.* Springer-Verlag, Berlin, 1998, pp. 226–228.

10. Sultan C, Terraza A, Devillier C, et al.: Inhibition of androgen metabolism and binding by a liposterolic extract of *Serenoa repens* in human foreskin fibroblasts. *J Steroid Biochem Molec Biol* 20:2041–2048, 1984.

11. Weisser H, Tunn S, et al.: Effects of the *Sabal serrulata* extract IDS 89 and its subfractions on 5α-reductase activity in human benign prostatic hyperplasia. *Prostate* 28:300–306, 1996.

12. Paubert-Braquet M, Cousse H, et al.: Effect of the lipidosterolic extract of *Serenoa repens* (Permixon®) and its major components on basic fibroblast growth factor-induced proliferation of cultures of human prostate biopsies. *Eur Urol* 33:340–347, 1998.

13. Di Silverio F, Monti S, et al.: Effects of long-term treatment with *Serenoa repens* (Permixon®) on the concentrations and regional distribution of androgens and epidermal growth factor in benign prostatic hyperplasia. *Prostate* 37:377–383, 1998.

14. Rhodes L, Primka RL, et al.: Comparison of finasteride, a 5α-reductase inhibitor, and various commercial plant extracts in in vitro and in vivo 5α-reductase inhibition. *Prostate* 22:43–51, 1993.

15. Iehlé C, Delos S, et al.: Human prostatic steroid 5α-reductase isoforms—a comparative study of selective inhibitors. *J Steroid Biochem Molec Biol* 54:273–279, 1995.

16. Bayne CW, Donnelly F, et al.: *Serenoa repens* (Permixon®): A 5α-reductase types I and II inhibitor—new evidence in a coculture model of BPH. *Prostate* 40:232–241, 1999.

17. Di Silverio F, Monti S, et al.: Effects of long-term treatment with *Serenoa repens* (Permixon®) on the concentrations and regional distribution of androgens and epidermal growth factor in benign prostatic hyperplasia. *Prostate* 37:377–383, 1998.

18. DiSilverio F, D'Eramo G, et al.: Evidence that *Serenoa repens* extract displays an antiestrogenic activity in prostatic tissue of benign prostatic hypertrophy patients. *Eur Urol* 21:309–314, 1992.

19. Breau W, Hagenlocher M, et al.: Antiphlogistic activity of an extract from *Sabal serrulata* fruits prepared by supercritical carbon dioxide: In vitro inhibition of the cyclooxygenase and 5-lipoxygenase metabolism. *Arzneim-Forsch Drug Res* 42:547–551, 1992.

20. Wilt TJ, Ishani A, et al.: Saw palmetto extracts for treatment of benign prostatic hyperplasia: A systematic review. *JAMA* 280:1604–1609, 1998.

21. Champault G, Bonnard AM, et al.: The medical treatment of prostatic adenoma—a controlled study: PA-109 versus placebo in 110 patients. *Ann Urol* 6:407–410, 1984.

22. Tasca A, Barulli M, et al.: Treatment of obstructive symptomology caused by prostatic adenoma with an extract of *Serenoa repens:* Double-blind clinical study vs. placebo. *Minerva Urolog Nefrol* 37:87–91, 1985.

23. Semino MA, Lozano JL, et al.: Symptomatic treatment of benign prostatic hypertrophy: Comparative study of prazosin and *Serenoa repens. Arch Esp Urol* 45:211–213, 1992.

References

24. Braeckman J: The extract of *Serenoa repens* in the treatment of benign prostatic hyperplasia: A multicenter open study. *Curr Ther Res* 55:776–785, 1994.

25. Carraro JC, Raynaud JP, et al.: Comparison of phytotherapy (Permixon®) with finasteride in the treatment of benign prostatic hyperplasia. *Prostate* 29:231–240, 1996.

26. Sökeland J, Albrecht J: A combination of Sabal and Urtica extracts versus finasteride in BPH (stage I to II acc. to Alken): A comparison of therapeutic efficacy in a one-year study. *Urologe [A]* 36:327–333, 1997.

27. Metzker H, Kieser M, Hölscher U. Efficacy of a combined *Sabal-Urtica* preparation in the treatment of benign prostatic hyperplasia. *Urologe [B]* 36:292–300, 1996.

28. Blumenthal M, Busse WR, et al., eds.: *The Complete German Commission E Monographs: Therapeutic Guide to Herbal Medicines.* Integrative Medicine Communications, Boston, Massachusetts, 1998, p. 201.

29. Braeckman J, Bruhwyler J, et al.: Efficacy and safety of the extract of *Serenoa repens* in the treatment of benign prostatic hyperplasia: Therapeutic equivalence between twice and once daily dosage forms. *Phytotherapy Res* 11:558–563, 1997.

30. Stepanov VN, Siniakova LA, et al.: Efficacy and tolerability of the lipidosterolic extract of *Serenoa repens* (Permixon®) in benign prostatic hyperplasia: A double-blind comparison of two dosage regimes. *Advances Ther* 16:231–241, 1999.

31. Bach D, Ebeling L: Long-term drug treatment of benign prostatic hyperplasia—results of a prospective 3-year multicenter study using Sabal extract IDS 89. *Phytomedicine* 3:105–111, 1996.

32. Bayne CW, Donnelly F, et al.: *Serenoa repens* (Permixon®): A 5α-reductase types I and II inhibitor—new evidence in a coculture model of BPH. *Prostate* 40:232–241, 1999.

33. Carraro JC, Raynaud JP, et al.: Comparison of phytotherapy (Permixon®) with finasteride in the treatment of benign prostatic hyperplasia. *Prostate* 29:231–240, 1996.

34. Braeckman J, Bruhwyler J, et al.: Efficacy and safety of the extract of *Serenoa repens* in the treatment of benign prostatic hyperplasia: Therapeutic equivalence between twice and once daily dosage forms. *Phytotherapy Res* 11:558–563, 1997.

35. Gerber GS, Zagaja GP, et al.: Saw palmetto (*Serenoa repens*) in men with lower urinary tract symptoms: Effects in urodynamic parameters and voiding symptoms. *Urology* 51:1003–1007, 1998.

VALERIAN

1. Hobbs C: Valerian—a literature review. *HerbalGram* 21:19–34, 1989.

2. Bradley PR, ed.: *British Herbal Compendium.* British Herbal Medicine Association, London, 1992, pp. 214–217.

3. Monograph, *Valerianae radix* (valerian root). *European Scientific Cooperative for Phytotherapy*, July, 1997.

4. Holzl J and Godau P: Receptor binding studies with *Valeriana officinalis* on the benzodiazepine receptor. *Planta Med* 55:642, 1989.

5. Mennini T, Bernasconi P, et al.: In vitro study on the interaction of extracts and pure compounds from *Valeriana officinalis* roots with GABA, benzodiazepine, and barbiturate receptors. *Fitoterapia* 64:291–300, 1993.

6. Santos MS, Ferreria F, et al.: Synaptosomal GABA release as influenced by valerian root extract—involvement of the GABA carrier. *Arch Int Pharmacodyn* 60:278–279, 1994.

7. Bixler EO, Kales A, et al.: Prevalence of sleep disorders in the Los Angeles metropolitan area. *Am J Psychiatr* 136:1257–1262, 1979.

References

8. Leathwood PD and Chauffard F: Aqueous extract of valerian reduces latency to fall asleep in man. *Planta Med* 51:144–148, 1985.

9. Leathwood PD, Chauffard F, et al.: Aqueous extract of valerian root (*Valeriana officinalis* L.) improves sleep quality in man. *Pharmacol Biochem Behav* 17:65–71, 1982.

10. Balderer G, Borbely AA: Effect of valerian on human sleep. *Psychopharmacology* 87:406–409, 1985.

11. Schulz H, Stoltz C, Müller J: The effect of valerian extract on sleep polygraphy in poor sleepers: A pilot study. *Pharmacopsychiatry* 27:147–151, 1994.

12. Lindahl O and Lindwall L: Double blind study of a valerian preparation. *Pharmacol Biochem Behav* 32:1065–1066, 1989.

13. Dressing H, Riemann D, et al.: Insomnia: Are valerian/balm combinations of equal value to benzodiazepine? *Therapiewoche* 42:726–736, 1992.

14. Dressing H, Köhler S, Müller WE: Improvement of sleep quality with a high-dose valerian/lemon balm preparation: A placebo controlled double-blind study. *Psychopharmako-therapie* 3:123–130, 1996.

15. Panijel M: The treatment of moderate states of anxiety: Randomized double-blind study comparing the clinical effectiveness of a phytomedicine with diazepam. *Therapiewoche* 41: 4659–4668, 1985.

16. Brown D: Valerian: A possible substitute for benzodiazepines. *Quart Rev Nat Med* Winter:17–18, 1993.

17. Blumenthal M, Busse WR, et al., eds.: *The Complete Commission E Monographs*. Integrative Medicine Communications, Boston, Massachusetts, 1998, pp. 226–227.

18. Monograph, *Valerianae radix* (Valerian root). *European Scientific Cooperative for Phyto-therapy*, July, 1997.

19. Blumenthal M, Busse WR, et al., eds.: *The Complete Commission E Monographs*. Integrative Medicine Communications, Boston, Massachusetts, 1998, pp. 226–227.

20. Albrecht M, Berger W, et al.: Psychopharmaceuticals and safety in traffic. *Z Allg Med* 71:1215–1221, 1995.

Vitex Agnus-Castus

1. Böhnert KJ and Hahn G: Phytotherapy in gynecology and obstetrics—*Vitex agnus-castus*. *Erfahrungsheilkunde* 39:494–502, 1990.

2. Blumenthal M, Busse WR, et al., eds.: *The Complete Commission E Monographs*. Integrative Medicine Communications, Boston, Massachusetts, 1998, p. 108.

3. Propping D, Katzorke T, and Belkien L: Diagnosis and therapy of corpus luteum insufficiency in general practice. *Therapiewoche* 38:2992–3001, 1988.

4. Muhlenstedt D, Bohnet JP, et al.: Short luteal phase and prolactin. *Int J Fertil* 23:213–217, 1978.

5. Weiss RF: *Herbal Medicine*. Ab Arcanum, Gothenburg, Sweden, 1988, pp. 317–318.

6. Amann W: Removing an obstipation using Agnolyt®. *Ther Gegenw* 104:1263–1265, 1965.

7. Sliutz G, Speiser P, et al.: *Agnus castus* extracts inhibit prolactin secretion of rat pituitary cells. *Horm Metab Res* 25:253–255, 1993.

8. Böhnert KJ: The use of *Vitex agnus castus* for hyperprolactinemia. *Quart Rev Nat Med* Spring:19–21, 1997.

9. Dittmar FW, Böhnert KJ, et al.: Premenstrual syndrome: Treatment with a phytopharmaceutical. *Ther Gynäkol* 5:60–68, 1992.

10. Peteres-Welte C and Albrecht M: Menstrual abnormalities and PMS: *Vitex agnus-castus. Ther Gynäkol* 7:49–52, 1994.

11. Lauritzen CH, Reuter HD, et al.: Treatment of premenstrual tension syndrome with *Vitex agnus castus:* Controlled, double-blind study versus pyridoxine. *Phytomedicine* 4:183–189, 1997.

12. Coeugniet E, Elek E, and Kühnast R: Premenstrual syndrome (PMS) and its treatment. *Ärztezeitschr Naturheilverf* 27:619–622, 1986.

13. Halaka M, Beles P, et al.: Treatment of cyclical mastalgia with a solution containing *Vitex agnus castus* extract: Results of a placebo-controlled double-blind study. *Breast* 8:175–181, 1999.

14. Loch EG and Kayser E: Diagnosis and treatment of dyshormonal menstrual periods in the general practice. *Gynäkol Praxis* 14:489–495, 1990.

15. Propping D and Katzorke T: Treatment of corpus luteum insufficiency. *Z Allg Med* 63:932–933, 1987.

16. Gerhard I, Patek A, et al.: Mastodynon® for female infertility. *Research Complement Med* 5:272–278, 1998.

17. Milewicz A, Gejdel E, et al.: *Vitex agnus-castus* in the treatment of luteal phase defects due to hyperprolactinemia: Results of a randomized placebo-controlled double-blind study. *Arzneim-Forsch Drug Res* 43:752–756, 1993.

18. Blumenthal M, Busse WR, et al., eds.: *The Complete Commission E Monographs.* Integrative Medicine Communications, Boston, Massachusetts, 1998, p. 108.

PART 6: HERBAL PRESCRIPTIONS FOR COMMON HEALTH CONDITIONS

CARDIOVASCULAR SYSTEM

Angina

1. Kamikawa T, Kobayashi A, et al.: Effects of coenzyme Q-10 on exercise tolerance in stable angina pectoris. *Am J Cardiol* 56:247, 1985.

2. Kamikawa T, Suzuki Y, et al.: Effects of L-carnitine on exercise tolerance in patients with stable angina pectoris. *Jpn Heart J* 25:587–597, 1984.

3. Cacciatore L, Cerio R, et al.: The therapeutic effect of L-carnitine in patients with exercise-induced stable angina: A controlled study. *Drugs Exp Clin Res* 17:225–235, 1991.

4. Motoyama T, Kawano H, et al.: Vitamin E administration improves impairment of endothelium-dependent vasodilation in patients with coronary spastic angina. *J Amer College Cardiol* 32:1672–1679, 1998.

5. Cohen L and Kitzes R: Magnesium sulfate in the treatment of variant angina. *Magnesium* 3:46–49, 1984.

6. Reichter A, Herlitz J, Hjalmarson A: Effect of acupuncture in patients with angina pectoris. *European Heart J* 12:175–178, 1991.

7. Ballegaard S, Norrelund S, Smith DF: Cost–benefit of combined use of acupuncture, Shiatsu, and lifestyle adjustment for treatment of patients with severe angina pectoris. *Acupunct Electrother Res* 21:187–197, 1996.

Bruising

1. Yarnell E: Review of clinical trials on oligomeric procyanidins. *Healthnotes Rev Comp Integrative Med* 6:92–94, 1999.
2. Reinhold U, Seiter S, et al.: Treatment of progressive pigmented purpurea with oral bioflavonoids and ascorbic acid: An open pilot study in 3 patients. *J Am Acad Dermatol* 41: 207–208, 1999.

Chronic Venous Insufficiency

1. Yarnell E: Review of clinical trials on oligomeric procyanidins. *Healthnotes Rev Comp Integrative Med* 6:92–94, 1999.
2. Cappelli R, Nicora M, and Di Perri T: Use of extract of *Ruscus aculeatus* in venous disease of the lower limbs. *Drugs Exp Clin Res* 14:277–283, 1988.
3. Unkauf M, Rehn D, et al.: Investigation of the efficacy of oxerutins compared to placebo in patients with chronic venous insufficiency treated with compression stockings. *Arzneim-Forsch Drug Res* 46:478–482, 1996.

Congestive Heart Failure

1. Morisco C, Trimarco C, and Condorelli M: Effect of coenzyme Q_{10} therapy in patients with congestive heart failure: A long-term multicenter randomized study. *Clin Invest* 71:S134–S136, 1993.
2. Soja AM, Mortensen SA: Treatment of chronic cardiac insufficiency with coenzyme Q_{10}—results of a meta-analysis of controlled clinical trials. *Ugeskr Laeger* 159:7302–7308, 1997.
3. Mancini M, Rengo F, et al.: Controlled study on the therapeutic efficacy of propionyl-L-carnitine in patients with congestive heart failure. *Arzneim-Forsch Drug Res* 42:1101–1104, 1992.
4. Caponetto S, Canale C, et al.: Efficacy of L-propionylcarnitine treatment in patients with left ventricular dysfunction. *European Heart J* 15:1267–1273, 1994.
5. Azuma J, Suwamura A, et al.: Therapeutic effect of taurine in congestive heart failure: A double blind crossover trail. *Clin Cardiol* 8:278–282, 1985.
6. Bashir Y, Sneddon JF, et al.: Effects of long-term oral magnesium chloride replacement in congestive heart secondary to coronary artery disease. *Am J Cardiol* 72:1156–1162, 1993.

Hypercholesterolemia (High Cholesterol)

1. Heber D, Yip I, et al.: Cholesterol-lowering effects of a proprietary Chinese red-yeast-rice dietary supplement. *Am J Clin Nutr* 69:231–236, 1999.
2. Verma SK and Bordia A: Effect of *Commiphora mukul* (gum guggul) in patients with hyperlipidemia with special reference to HDL-cholesterol. *Indian J Med Res* 87:356–360, 1988.
3. Olson BH, Anderson SM, et al.: Psyllium-enriched cereals lower blood total cholesterol and LDL cholesterol, but not HDL cholesterol, in hypercholesterolemic adults: Results of a meta-analysis. *J Nutr* 127:1973–1980, 1997.
4. Sharma RD, Raghuram TC, and Rao VD: Hypolipidemic effect of fenugreek seeds. A clinical study. *Phytother Res* 5:145–147, 1991.
5. Brown WV: Niacin for lipid disorders. *Postgrad Med* 98:185–193, 1995.
6. McKenney JM, Proctor JD, et al.: A comparison of the efficacy and toxic effects of sustained- vs. immediate-release niacin in hypercholesterolemic patients. *JAMA* 271:672–677, 1994.
7. Murray M: Lipid-lowering drugs vs. inositol hexaniacinate. *J Natural Med* 2:9–12, 1995.
8. Ubbink JB, Hayward WJ, et al.: Vitamin requirements for the treatment of hyperhomocysteinemia in humans. *J Nutr* 124:1927–1933, 1994.

References

9. Lobo A, Naso A, et al.: Reduction of homocysteine levels in coronary artery disease by low-dose folic acid combined with vitamins B_6 and B_{12}. *Am J Cardiol* 83:821–825, 1999.

10. Roeback JR, Hla KM, et al.: Effects of chromium supplementation on serum high-density lipoprotein cholesterol levels in men taking beta-blockers. *Annals Internal Med* 115:917–924, 1991.

11. Rimm EB, Stampfer MJ, et al.: Vitamin E consumption and the risk of coronary heart disease. *New Engl J Med* 328:1444–1449, 1993.

12. Galeone F, Scalabrino A, et al.: The lipid-lowering effect of pantethine in hyperlipidemic patients: A clinical investigation. *Current Ther Res* 34:383–390, 1983.

13. Prichard BN, Smith CCT, et al.: Fish oils and cardiovascular disease. *BMJ* 310:819–820, 1995.

Intermittent Claudication

1. Drabaek H, Mehlsen J, et al.: A botanical compound, Padma 28, increases walking distance in stable intermittent claudication. *Angiology* 44:863–867, 1993.

2. Haeger K: Long-term study of α-tocopherol in intermittent claudication. *Ann NY Acad Sci* 393:369–375, 1982.

3. O'Hara J, Jolly PN, and Nicol CG: The therapeutic efficacy of inositol nicotinate (Hexopal®) in intermittent claudication: A controlled trial. *Br J Clin Pract* 42:377–383, 1988.

4. Brevetti G, Chiariello M, et al.: Increases in walking distance in patients with peripheral vascular disease treated with L-carnitine: A double-blind, cross-over study. *Circulation* 77:767–773, 1988.

5. Brevetti G, Diehm C, Lambert D: European multicenter study on propionyl-L-carnitine in intermittent claudication. *J Am Coll Cardiol* 34:1618–1624, 1999.

Raynaud's Disease

1. Belch JJF, et al.: Evening primrose oil (Efamol®) as a treatment for cold-induced vasospasm (Raynaud's phenomenon). *Prog Lipid Res* 25:335–340, 1986.

2. Sunderland GT, Belch JJF, et al.: A double-blind randomized placebo-controlled trial of Hexopal in primary Raynaud's disease. *Clin Rheum* 7:46–49, 1988.

3. DiGiacomo RA, Kremer JM, Shah DM: Fish-oil dietary supplementation in patients with Raynaud's phenomenon: A double-blind, controlled, prospective study. *Am J Med* 86:158–164, 1989.

DIGESTIVE SYSTEM

Alcohol-Related Liver Disease

1. Bulanov AE, Polozhentseva MI, and Yatskov LP: Anti-alcoholic effect of *Eleutherococcus*. In: *New Data on Eleutherococcus, Proceedings of the 2nd International Symposium on Eleutherococcus.* Moscow, 1984, pp. 175–183.

2. Kubo S, Ohkura Y, et al.: Effect of Gomisin A (TJN-101) on liver regeneration. *Planta Med* 58:489–492, 1992.

Constipation

1. Kinnunen O and Salokannel J: Constipation in elderly long-term stay patients: Its treatment by magnesium hydroxide and bulk-laxative. *Ann Clin Res* 19:321–323, 1987.

Diarrhea

1. Dicesare D, DuPont HL, et al.: A double-blind, randomized, placebo-controlled study of SP-303 (Provir™) in the symptomatic treatment of acute diarrhea among travelers to Mexico and Jamaica. Infectious Diseases Society of America—36th Annual Meeting, Denver, Colorado, 1998.
2. Holodniy M, Koch J, et al.: A double blind, randomized, placebo-controlled phase II study to assess the safety and efficacy of orally administered SP-303 for the symptomatic treatment of diarrhea in patients with AIDS. *Am J Gastroenterol* 94:3267–3273, 1999.
3. Koch J, Tuveson J, Carlson T, Schmidt JM: SB-300: A new and effective therapy for HIV-associated diarrhea. Poster presentation, Seventh European Conference on Clinical Aspects and Treatment of HIV-Infection, Lisbon, Portugal, October 23–27, 1999.
4. Loeb H, Vandenplas Y, et al.: Tannin-rich pod for treatment of acute-onset diarrhea. *J Pediatr Gastroenterol Nutr* 8:480–485, 1989.
5. Robbers JE, Tyler VE: *Tyler's Herbs of Choice: The Therapeutic Use of Phytomedicinals.* Haworth Herbal Press, Binghamton, New York, 1999, pp. 62–65.
6. Eherer AH, Santa Ana CA, et al.: Effect of psyllium, calcium polycarbophil, and wheat bran on diarrhea induced by phenolphthalein. *Gastroenterol* 104:1007–1012, 1993.
7. Khin-Maung U, Khin M, et al.: Clinical trial of berberine in acute watery diarrhea. *BMJ* 291:1601–1605, 1985.
8. Isolauri E, Juntunen M, et al.: A human *Lactobacillus* strain (*Lactobacillus casei* sp. strain GG) promotes recovery from acute diarrhea in children. *Pediatrics* 88:90–97, 1991.
9. Oksanen PJ, Salminen S, et al.: Prevention of travelers' diarrhea by *Lactobacillus* GG. *Ann Med* 23:53–56, 1990.
10. Vanderhoof JA, Whitney DB, et al.: *Lactobacillus GG* in the prevention of antibiotic-associated diarrhea in children. *J Pediatrics* 135:564–568, 1999.

Heartburn

1. Segal I, Hale M, et al.: Pathological effects of pellagra on the esophagus. *Nutr Cancer* 14: 233–238, 1990.

Irritable Bowel Syndrome

1. Somerville K, Richmond C, and Bell G: Delayed response peppermint oil capsules (Colpermin®) for the spastic colon syndrome: A pharmacokinetic study. *Br J Pharm* 18:638–640, 1984.
2. Dew MJ, Evans BK, and Rhodes J: Peppermint oil for the irritable bowel syndrome: A multicenter trial. *Br J Clin Pract* 38:394–398, 1984.
3. May B, Kuntz HD, et al.: Efficacy of a fixed peppermint/caraway oil combination in non-ulcer dyspepsia. *Arzneim-Forsch Drug Res* 46:1149–1153, 1996.
4. Friese J, Köhler S: Peppermint oil/caraway oil fixed combination in non-ulcer dyspepsia: equivalent efficacy of the drug combination in an enteric-coated or enteric-soluble formula. *Pharmazie* 54:210–215, 1999.
5. Jalihal A, Kurian G: Ispaghula therapy in irritable bowel syndrome: improvement in overall well-being is related to reduction in bowel dissatisfaction. *J Gastroenterol Hepatol* 11: 1510–1513, 1990.
6. Bensoussan A, Talley NJ, et al.: Treatment of irritable bowel syndrome with Chinese herbal medicine. A randomized controlled trial. *JAMA* 280:1585–1589, 1998.
7. Whorwell PJ, Prior A, and Feregher EB: Controlled trial of hypnotherapy in the treatment of severe refractory irritable bowel syndrome. *Lancet* ii:1232–1234, 1984.

8. Blanchard EB, Grenne B, et al.: Relaxation training as a treatment for irritable bowel syndrome. *Biofeedback Self-Regul* 18:125–132, 1993.
9. Shaw G, Srivastava ED, et al.: Stress management for irritable bowel syndrome: A controlled trial. *Digestion* 50:36–42, 1991.

Peptic Ulcer Disease

1. Wilson JAC: A comparison of carbenoxolone sodium and deglycyrrhizinated licorice in the treatment of gastric ulcer in the ambulant patient. *Br J Clin Pract* 25:563–566, 1972.
2. Brogden RN, Speight TM, and Avery GS: Deglycyrrhizinated licorice: A report of its pharmacological properties and therapeutic efficacy in peptic ulcer. *Drugs* 8:330–339, 1974.
3. Wendt P, Reiman H, et al.: The use of flavonoids as inhibitors of histidine decarboxylase in gastric diseases: Experimental and clinical studies. *Naunyn-Schmeidebergs Arch Pharmakol* 313(Suppl.):238, 1980.
4. Al-Habbal MJ, Al-Habbal Z, Huwez FU: A double-blind controlled clinical trial of mastic and placebo in the treatment of duodenal ulcer. *Clin Experimental Pharmacol Physiol* 11:541–544, 1984.
5. Frommer DJ: The healing of gastric ulcers by zinc sulphate. *Med J Aust* 2:793, 1975.
6. Jimenez E, Bosch F, et al.: Meta-analysis of efficacy of zinc acexamate in peptic ulcer. *Digestion* 51:18–26, 1992.
7. Patty I, Benedek S, et al.: Controlled trial of vitamin A therapy in gastric ulcer [Letter]. *Lancet* ii:876, 1982.
8. Sobala GM, Schorah CJ, et al.: Ascorbic acid in the human stomach. *Gastroenterology* 97:357–363, 1989.
9. Al-Somal N, Coley KE, et al.: Susceptibility of *Helicobacter pylori* to the antibacterial activity of manuka honey. *J R Soc Med* 87:9–12, 1994.

Ulcerative Colitis

1. Gupta I, Parihar A, et al.: Effects of *Boswellia serrata* gum resin in patients with ulcerative colitis. *Eur J Med* 2:37–43, 1997.
2. Fernádez-Banares F, Hinojosa J, et al.: Randomized clinical trial of *Plantago ovata* seeds (dietary fiber) as compared with mesalamine in maintaining remission in ulcerative colitis. *Amer J Gastroenterol* 94:427–433, 1999.
3. Stenson WF, Cort D, et al.: Dietary supplementation with fish oil in ulcerative colitis. *Annals Internal Med* 116:609–614, 1992.
4. Lashner BA, Provencher KS, et al.: The effect of folic acid supplementation on the risk for cancer or dysplasia in ulcerative colitis. *Gastroenterol* 112:29–32, 1997.
5. Scheppach W, Sommer H, et al.: Effect of butyrate enemas on the colonic mucosa in distal ulcerative colitis. *Gastroenterol* 103:51–56, 1992.

EARS, NOSE, THROAT, AND RESPIRATORY TRACT

Asthma

1. Lindahl O, Lindwall L, et al.: Vegan regimen with reduced medication in the treatment of bronchial asthma. *J Asthma* 22:45–55. 1985.
2. Wickens K, Pearce N, et al.: Antibiotic use in early childhood and the development of asthma. *Clin Exp Allergy* 29:766–771, 1999.

References

3. Spitzer WO, Suissa S, et al.: The use of beta-agonists and the risk of death and near death from asthma. *New Engl J Med* 326:501–506, 1992.

4. Pearce N, Crane J, et al.: Beta agonists and asthma mortality: Déjà vu. *Clin Exp Allergy* 21:401–410, 1991.

5. Crane J, Pearce N, et al.: Worldwide worsening of wheezing—is the cure the cause? *Lancet* 339:814, 1992.

6. Wilkens JH, Wilkens H, et al.: Effect of PAF-antagonist (BN 52063) on bronchoconstriction and platelet activation during exercise-induced asthma. *Br J Clin Pharm* 29:85–101, 1990. Guinot P, Brambilla C, et al.: Effect of BN 52063, a specific PAF-acether antagonist, on bronchial provocation test to allergens in asthmatic patients: A preliminary test. *Prostaglandins* 34:723–731, 1987.

7. Li M, Yang B, et al.: Clinical observation of the therapeutic effect of ginkgo leaf concentrated oral liquor on bronchial asthma. *Chinese J Integrative Western Med* 3:264–267, 1997.

8. Mansfeld HJ, Höhre H, et al.: Therapy of bronchial asthma with dried ivy leaf extract. *Münch Med Wschr* 140:32–36, 1998.

9. Reichert R: Ivy leaf extract and asthma reduction in children. *Healthnotes Rev Comp Integrative Med* 6:154–155, 1999.

10. Robbers JE, Tyler VE: *Tyler's Herbs of Choice: The Therapeutic Use of Phytomedicinals.* Haworth Herbal Press, Binghamton, New York, 1999, pp. 112–116.

11. Shipura DN, Menon MPS, Prakash D: A crossover, double-blind study on *Tylophora indica* in the treatment of asthma and allergic rhinitis. *J Allergy* 43:145–150, 1969.

12. Thiruvengadam KV, Haranatii K, et al.: *Tylophora indica* in bronchial asthma: A controlled comparison with a standard anti-asthmatic drug. *J Indian Med Assoc* 71:172–176, 1978.

13. Bone K: *Clinical Applications of Ayurvedic and Chinese Herbs.* Phytotherapy Press, Warwick, Queensland, Australia, 1996, pp. 134–136.

14. Middleton E and Drzewiecki G: Naturally occurring flavonoids and human basophil histamine release. *Int Arch Allergy Appl Immunol* 77:155–157, 1985.

15. Collipp PJ, Goldzier S, et al.: Pyridoxine treatment of childhood bronchial asthma. *Ann Allergy* 35:93–97, 1975.

16. Anah CO, Jarike LN, and Baig HA: High dose ascorbic acid in Nigerian asthmatics. *Trop Geogr Med* 32:132–137, 1980.

17. Hasselmark L, Malmgren R, et al.: Selenium supplementation in intrinsic asthma. *Allergy* 48:30–36, 1993.

18. Dorsh W, Wagner H, et al.: Antiasthmatic effects of onions: Alk(en)ylsulfinothic acid alk(en)ylesters inhibit histamine release, leukotriene and thromboxane biosynthesis in vitro and counteract PAF- and allergen-induced bronchial obstruction in vivo. *Biochem Pharmacol* 37:4479–4485, 1988.

19. Wright AL, Holberg CJ, et al.: Breast feeding and lower respiratory tract illness in the first year of life. *Br Med J* 299:946–949, 1989.

20. Singh V, Wisniewski A, et al.: Effect of yoga breathing exercises (pranayama) on airway reactivity in subjects with asthma. *Lancet* 335:1381–133, 1990.

21. Chilmonczyx BA, Salmun LM, et al.: Association between exposure to environmental tobacco smoke and exacerbations of asthma in children. *New Engl J Med* 328:1665–1669, 1993.

Coughs

1. Robbers JE, Tyler VE: *Tyler's Herbs of Choice: The Therapeutic Use of Phytomedicinals.* Haworth Herbal Press, Binghamton, New York, 1999, pp. 116–120.

References

2. Schilcher H and Elzer M: *Drosera* (Sundew): A proven antitussive. *Zeits Phytother* 14:50–54, 1993.

3. Czygan FC and Hansel R: Thyme species as cough medicines. *Zeits Phytother* 14:104–110, 1993.

4. Blumenthal M, Goldberg A, et al., eds.: *The Complete German Commission E Monographs: Therapeutic Guide to Herbal Medicines.* Integrative Medical Communications, Boston, Massachusetts, 1998, p. 153.

5. März RW, Ismail C, Popp MA: Action profile and efficacy of a herbal combination preparation for the treatment of sinusitis. *Wien Med Wschr* 149:202–208, 1999.

Ear Infections (Recurrent)

1. Diamant M and Diamant B: Abuse and timing of use of antibiotics in acute otitis media. *Arch Otolaryngol* 100:226–232, 1974.

2. Strachan DP, Jarvis MJ, and Feyerabend C: Passive smoking, salivary cotinine concentrations, and middle ear effusion in 7 year old children. *Br Med J* 298:1549–1552, 1989.

3. Jackson JM, Mourino AP: Pacifier use and otitis media in infants twelve months of age and younger. *Pediatr Dent* 21:256–261, 1999.

4. Balli R: Controlled trial on the use of oral acetylcysteine in the treatment of glue-ear following drainage. *Eur J Respir Dis* 61(Suppl. 111):158, 1980.

5. Backon J: Prolonged breastfeeding for at least 4 months protects against otitis media. *Pediatrics* 91:867–872, 1993.

6. Saarinen UM: Prolonged breast feeding as prophylaxis for recurrent otitis media. *Acta Pediatr Scand* 71:567–571, 1982.

7. Hurst DS: Allergy management of refractory serous otitis media. *Otolaryngol Head Neck Surg* 102:664–669, 1990.

Sinus Infections (Recurrent)

1. März RW, Ismail C, Popp MA: Action profile and efficacy of a herbal combination preparation for the treatment of sinusitis. *Wien Med Wschr* 149:202–208, 1999.

2. Schulz V, Hänsel R, Tyler VE: *Rational Phytotherapy: A Physicians' Guide to Herbal Medicine.* Springer-Verlag, Berlin, 1998, pp. 288–292.

3. Panosetti E, Pidoux JM, and Lehmann W: Clinical trial with oral acetylcysteine in chronic sinusitis. *Eur J Respir Dis* 61(Suppl. 111):159, 1980.

4. Ryan R: A double-blind clinical evaluation of bromelains in the treatment of acute sinusitis. *Headache* 7:13–17, 1967.

Tinnitus and Hearing Loss

1. Moller AR: Pathophysiology of tinnitus. *Ann Otol Rhinol Laryngol* 93:39–44, 1984.

2. Coles R: Trial of an extract of *Ginkgo biloba* for tinnitus and hearing loss. *Clin Otolaryngol* 13:501–502, 1988.

3. Shemesh Z, Attias J, et al.: Vitamin B_{12} deficiency in patients with chronic tinnitus and noise-induced hearing loss. *Am J Otolaryngol* 14:94–99, 1993.

4. Shambaugh GE: Zinc for tinnitus, imbalance, and hearing loss in the elderly. *Am J Otolaryngol* 7:467–467, 1986.

5. Brown DJ: Alternative approaches to tinnitus, Meniere's disease and hearing loss. *Let's Live* October:80, 1993.

6. Marion MS and Cevette MJ: Tinnitus. *Mayo Clin Proc* 66:614–620, 1991.

Hay Fever

1. Mittman P: Randomized double-blind study of freeze-dried *Urtica diocia* in the treatment of allergic rhinitis. *Planta Med* 56:44–47, 1990.
2. Middleton E and Drzewicki G: Effect of ascorbic acid and flavonoids on human basophil release. *J Allerg Clin Immunol* January:278, 1992.
3. Clemetson CA: Histamine and ascorbic acid in human blood. *J Nutr* 110: 662–668, 1980.

ENDOCRINE SYSTEM

Diabetes

1. Madar Z, Abel R, et al.: Glucose-lowering effect of fenugreek in non-insulin-dependent diabetics. *Eur J Clin Nutr* 42:51–54, 1988.
2. Sharma RD, Raghuram TC, and Rao NS: Effect of fenugreek seed on blood glucose and serum lipids in type I diabetes. *Eur J Clin Nutr* 44:301–306, 1990.
3. Shanmugasundaram ERB, Rajeswari G, et al.: Use of *Gymnema sylvestre* leaf extract in the control of blood glucose in insulin-dependent diabetes mellitus. *J Ethnopharmacol* 30:281–294, 1990.
4. Baskaran K, Ahamath BK, et al.: Antidiabetic effect of a leaf extract from *Gymnema sylvestre* in non-insulin dependent diabetes mellitus patients. *J Ethnopharmacol* 30:295–305, 1990.
5. Bunyapraphatsara N, Yongchaiydha S, et al.: Antidiabetic activity of *Aloe vera* L. juice. II. Clinical trial in diabetes mellitus patients in combination with glibenclamide. *Phytomedicine* 3:245–248, 1996.
6. Yongchaiydha S, Rungpitarangsi V, et al.: Antidiabetic activity of *Aloe vera* L. juice. I. Clinical trial in new cases of diabetes mellitus patients in combination with glibenclamide. *Phytomedicine* 3:241–243, 1996.
7. Varma SD: Diabetic cataracts and flavonoids. *Science* 1985:205, 1977.
8. Lysy J and Zimmerman J: Ascorbic acid status in diabetes mellitus. *Nutr Res* 12:713–20, 1992.
9. Will JC, Tyers T: Does diabetes mellitus increase the requirement for vitamin C? *Nutrition Rev* 54:193–202, 1996.
10. Evans GW: The effect of chromium picolinate on insulin controlled parameters in humans. *Int J Biosocial Med Res* 11:163–180, 1989.
11. Anderson RA, Polansky MM, et al.: Supplemental chromium effects glucose, insulin, glucagon, and urinary chromium losses in subjects consuming controlled low-chromium diets. *Am J Clin Nutr* 54:909–916, 1991.
12. Rude RK: Magnesium deficiency and diabetes mellitus. *Postgrad Med* 92:217–224, 1992.
13. McNair P, Christiansen C, et al.: Hypomagnesemia, a risk factor in diabetic retinopathy. *Diabetes* 27:1075–1077, 1978.
14. Mocchegiani E, Boemi M, et al.: Zinc-dependent low thymic hormone level in type I diabetes. *Diabetes* 12:932–937, 1989.
15. Ceriello A, Giugliano D, et al.: Vitamin E reduction of protein glycosylation in diabetes. *Diabetes Care* 14:68–72, 1991.
16. Tütüncü NB, Bayraktar M, Varli K: Reversal of defective nerve condition with vitamin E supplementation in type 2 diabetes. *Diabetes Care* 21:1915–1918, 1998.
17. Maebashi M, Makino Y, et al.: Therapeutic evaluation of the effect of biotin on hyperglycemia in patients with non-insulin-dependent diabetes mellitus. *J Clin Biochem Nutr* 14:211–218, 1993.

18. Ziegler D, Schatz H, et al.: Effects of treatment with the antioxidant alpha-lipoic acid on cardiac autonomic neuropathy in NIDDM patients: A 4-month randomized controlled multicenter trial (DEKAN Study). *Diabetes Care* 20:369–373, 1997.

Stress and Fatigue (Adrenal Exhaustion)

1. Selye H: The general adaptation syndrome and the diseases of adaptation. *J Clin Endocrinol* 6:117, 1946.
2. Tintera JW: The hypoadrenocortical state and its management. *NY State Med J* 55:1869–1876, 1955.

EYES

Cataracts

1. Leske MC and Sperduto RD: The epidemiology of senile cataracts: A review. *Am J Epidemiol* 118:152–165, 1983.
2. U.S. Department of Health and Human Services: Report of the Cataract Panel, Vol. 2, part 3. *Vision Research, a National Plan.* NIH Publication No. 83-2473. U.S. Department of Health and Human Services, Washington, D.C., 1983.
3. Bravetti G: Preventive medical treatment of senile cataract with vitamin E and anthocyanosides: Clinical evaluation. *Ann Ottamol Clin Ocul* 115:109, 1989.
4. Robertson JM, Donner AP, and Trevithick JR: A possible role for vitamins C and E in cataract prevention. *Am J Clin Nutr* 53(Suppl.):346–351, 1991.
5. Leske MC, Chylack LT, et al.: Antioxidant vitamins and nuclear opacities. The Longitudinal Study of Cataract. *Ophthalmology* 105:831–836, 1998.
6. Sperduto RD, HU, et al.: The Linixian cataract studies. *Arch Ophthalmol* 111:1246–1253, 1993.

Diabetic Retinopathy

1. Droy-Lefaix MT and Doly M: EGb 761, a retina free-radical scavenger. In: *Effects of* Ginkgo biloba *Extract (EGb 761) on the Central Nervous System* (Christen Y, Costentin M, and Lacour M, eds.). Elsevier, Paris, 1992, pp. 7–17.

Macular Degeneration

1. Farber ME and Farber AS: Macular degeneration: A devastating but treatable disease. *Postgrad Med* 88:181–183, 1990.
2. Lebuisson DA, Leroy L, and Reigal G: Treatment of senile macular degeneration with *Ginkgo biloba* extract: A preliminary double-blind study versus placebo. In: *Rökan* (Ginkgo biloba)*: Recent Results in Pharmacology and Clinic* (Fünfgeld EW, ed.). Springer-Verlag, Berlin, 1988, pp. 231–236.
3. Yarnell Y: Review of clinical trials on oligomeric proanthocyanidins. *Healthnotes Rev Comp Integrative Med* 6:92–94, 1999.
4. Seddon JM, Ajani UA, et al.: Dietary carotenoids, vitamins A, C, E, and advanced age-related macular degeneration. *JAMA* 272:143–20, 1994.
5. Newsome DA, Swartz M, et al.: Oral zinc in macular degeneration. *Arch Ophthamol* 106:192–198, 1988.

References

6. Seddon JM, Ajani UA, et al.: Dietary carotenoids, vitamins A, C, E, and advanced age-related macular degeneration. *JAMA* 272:143–20, 1994.

7. Mares-Perlman JA, Brady WE, et al.: Dietary fat and age-related maculopathy. *Arch Opthalmol* 113:743–748, 1995.

Dry Eyes Associated with Sjögren's Syndrome

1. Campbell A and MacEwen CG: Systemic treatment of Sjögren's syndrome and the sicca syndrome with Efamol (evening primrose oil), vitamin C, and pyridoxine. In: *Clinical Uses of Essential Fatty Acids* (Horrobin DF, ed.). Eden Press, London, 1982, pp. 129–137.

Uveitis (Chronic and Acute)

1. Lavine JB: Suppression of chronic uveitis with the platelet-activating factor antagonist *Ginkgo biloba*. *Quart Rev Nat Med* Summer:5–6, 1993.

2. Lal B, Kapoor AK, et al.: Efficacy of curcumin in the management of chronic anterior uveitis. *Phytotherapy Res* 13:318–322, 1999.

3. van Rooij J, Schwartzenberg GWS, et al.: Oral vitamins C and E as additional treatment in patients with acute anterior uveitis: a randomized double masked study in 145 patients. *British J Opthalmol* 83:1277–1282, 1999.

FEMALE HEALTH CONDITIONS

Fibrocystic Breast Disease/Cyclical Breast Pain

1. Minton JP, Foecking MK, et al.: Caffeine, cyclic nucleotides, and breast disease. *Surgery* 86:105–109, 1979.

2. Minton JP and Abou-Issa H: Clinical and biochemical studies on methylxanthine-related fibrocystic breast disease. *Surgery* 90:299–304, 1981.

3. Prior JC, Vigna Y, et al.: Conditioning exercise decreases premenstrual symptoms: A prospective, controlled 6-month trial. *Fertil Steril* 47:402–408, 1987.

Hot Flashes (Associated with Menopause)

1. Smith CJ: Non-hormonal control of vasomotor flushing in menopausal patients. *Chicago Med* 67:193–195, 1964.

2. Barton DL, Loprinzi CL, et al.: Prospective evaluation of vitamin E for hot flashes in breast cancer survivors. *Arch Internal Med* 16:495–500, 1998.

3. Ohta H, Komukai S, et al.: Effects of 1-year ipriflavone treatment on lumbar bone mineral density and bone metabolic markers in postmenopausal women with low bone mass. *Hormone Res* 51:178–183, 1999.

4. Messina M and Barnes S: The roles of soy products in reducing risk of cancer. *J Natl Cancer Inst* 83:541–546, 1991.

5. Albertazzi P, Pasini F, et al.: The effect of dietary soy supplementation on hot flushes. *Obstet Gynecol* 91:6–11, 1998.

6. Reichert R: Phytoestrogens. *Quart Rev Nat Med* Spring:27–33, 1994.

7. Nestel PJ, Pomeroy S, et al.: Isoflavones from red clover improve systemic arterial compliance but not plasma lipids in menopausal women. *J Clin Endocrinol Metab* 84:895–898, 1999.

8. Knight D, Howes J, Eden J: The effect of Promensil, an isolfavone extract on menopausal symptoms. *Climacteric* 2:79–84, 1999.

Infertility

1. Judd AM, MacLeod RM, and Login IS: Zinc acutely, selectively and reversibly inhibits prolactin secretion. *Brain Res* 294:190–192, 1984.
2. MacIntosh EN: Treatment of women with galactorrhea–amenorrhea syndrome with pyridoxine. *J Clin Endocrinol Metab* 42:1192–1195, 1976.
3. Gerhard I, Postneek F: Auricular acupuncture in the treatment of female infertility. *Gynecol Endocrinol* 6:171–181, 1992.

Morning Sickness during Pregnancy

1. Vutyavanich T, Wongtrangan S, Ruangsri R: Pyridoxine for nausea and vomiting of pregnancy: A randomized, double-blind, placebo-controlled trial. *Am J Obstet Gynecol* 173:881–884, 1995.
2. The use of menadione bisulfite and ascorbic acid in the treatment of nausea and vomiting of pregnancy. *Am J Obstet Gynecol* 64:416–418, 1952.

Premenstrual Syndrome

1. Qi-bing M, Jing-yi T, and Bo C: Advances in the pharmacological studies of radix *Angelica sinensis* (oliv) diels (Chinese danggui). *Chin Med J* 104:776–781, 1991.
2. London RS, Bradley L, and Chiamori NY: Effect of nutritional supplement on premenstrual symptomology in women with premenstrual syndrome: A double-blind longitudinal study. *J Am Coll Nutr* 10:494–499, 1991.
3. Abraham GE and Hargrove JT: Effect of vitamin B_6 on premenstrual symptomology in women with premenstrual tension syndrome: A double-blind crossover study. *Infertility* 3:155–165, 1980.
4. Wyatt KM, Dimmock PW, et al.: Efficacy of vitamin B6 in the treatment of premenstrual syndrome: A systematic review. *BMJ* 318:1375–1381, 1999.
5. Thys-Jacobs S, Starkey P, et al.: Calcium carbonate and the premenstrual syndrome: Effects on premenstrual and menstrual symptoms. *Am J Obstet Gynecol* 179:444–452, 1998.
6. Facchinetti F, Borella P, et al.: Oral magnesium successfully relieves premenstrual mood changes. *Obstet Gynecol* 78:177–181, 1991.
7. London RS, Murphy L, et al.: Efficacy of α-tocopherol in the treatment of the premenstrual syndrome. *J Reprod Med* 32:400–404, 1987.

Vaginal Yeast Infections (Recurrent)

1. Belaiche P: Treatment of vaginal yeast infections of *Candida albicans* with the essential oil of *Malaleuca alternifolia*. *Phytotherapie* 15:15–16, 1985.
2. Blackwell AL: Tea tree oil and anaerobic (bacterial) vaginosis. *Lancet* 337:300, 1991.
3. Jovanovic R, Congema E, Nguyen HT: Antifungal agents versus boric acid for treating chronic mycotic vulvovaginitis. *J Reproductive Med* 36:593–597, 1977.
4. Hilton E, Isenberg HD, et al.: Ingestion of yogurt containing *Lactobacillus acidophilus* as prophylaxis for candidal vaginitis. *Ann Intern Med* 116:353–357, 1992.

IMMUNE SYSTEM

Chronic Fatigue Immunodeficiency Syndrome

1. Demitrack MA, Dale JK, et al.: Evidence for impaired activation of the hypothalamic–pituitary–adrenal axis in patients with chronic fatigue syndrome. *J Clin Endocrinol Metab* 73:1224–1234, 1991.

2. Jeffries WM: Mild adrenocortical deficiency, chronic allergies, autoimmune disorders and the chronic fatigue syndrome: A continuation of the cortisone story. *Med Hypotheses* 42:183–189, 1994.

3. Tintera JW: The hypoadrenocortical state and its management. *NY State J Med* 55:1869–1876, 1955.

4. Buchwald D, Garrity D: Comparison of patients with chronic fatigue syndrome, fibromyalgia, and multiple chemical sensitivities. *Arch Inter Med* 154:2049–2053, 1994.

5. Griep EN, Boersma JW, et al.: Function of the hypothalamic–pituitary–adrenal axis in patients with fibromylagia and low back pain. *J Rheumatol* 25:1374–1381.

6. Lloyd A, Hickie I, et al.: Cell-mediated immunity in patients with chronic fatigue syndrome, healthy control subjects, and patients with major depression. *Clin Exp Immunol* 87:76–79, 1992.

7. Klimas NG, Slavato FR, et al.: Immunologic abnormalities in chronic fatigue syndrome. *J Clin Microbiol* 28:1403–1410, 1990.

8. Brown D: Licorice root—potential early intervention for chronic fatigue syndrome. *Quart Rev Nat Med* Summer:95–97, 1996.

9. Whorwood CR, Sheppard MC, Stewart PM: Licorice inhibits 11β-hydroxysteroid dehydrogenase messenger ribonucleic acid levels and potentiates glucocorticoid hormone action. *Endocrinology* 132: 2287–2292, 1993.

10. Cox IM, Campbell MJ, and Dowson D: Red blood cell magnesium and chronic fatigue syndrome. *Lancet* 337:757–760, 1991.

11. Plioplys AV, Plioplys S: Amantadine and L-carnitine treatment of chronic fatigue syndrome. *Neuropsychobiol* 35:16–23, 1997.

12. Diet may be the key to beating chronic fatigue syndrome. *Seattle Post–Intelligencer* September 9, 1992, p. C6.

13. Lathan SR: Chronic fatigue? Consider hypothyroidism. *Phys Sports Med* 19:67–70, 1991.

14. Fulcher KY, White PD: Randomized controlled trial of graded exercise in patients with the chronic fatigue syndrome. *BMJ* 314:1647–1652, 1997.

Colds and Flu

1. Cáceres DD, Hancke JL, et al.: Use of visual analogue scale measurements (VAS) to assess the effectiveness of standardized *Andrographis paniculata* extract SHA-10 in reducing the symptoms of common cold. A randomized double-blind placebo study. *Phytomedicine* 6:217–223, 1999.

2. Zakay-Rones Z, Varsano N, et al.: Inhibition of several strains of influenza virus in vitro and reduction of symptoms by an elderberry extract (*Sambucus nigra* L.) during an outbreak of influenza B Panama. *J Altern Complement Med* 1:361–369, 1995.

3. Hemilä H: Does vitamin C alleviate the symptoms of the common cold?—a review of current evidence. *Scand J Infect Dis* 26:1–6, 1994.

4. Macknin ML: Zinc lozenges for the common cold. *Cleveland Clin J Med* 66:27–32, 1999.

HIV Infection/AIDS

1. Durant J, Cahntre PH, et al.: Efficacy and safety of *Buxus sempervirens* L. preparations (SPV 30) in HIV-infected asymptomatic patients: A multicenter, randomized, double-blind, placebo-controlled trial. *Phytomedicine* 5:1–10, 1998.

2. Bohn B, Nebe CT, and Birr C: Flow-cytometric studies with *Eleutherococcus senticosus* as an immunomodulatory agent. *Arzneim-Forsch Drug Res* 37:1193–1196, 1987.

3. Lau BHS, Ong PY, et al.: Chinese medicinal herbs for immunodeficiency. *Int Clin Nutr Rev* 10:430–434, 1990.

4. Ikehara S, Kawamura H, et al.: Effects of medicinal plants on hemopoietic cells. In: *Microbial Infections* (Friedman H, ed.). Plenum Press, New York, 1992, pp. 319–330.

5. Nai-lan G, Dao-pei L, et al.: Demonstrations of the anti-viral activity of garlic extract against human cytomegalovirus in vitro. *Chin Med J* 106:93–96, 1993.

6. Ghannoum MA: Studies on the anticandidal mode of action of *Allium sativum* (garlic). *J Gen Microbiol* 134:2917–2924, 1988.

7. Despande RG, Kahn MG, et al.: Inhibition of *Mycobacterium avium* complex isolates from AIDS patients by garlic (*Allium sativum*). *J Antimicrob Chemother* 32:623–626, 1993.

8. Jandourek A, Vaishampayan JK, Vazquez JA: Efficacy of melaleuca oral solution for the treatment of fluconazole refractory oral candidiasis in AIDS patients. *AIDS* 12:1033–1037, 1998.

9. Koch J, Tuveson J, Carlson T, Schmidt JM: SB-300: A new and effective therapy for HIV-associated diarrhea. Poster presentation, Seventh European Conference on Clinical Aspects and Treatment of HIV-Infection, Lisbon, Portugal, October 23–27, 1999.

10. Holondy M, Koch J, Mistal M, et al.: A double-blind, randomized, placebo-controlled, phase II study to assess the safety and efficacy of orally administered SP-303 for the symptomatic treatment of diarrhea in AIDS patients. *Am J Gastroenterol* 94:3267–3273, 1999.

11. Dworkin BM: Selenium deficiency in HIV infection and the acquired immunodeficiency syndrome. *Chemico Biol Interact* 91:199–205, 1994.

12. Wang Y and Watson RR: Is vitamin E supplementation a useful agent in AIDS therapy? *Prog Food Nutr Sci* 17:351–375, 1993.

13. Semba RD, Graham NMH, et al.: Increased mortality associated with vitamin A deficiency during human immunodeficiency virus type 1 infection. *Arch Inter Med* 153:2149–2154, 1993.

14. Harakeh S, Niedzwiecki A, and Jariwalla RJ: Mechanistic aspects of ascorbate inhibition of human immunodeficiency virus. *Chemico Biol Interact* 91:207–215, 1994.

15. Remacha AF, Riera A, et al.: Vitamin B_{12} abnormalities in HIV-infected patients. *Eur J Hematol* 47:60–64, 1991.

16. Boudes P, Zittoun J, and Sobel A: Folate, vitamin B_{12}, and HIV infection. *Lancet* 335:1401–1402, 1990.

MALE HEALTH CONDITIONS

Benign Prostate Enlargement/Prostate Cancer Prevention

1. Geller J: Overview of benign prostatic hypertrophy. *Urology* 34(Suppl.):57–68, 1989.

2. Berges RR, Windler J, et al.: Randomized, placebo-controlled, double-blind clinical trial of β-sitosterol in patients with benign prostatic hyperplasia. *Lancet* 345:1529–1532, 1995.

3. Wilt TJ, MacDonald R, Ishani A: β-sitosterol for the treatment of benign prostatic hyperplasia: A systematic review. *BJU International* 83:976–983, 1999.

4. Zahradnik HP, Schillifahrt R, et al.: Prostaglandin content in prostate adenomas following treatment with a sterol. *Fortschr Med* 98:69–72, 1980.

5. Murray MT: *The Healing Power of Herbs*. Prima Publishing, Rocklin, California, 1995, pp. 286–293.

6. Koch E and Biber A: Pharmacological effects of sabal and urtica extracts as a basis for a rational medication of benign prostatic hyperplasia. *Urologe B* 334:90–95, 1994.

7. Buck AC, Cox R, et al.: Treatment of outflow tract obstruction due to benign prostatic hyperplasia with the pollen extract, Cernilton: A double-blind, placebo-controlled study. *British J Urology* 66:398–404, 1990.

8. Clark LC, Dalkin B, et al.: Decreased incidence of prostate cancer with selenium supplementation: Results of a double-blind cancer prevention trial. *British J Urology* 81:730–734, 1998.

9. Heinonen OP, Albanes D, et al.: Prostate cancer and supplementation with α-tocopherol and β-carotene: Incidence and mortality in a controlled trial. *J National Cancer Inst* 90:440–446, 1998.

10. Giovannucci E: Tomatoes, tomato-based products, lycopene, and cancer: Review of the epidemiologic literature. *J National Cancer Inst* 91:317–331, 1999.

11. Liang JY, Liu YY, et al.: Inhibitory effect of zinc on human prostatic carcinoma cell growth. *Prostate* 40:200–207, 1999.

12. Ross JK, Pusateri DJ, and Schultz TD: Dietary and hormonal evaluation of men at different risks for prostate cancer: Fiber intake, excretion, and composition, with in-vitro evidence for an association between steroid hormones and specific fiber components. *Am J Clin Nutr* 51: 365–370, 1990.

13. Pusateri DJ, Roth WT, et al.: Dietary and hormonal evaluation of men at different risks for prostate cancer: Plasma and fecal hormone–nutrient interrelationships. *Am J Clin Nutr* 51:371–377, 1990.

14. Aldercreutz H, Markkanen H, and Watanabe S: Plasma concentrations of phytoestrogens in Japanese men. *Lancet* 342:1209–1210, 1993.

15. Gupta S, Ahmad N, Mukhtar H: Prostate cancer chemoprevention by green tea. *Seminars Urologic Oncology* 17:70–76, 1999.

16. Buck AC, Rees RW, Ebeling L: Treatment of chronic prostatitis and prostatodynia with pollen extract. *British J Urology* 64:496–499, 1989.

Impotence (Erectile Dysfunction)

1. Sohn M and Sikora R: *Ginkgo biloba* extract in the therapy of erectile dysfunction. *J Sex Educ Ther* 17:53–61, 1991.

2. Sikora R, Sohn M, et al.: *Ginkgo biloba* extract in the therapy of erectile dysfunction. *J Urol* 141:188A, 1989.

3. Riley AJ, Goodman RE, et al.: Double-blind trial of yohimbine hydrochloride in the treatment of erection inadequacy. *Sex Marital Ther* 4:17–26, 1989.

4. Southwick SM, Morgan CA, et al.: Yohimbine use in a natural setting: Effects on posttraumatic stress disorder. *Biol Psychiatry* 46:442–444, 1999.

5. Waynberg J: Aphrodisiacs: Contribution to the clinical validation of the traditional use of *Ptychopetalum guyanna*. Presented at the First International Congress on Ethnopharmacology, Strasbourg, France, June 5–9, 1990.

6. Reiter WJ, Pycha A, et al.: Dehydroepiandrosterone in the treatment of erectile dysfunction: A prospective, double-blind, randomized, placebo-controlled study. *Urology* 53:590–595, 1999.

7. Zorgniotti AW, Lizza EF: Effect of large doses of the nitric oxide precursor, L-arginine, on erectile dysfunction. *Int J Impot Res* 6:33–36, 1994.

Infertility

1. Salvati G, Genovesi G, et al.: Effects of *Panax ginseng* C.A. Meyer saponins on male fertility. *Panminerva Med* 38:249–254, 1996.

References

2. ADIS International: L-carnitine and acetylcarnitine in male fertility. *Healthnotes Rev Comp Integrative Med* 6:189–200, 1999.

3. Hunt CD, Johnson PE, et al.: Effects of dietary zinc depletion on seminal volume and zinc loss, serum testosterone concentrations, and sperm morphology in young men. *Am J Clin Nutr* 56:148–157, 1992.

4. Dawson EB, Harris WA, Powell LC: Relationship between ascorbic acid and male fertility [Review]. In: *Aspects of Some Vitamins, Minerals, and Enzymes in Health and Disease* (Bourne GH, ed.). *World Rev Nutr Diet* 62:1–26, 1990.

5. Bayer R: Treatment of infertility with vitamin E. *Int J Fertil* 5:70–78, 1960.

6. Scott R, MacPherson A, et al.: The effect of oral selenium supplementation on human sperm motility. *Br J Urol* 82:76–80, 1998.

MOUTH AND GUMS

Canker Sores

1. Das SK, Gulati AK, and Singh VP: Deglycyrrhizinated licorice in aphthous ulcers. *J Assoc Physicians India* 37:647, 1989.

2. Wray DW, Ferguson MM, et al.: Nutritional deficiencies in recurrent aphthae. *J Oral Pathol* 7:418–423, 1978.

3. Nolan A, McIntosh WB, et al.: Recurrent aphthous ulceration: Vitamin B_1, B_2, and B_6 status and response to replacement therapy. *J Oral Pathol Med* 20:389–391, 1991.

4. Wray D: A double-blind trial of systemic zinc sulfate in recurrent aphthous stomatitis. *Oral Surg* 53:469, 1982.

5. Gerenrich RL, Hart RW. Treatment of oral ulcerations with Bacid (*Lactobacillus acidophilus*). *Oral Surg* 30:196–200, 1970.

6. Wray D: Gluten-sensitive recurrent aphthous stomatitis. *Digest Dis Sci* 26:737, 1981.

7. Herlosfson BB, Barkvoll P: The effect of two toothpaste detergents on the frequency of recurrent aphthous ulcers. *Acta Odontol Scand* 54:150–153, 1996.

8. Andrews VH and Hall HR: The effects of relaxation/imagery training on recurrent aphthous stomatitis: A preliminary study. *Psychosom Med* 52:526–535, 1990.

Cold Sores

1. Wöbling RH and Leonhardt K: Local therapy of herpes simplex with dried extract from *Melissa officinalis*. *Phytomedicine* 1:25–31, 1994.

2. Koytchev R, Alken RG, Dundarov S: Balm mint extract (Lo-701) for topical treatment of recurring *Herpes labialis*. *Phytomedicine* 6:225–230, 1999.

3. Griffith RS, et al.: Success of L-lysine therapy in frequently recurrent herpes simplex infection. *Dermatologica* 175:183–190, 1987.

4. Terezhealmy G, Bottomley W, and Pellu G: The use of water-soluble bioflavonoid–ascorbic acid complex in the treatment of recurrent *Herpes labialis*. *Oral Surg* 45:56–62, 1978.

Periodontal Disease

1. Serfaty R and Itic J: Comparative trial with natural herbal mouthwash versus chlorhexidine in gingivitis. *J Clin Dent* 1:A34, 1988.

2. Yamnkell S and Emling RC: Two-month evaluation of Parodontax dentifrice. *J Clin Dent* 1:A41, 1988.

3. Pack ARC: Folate mouthwash: Effects on established gingivitis in periodontal patients. *J Clin Periodontol* 11:619–628, 1984.

4. Leggott PJ, Robertson PB, et al.: Effects of ascorbic acid depletion and supplementation on periodontal health and subgingival microflora in humans. *J Dent Res* 70:1531–1536, 1991.

5. Wilkinson EG: Adjunctive treatment of periodontal disease with coenzyme Q_{10}. *Res Commun Chem Pathol Pharmacol* 14:715, 1978.

6. You SQ: Study on feasibility of Chinese green tea polyphenols (CTP) for preventing dental caries. *Chin J Stom* 28:197–199, 1993.

MUSCULOSKELETAL SYSTEM

Osteoarthritis

1. Deal CL, Schnitzer TJ, et al.: Treatment of arthritis with topical capsaicin: A double-blind trial. *Clin Ther* 13:383–395, 1991.

2. Qiu GX, Gao SN, et al.: Efficacy and safety of glucosamine sulfate versus ibuprofen in patients with knee osteoarthritis of the knee. *Arzneim-Forsch Drug Res* 48:469–474, 1998.

3. Drovanti A, Bignamini AA, Rovati AL: Therapeutic activity of oral glusoamine sulfate in osteoarthrosis: A placebo-controlled double-blind investigation. *Clin Ther* 3:260267, 1980.

4. Buscih L, Poór G: Efficacy and tolerability of oral chondroitin sulfate as a symptomatic, slow-acting drug for osteoarthritis in the treatment of knee osteoarthritis. *Osteoarthritis Cartilage* 6(Suppl A):31–36, 1998.

5. Marcolongo R, Giordano N, et al.: Double-blind multicenter study of the activity of s-adenosylmethionine in hip and knee osteoarthritis. *Curr Ther Res* 37:82–94, 1985.

6. Scherak O, Kolarz G, et al.: Vitamin E therapy for patients with osteoarthritis. *Z A Rheumatol* 49:369–373, 1990.

Rheumatoid Arthritis

1. Etzel R: Special extract of *Boswellia serrata* (H15) in the treatment of rheumatoid arthritis. *Phytomedicine* 3:91–94, 1996.

2. Singh BH, Bani S, Singh S: Toxicity and safety evaluation of boswellic acids. *Phytomedicine* 3:87–90, 1996.

3. Belch JJF, Ansell D, et al.: Effects of altering dietary essential fatty acids on requirements for non-steroidal anti-inflammatory drugs in patients with rheumatoid arthritis: A double-blind, placebo-controlled study. *Ann Rheum Dis* 47:96–104, 1988.

4. Leventhal LJ, Boyce EG, et al.: Treatment of rheumatoid arthritis with gammalinolenic acid. *Arch Intern Med* 119:867–873, 1993.

5. Deal CL, Schnitzer TJ, et al.: Treatment of arthritis with topical capsaicin: A double-blind trial. *Clin Ther* 13:383–395, 1991.

6. Deodhar SD, Sethi R, Srimal RC: Preliminary studies on the antirheumatic activity of curcumin (difereuloyl methane). *Indian J Med Res* 71:632–634, 1980.

7. Heliövaara M, Knekt P, et al.: Serum antioxidants and risk of rheumatoid arthritis. *Ann Rheum Dis* 53:51–53, 1994.

8. Cohen A, Goldman J: Bromelains therapy in rheumatoid arthritis. *Pennsylvania Med J* 67:27–30, 1964.

9. van der Tempel H, Tulleken JE, et al.: Effects of fish oil supplementation in rheumatoid arthritis. *Ann Rheumatol Dis* 49:76–80, 1990.

10. Edmonds SE, Winyard PG, et al.: Putative analgesic activity of repeated oral doses of vitamin E in the treatment of rheumatoid arthritis. Results of a prospective placebo-controlled double-blind trial. *Ann Rheum Dis* 56:649–655, 1997.

11. Peretz A, Neve J, et al.: Adjuvant treatment of recent onset of rheumatoid arthritis by selenium supplementation: Preliminary observations [Letter]. *British J Rheumatol* 31:281–282, 1992.

12. Kjeldsen-Kragh J, Haugen M, et al.: Controlled trial of fasting and one-year vegetarian diet in rheumatoid arthritis. *Lancet* ii:899–902, 1991.

13. Peltonen R, Kjeldsen-Kragh J, et al.: Changes of fecal flora in rheumatoid arthritis during fasting and one-year vegetarian diet. *Br J Rheum* 33:638–643, 1994.

Sprains and Strains

1. Rothhaar J and Thiel W: Percutaneous gel therapy for blunt sports injuries. *Med Welt* 33:1006–1010, 1982.

2. Calabrese C and Preston P: Report of the results of a double-blind, randomized, single-dose trial of topical 2% escin gel versus placebo in the acute treatment of experimentally induced hematoma in volunteers. *Planta Med* 59:394–397, 1993.

3. Cirelli MG: Five years of experience with bromelains in therapy of edema and inflammation in postoperative tissue reaction, skin infections and trauma. *Clin Med* 74:55–59, 1967.

4. Srimal R and Dhawan B: Pharmacology of diferuloyl methane (curcumin), a non-steroidal anti-inflammatory agent. *J Pharm Pharmacol* 25:447–452, 1973.

NERVOUS SYSTEM

Age-Related Cognitive Decline and Early-Stage Alzheimer's Disease

1. Petkov VD, Belcheva S, et al.: Participation of the serotonergic system in the memory effects of *Ginkgo biloba* L. and *Panax ginseng* C.A. Meyer. *Phytother Res* 8:470–477, 1994.

2. Xu SS, Gao ZX, et al.: Efficacy of tablet hyuperizine A on memory, cognition, and behavior in Alzheimer's disease. *Chung Kuo Yao Li Hsueh Pao* 16:391–395, 1995.

3. Spagnoli A, Lucca U, et al.: Long-term acetyl-L-carnitine treatment in Alzheimer's disease. *Neurology* 41:1726–1732, 1991.

4. Rai G, Wright G, et al.: Double-blind, placebo controlled study of acetyl-L-carnitine in patients with Alzheimer's disease. *Current Med Res Opinion* 11:638–647, 1990.

5. Crook T, Petrie W, et al.: Effects of phosphatidylserine in Alzheimer's disease. *Psychopharmacol Bull* 28:61–66, 1992.

6. Gold M, Chen MF, Johnson K: Plasma and red blood cell thiamine deficiency in patients with dementia of the Alzheimer's type. *Arch Neurol* 52:1081–1086, 1995.

7. Bottiglieri T, Hyland K, et al.: Enhancement of recovery from psychiatric illness by methyl-folate. *Lancet* 336:1579–1580, 1990.

8. Lowinger P: Cobalamin and organic mood syndrome. *J Neuropsychiatr* 2:467, 1991.

9. Joosten E, van den Berg A, et al.: Metabolic evidence that deficiencies of vitamin B_{12}, folate, and vitamin B_6 occur commonly in elderly people. *Am J Clin Nutr* 58:468–476, 1993.

10. Behl C, Davis J, et al.: Vitamin E protects nerve cells from amyloid beta-protein toxicity. *Biochem Biophys Res Commun* 186:944–950, 1992.

11. Sano M, Ernesto C, et al.: A controlled trial of selegine, alpha-tocopherol, or both as treatments for Alzheimer's disease. *New Engl J Med* 336:1216–1222, 1997.

Attention Deficit–Hyperactivity Disorder

1. Pihl RO and Peterson JB: Attention deficit hyperactivity disorder, childhood conduct disorder, and alcoholism. *Alcohol Health Research World* 15:25–31, 1991.
2. Bhagavan HH, Coleman M, and Coursin DB: The effect of pyridoxine hydrochloride on blood serotonin and pyridoxil phosphate contents in hyperactive children. *Pediatrics* 55:437–441, 1975.
3. Starobrat-Hermelin B, Kozielec T: The effects of magnesium physiological supplementation on hyperactivity in children with attention deficit–hyperactivity disorder (ADHD). Positive response to magnesium oral loading test. *Magnesium Res* 10:149–156.
4. Mertz W: Chromium occurrence and function in biological systems. *Physiol Rev* 49:163–239, 1969.
5. Colquhoun I and Bunday S: A lack of essential fatty acids as a possible cause of hyperactivity in children. *Med Hypotheses* 7:673–679, 1981.
6. Zametkin AJ, Nordahl TE, et al.: Cerebral glucose metabolism in adults with hyperactivity of childhood onset. *New Engl J Med* 323:1361–1366, 1990.
7. Swain A, Soutter V, et al.: Salicylates, oligoantigenic diets and behavior. *Lancet* iii, July 6:41–42, 1985.
8. Egger J, Stolla A, and McEwen LM: Controlled trial of hyposensitisation in children with food-induced hyperkinetic syndrome. *Lancet* 339:1150–1153, 1992.

Depression

1. Wheatley D: *Hypericum* in seasonal affective disorder (SAD). *Current Med Res Opinion* 15: 33–37, 1999.
2. Bell IR, Edman JS, et al.: Brief communication: Vitamin B_1, B_2, and B_6 augmentation of tricyclic antidepressant treatment in geriatric depression with cognitive dysfunction. *J Am Coll Nutr* 11:159–163, 1992.
3. Bottiglieri T, Hyland K, et al.: Enhancement of recovery from psychiatric illness by methylfolate. *Lancet* 336:1579–1580, 1990.
4. Lowinger P: Cobalamin and organic mood syndrome. *J Neuropsychiatr* 2:467, 1991.
5. Joosten E, van den Berg A, et al.: Metabolic evidence that deficiencies of vitamin B_{12}, folate, and vitamin B_6 occur commonly in elderly people. *Am J Clin Nutr* 58:468–476, 1993.
6. Adams PW, Wynn V, et al.: Effect of pyridoxine hydrochloride (vitamin B6) upon depression associated with oral contraception. *Lancet* i:897–904, 197 3.
7. Bell IR, Edman JS, et al.: Plasma homocysteine in vascular disease and in nonvascular dementia of depressed elderly people. *Acta Psychiatr Scand* 86:386–90, 1992.
8. Wolkowitz OM, Reus VI, et al.: Double-blind treatment of major depression with dehydroepiandrosterone. *Am J Psychiatry* 156:646–649, 1999.

Insomnia

1. Wichtl M: *Herbal Drugs and Phytopharmaceuticals*. CRC Press, Boca Raton, Florida, 1994, pp. 363–365.
2. Zhdanova IV, Wurtman RJ, et al.: Sleep-inducing effects of low doses of melatonin ingested in the evening. *Clin Pharmacol Ther* 57:552–558, 1995.
3. Montakab H: Acupuncture and insomnia. *Forsch Komplementarmed* 6:29–31, 1999.

Migraine Headache

1. DeFeudis FV: Ginkgo biloba *Extract (EGb 761): From Chemistry to the Clinic*. Ullstein Medical, Wiesbaden, Germany, 1998, p. 195.

2. Gallai V, Sarchielli P, et al.: Red blood cell magnesium levels in migraine patients. *Cephalagia* 13:94–98, 1993.

3. Peikert A, Wilimzig C, Kohne-Volland R: Prophylaxis of migraine with oral magnesium: Results from a prospective, multi-center, placebo-controlled, and double-blind randomized study. *Cephalagia* 16:257–263, 1996.

4. Schonen J, Jacquy J, Lenaerts M: Effectiveness of high-dose riboflavin in migraine prophylaxis. A randomized controlled trial. *Neurology* 50:466–470, 1998.

5. McCarren T, Hitzemann R, et al.: Amelioration of severe migraine by fish oil (omega-3) fatty acids. *Am J Clin Nutr* 41:874a, 1985.

6. De Benedittis G, Massei R: 5-HT precursors in migraine prophylaxis: A double-blind cross-over study with L-5-hydroxytryptophan versus placebo. *Clin J Pain* 3:123–129, 1986.

7. Egger J, Carter CM, et al.: Is migraine food allergy? A double-blind controlled trial of oligoantigenic diet treatment. *Lancet* October 15:865–869, 1983.

8. Shuyuan G, Donglan Z, Yanguang X: A comparative study on the treatment of migraine headache with combined distant and local acupuncture points versus conventional drug therapy. *Am J Acupuncture* 27:27–30, 1999.

Neuropathy (Diabetic)

1. Capsaicin Study Group: Effect of treatment with capsaicin on daily activities of patients with painful diabetic neuropathy. *Diabetes Care* 15:159–165, 1992.

2. Ziegler D, Schatz H, et al.: Effects of treatment with the antioxidant alpha-lipoic acid on cardiac autonomic neuropathy in NIDDM patients. A 4-month randomized controlled multicenter trial (DEKAN Study). *Diabetes Care* 20:369–373, 1997.

3. Levin ER, Hanscom TA, et al.: The influence of pyridoxine in diabetic peripheral neuropathy. *Diabetes Care* 4:606–609, 1981.

4. Sancetta SM, Ayres PR, Scott RW: The use of vitamin B12 in the management of the neurologic manifestations of diabetes mellitus, with notes on the administration of massive doses. *Annals Intern Med* 35:1028–1048, 1951.

SKIN CONDITIONS

Acne

1. Bassett IB, Pannowitz DL, and Barnetson RSC: A comparative study of tea-tree oil versus benzoyl peroxide in the treatment of acne. *Med J Aust* 153:455–458, 1990.

2. Michaelsson G, Juhlin L, and Vahlquist A: Effects of oral zinc and vitamin A in acne. *Arch Dermatol* 113:31–36, 1977.

3. Michaelsson G, Juhlin L, and Ljunghall K: A double-blind study of the effect of zinc and oxytetracycline in acne vulgaris. *Br J Dermatol* 97:561–565, 1977.

4. Michaelsson G and Edqvist LE: Erythrocyte glutathione peroxidase activity in acne vulgaris and the effect of selenium and vitamin E treatment. *Acta Derm Venereol* 64:9–14, 1984.

5. Snider BL and Dieteman DF: Pyridoxine therapy for premenstrual acne flare. *Arch Dermatol* 110:130–131, 1974.

Eczema

1. Sheehan MP and Atherton DJ: One-year follow up of children treated with Chinese medical herbs for atopic eczema. *Br J Dermatol* 130:488–493, 1994.

2. Sheehan MP, Rustin MHA, et al.: Efficacy of traditional Chinese herbal therapy in adult atopic dermatitis. *Lancet* 340:13–17, 1992.

3. Aergeerts P, Albring M, et al.: Vergleichende Prüfung von Kamillosan®-crème gegenüber steroidalen (0.25% hydrocortisone, 0.75% flucortin butyl ester) und nichsteroidsalen (5% bufexamac) Externa in der Erhaltungstherapie von Ekzemerkrankugen. *Z Hautkr* 60:270–277, 1985.

4. Pfister R: Problems in the treatment and after care of chronic dermatoses. A clinical study on Hametum ointment. *Fortschr Med* 99:1264–1268, 1981.

5. Evans FQ: The rational use of glycyrrhetinic acid in dermatology. *Br J Clin Pract* 12:269–279, 1958.

6. Teelucksingh S, Mackie ADR, et al.: Potentiation of hydrocortisone activity in the skin by glycyrrhetinic acid. *Lancet* 335:1060–1063, 1990.

7. Burks AW, Mallory SB, et al.: Atopic dermatitis: clinical relevance of food hypersensitivity. *J Pediatrics* 113:447–451, 1988.

8. Sloper KS, Wadsworth J, and Brostoff J: Children with atopic eczema. I. Clinical response to food elimination and subsequent double-blind food challenge. *Q Rev Med* 292:677–693, 1991.

Psoriasis

1. Ellis CN, Berberian B, et al.: A double-blind evaluation of topical capsaicin in pruritic psoriasis. *J Am Acad Dermatol* 29:438–442, 1993.

2. Bernstein JE, Parish LC, et al.: Effects of topically applied capsaicin on moderate and severe psoriasis vulgaris. *J Am Acad Dermatol* 15:504–507, 1986.

3. Syed TA, Ahmed SA, et al.: Management of psoriasis with *Aloe vera* in a hydrophilic cream: A placebo-controlled, double-blind study. *Tropical Med Inter Health* 1:505–509, 1996.

4. Wiesenauer M, Lüdtke R: *Mahonia aquifolium* in patients with psoriasis vulgaris—an intraindividual study. *Phytomedicine* 3:231–235, 1996.

5. Werbach MR and Murray MT: *Botanical Influences on Illness*. Third Line Press, Tarzana, California, 2000, p. 548.

6. Kragballe K and Fogh K: A low-fat diet supplemented with dietary fish oil (Max-EPA) results in improvement of psoriasis and in formation of leukotriene B5. *Acta Derm Venereol* 69:23–28, 1989.

7. Kojiima T, Terano T, et al.: Long-term administration of highly purified eicosapentaenoic acid provides improvements in psoriasis. *Dermatologica* 182:225–230, 1991.

8. Donadini A, et al.: Plasma levels of zinc, copper, and nickel in healthy controls and in psoriatic patients. *Acta Vitaminol Enzymol* 2:9–16, 1980.

9. Michaelsson G, Berne B, et al.: Selenium in whole blood and plasma is decreased in patients with moderate and severe psoriasis. *Acta Derm Venereol* 69:29–34, 1989.

10. Fry L, McDonald A, et al.: The mechanism of folate deficiency in psoriasis. *Br J Dermatol* 84:539–544, 1971.

Vitiligo

1. Abdel-Fattah A, Aboul-Enein MN, et al.: An approach to the treatment of vitiligo by khellin. *Dermatologica* 165:136–140, 1982.

2. Montes LF, Diaz ML, et al.: Folic acid and vitamin B12 in vitiligo: A nutritional approach. *Cutis* 50:39–42, 1992.

3. Juhlin L, Olsson MJ: Improvement of vitiligo after oral treatment with vitamin B12 and folic acid and the importance of sun exposure. *Acta Derm Venereol* 77:460–462, 1997.

4. Siddiqui AH, Stolk LM, et al.: L-phenylalanine and UVA irradiation in the treatment of vitiligo. *Dermatology* 188:215–218, 1994.

5. Camacho F, Mazuecos J: Treatment of vitiligo with oral and topical phenylalanine: 6 years of experience. *Arch Dermatol* 135:216–217, 1999.

6. Howitz J and Schwartz M: Vitiligo, acholrhydria, and pernicious anemia. *Lancet* 1:1331–1335, 1971.

Athlete's Foot (Tinea Pedis)

1. Tong MM, Altman PM, and Barnetson RSC: Tea tree oil in the treatment of tinea pedis. *Austr J Dermatol* 33:145–149, 1992.

Fungal Infection of the Nails (Onychomycosis)

1. Buck DS, Nidorf DM, and Addino JG: Comparison of two topical preparations for the treatment of onychomycosis: *Malaleuca alternifolia* (tea tree) oil and clotrimazole. *J Family Pract* 38:601–605, 1994.

Shingles (Herpes zoster)

1. Peikert A, et al.: Topical 0.025% capsaicin in chronic post-herpetic neuralgia: Efficacy, predictors of response, and long-term course. *J Neurol* 238:452–456, 1991.

2. Watson CP, et al.: Post-herpetic neuralgia and topical capsaicin. *Pain* 33:333–340, 1988.

3. Baba M and Shigeta S: Antiviral activity of glycyrrhizin against varicella-zoster virus in vitro. *Antiviral Res* 7:99–107, 1987.

URINARY TRACT

Recurrent Urinary Tract Infections

1. Stamm WE and Turck M: Urinary tract infection, pyelonephritis, and related conditions. In: *Harrison's Principles of Internal Medicine* (Braunwald E, Isselbacher KJ, et al., eds.). McGraw-Hill, New York, 1987, pp. 1189–1194.

2. Meares EM: Nonspecific infections of the genitourinary tract. In: *General Urology* (Smith DR, ed.). Lange Medical Publications, Los Altos, California, 1981, pp. 177–227.

3. Krieger JN: Complications and treatment of urinary tract infections during pregnancy. *Urol Clin North Am* 13:685–693, 1986.

4. Sun D, Abraham SN, and Beachey EH: Influence of berberine sulfate on synthesis and expression of pap fimbrial adhesion in uropathogenic *Escherichia coli*. *Antimicrob Agents Chemother* 32:1274–1277, 1988.

5. Bruce AW and Reid G: Intravaginal instillation of lactobacilli for prevention of recurrent urinary tract infections. *Can J Microbiol* 34:339–343, 1988.

6. Aune A, Alraek T, et al.: Acupuncture in the prophylaxis of recurrent lower urinary tract infection in adult women. *Scand J Prim Health Care* 16:37–39, 1998.

Support for Kidney Function While Taking Immune-Suppressive Drugs

1. Pirotzky E, Colliez P, et al.: Cyclosporin-induced nephrotoxicity: Preventive effect of a PAF-acether antagonist, BN 5206 3. *Transplant Proceed* 20(Suppl. 3):665–669, 1988.

2. van der Heide JJ, Bilo HJ, et al.: Effect of dietary fish oil on renal function and rejection in cyclosporine-treated recipients of renal transplants. *New Engl J Med* 329:769–773, 1993.

References

Index

D

E

European health care, 29–30
European Scientific Cooperative on
        Phytotherapy, 29–30
Euvegal, 228, 231
Evening primrose oil
    key facts, summary, 95–96
    medical applications,
        101–105
    physiological effects, 97–99
    side effects, 105–106
    using, 105–106
Exercise. *See* Physical performance
Extracts, 23

F

Fatigue, 161, 293–296
Fats. *See* Dietary fats
FDA. *See* Food and Drug
        Administration
Felter, H. W., 195
Femaprin, 239
Fenugreek seeds, 289
Feverfew
    active constituents, 109–110
    history, 109
    key facts, summary,
        107–108
    medical applications,
        110–112
    physiological effects, 110
    plant facts, 108
    using, 112–113
Fibrosis, 197–198
Flavonoids
    in bilberry, 49–50
    description, 36–37
    ginkgo, 145
    milk thistle, 193, 196
    venous insufficiency, 250
Flu, 316–319
Fluids, 23
Folic acid, 272
Food and Drug Administration

DSHEA, 14
    St. John's wort, 212–213
    supplement claims, 7, xvii
Forster, Johann Georg, 186
Foster, Steven, 159
Free radicals, 36

G

Galen, 225
Gamma-linolenic acid.
        See Evening primrose oil
Garlic
    active constituents, 117–119
    history, 117
    key facts, summary, 114–115
    medical applications, 123–127
    physiological effects, 119–123
    plant facts, 116–117
    using, 128
Gastrointestinal tract, 66–67
Gay Men's Health Crisis, 320
German chamomile. *See* Chamomile
Ginger
    active constituents, 132–133
    history, 132
    key facts, summary, 130–131
    medical applications, 135–139
    physiological effects, 133–135
    plant facts, 132
    side effects, 139
    using, 139
Gingivitis. *See* Periodontal disease
Ginkgo biloba
    active constituents, 145
    history, 144
    key facts, summary, 141–142
    medical applications, 149–153
    modern development, 144
    physiological effects, 145–148
    plant facts, 143–144
    side effects, 153
    using, 153–154
Ginsenosides, 160

Irritable bowel syndrome,
267–269
Ivy leaf extract, 276, 280

J

James, John, 321
Jartoux, Petrus, 159
*Journal of the American Medical
Association*, 167

K

Kaempfer, Dr. Englebert, 144
Kava: The Pacific Drug, 186
Kava-kava
active constituents, 188
history, 186–187
key facts, summary, 184–185
medical applications, 189–190
physiological effects, 188–189
plant facts, 186
side effects, 191
using, 191–192
Khella, 367
Kidney function, 372
Kind of Blue, 247
Kloss, Jethro, xvi
Kupperman Index, 60
Kwai, 123–125

L

Labels, 6–7, 13–14
Lactation, 18–19
Lactobacillus, 265
Lancet, 181
L-arginine, 331
Laxatives, 43–44, 262–263
L-carnitine, 332
Lebot, Vincent, 186
Legalon, 196, 202
Lehrbuch der Phytoterapie, 28
Leigh, Evelyn, 1
Lemon balm, 336
LH. *See* Luteinizing hormone
LI 132, 173, 175

LI 160, 210–211
Lichtwer Pharma, 206
Licorice
deglycyrrhizinated
canker sores, 334
heartburn, 266–267
ulcers, 270
root, 315
Lindstrom, Lamont, 186
Linnaeus, 144
Linoleic acid. *See* Evening primrose oil
Lipoproteins, 120–121
Liver disease
alcohol-related, 198–199, 258–260
cirrhosis, 199–200
hepatitis, 198, 200–201
protection, 196–197
Lloyd J. U., 195
L-lysine, 337
Low-density lipoproteins, 120–121
Luteinizing hormone, 58–59, 236

M

Macular degeneration, 299–301
Madaus, Dr. Gerhard, 79–80
Magnesium
CFIDS, 316
CHF, 252
insulin and, 292
Ma Huang, 276, 280
Marshmallow root, 277
Martin, Steve, 143
Maslow, Dr. Abraham H., 2
Mastodynon, 235, 237–238
Matricaria recutita. *See* Chamomile
Matricin, 65
Maximowicz, Karl Johann, 88
McCaleb, Rob, 1
Melatonin, 358–359
Melissa officinalis, 336
Memory. *See* Cognitive activity
Menopause, 304–307
Merlin, Mark, 186
Mevacor, 253

Migraines
 description, 359
 ginger effects, 139
 treatments, 359–360
Milk thistle
 active constituents, 196
 history, 195
 key facts, 193–194
 modern development, 196
 physiological effects,
  196–198
 plant facts, 195
 side effects, 202
 using, 202
Ming Yi Bie Lu, 117
A Modern Herbal, 171
Monascus pupureas. See Red yeast
Monk, Thelonius, 337
Monk's Dream, 337
Monk's pepper. *See* Vitex agnus-castus
Morien, Krista, 1
Morning sickness, 137–138, 308
Mouth irritations, 67–68
Mowrey, Daniel, 135
Müller, Dr. Walter, 207–208
Muria puama, 330–331
Mutiny on the Bounty, 135

N

Nails, infection, 368
NASA. *See* National Aeronautics and
  Space Administration
National Aeronautics and Space
  Administration, 136–137
National Institutes of Health,
  350, xvii
Nausea, 133–134, 137
Nerves, 147
Nestlé, 228
Nettle root extract, 328
Neuropathy
 description, 360–361
 EPO effects, 103–104
 treatments, 361

Niacin
 cataracts, 298
 deficiency, 267
 hypercholesterolemia, 252
 intermittent claudication, 255
 PMS, 236
 time-release, 254
Night vision, 301
NIH. *See* National Institutes of Health
Nonsteroidal anti-inflammatory
  drugs, 341
NSAIDs. *See* Nonsteroidal
  anti-inflammatory drugs
Nutraceuticals, 21

O

Oenothera biennis.
  See Evening primrose
Oligomeric proanthocyanidins, 300
Omeprazole, 76
Onychomycosis, 368
Organic herbs, 25–26
Osteoarthritis, 138, 240–242

P

Padma 28, 255
Pain, 134–135, 138
Panax ginseng. See Asian Ginseng
Parkinson, Sydney, 186
Pasteur, Louis, 117, 121
Peppermint oil, 268
Peppermint tea, 261
Peptic ulcer disease, 269–271
Periodontal disease, 337–339
Phosphatidylserine, 351
Physical performance,
  90, 163
Physicians, 12–13
Phytoestrogens, 306–307
Phytotherapy
 definition, 27–28
 history, 28
 medicine, 29–32
 regulation, 29–30